Derived from *The Merck Manual—Second Home Edition*, a bestselling medical reference, *The Merck Manual of Women's and Men's Health* isn't over your head—or below your doctor's standards. Here's what critics had to say about *The Merck Manual—Home Edition*.

"[A] very valuable resource . . . for any home."

—*Publishers Weekly*

"Doctors should encourage their patients to own [the Home Edition]."

—Dr. Sherwin Nuland, Clinical Professor of Surgery, Yale School of Medicine; author of *How We Die, Doctors,* and *The Wisdom of the Body*

"Essential for all medical, consumer health and public libraries."

—*Library Journal*

"Anyone interested in health should have this book."

—Ellen Levine, Editor-in-Chief, *Good Housekeeping*

"Devoid of doctor double talk . . . it should help put you and your doctor on the same wavelength."

—*USA Today*

"Well written and comprehensive, this book makes the patient a better partner."

—American Lung Association

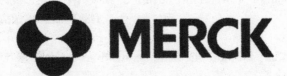

The Merck Manual of Women's and Men's Health

Justin L. Kaplan, MD
Robert S. Porter, MD
Editors

Susan L. Hendrix, DO
Consulting Editor, Women's Health

Ralph E. Cutler, MD
Consulting Editor, Men's Health

Mark H. Beers, MD
Editor Emeritus

POCKET BOOKS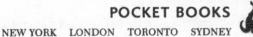
NEW YORK   LONDON   TORONTO   SYDNEY

POCKET BOOKS, a division of Simon & Schuster, Inc.
1230 Avenue of the Americas, New York, NY 10020

Copyright © 2003, 2007, by Merck & Co., Inc.

Published by arrangement with Merck & Co., Inc.

A previous version of this work was published as part of *The Merck Manual of Medical Information, Second Home Edition*.

ISBN-13: 978-1-5011-0453-4

This Pocket Books paperback edition January 2007

10 9 8

POCKET and colophon are registered trademarks of Simon & Schuster, Inc.

Manufactured in the United States of America

For information regarding special discounts for bulk purchases, please contact Simon and Schuster Special Sales at 1-800-456-6798 or business@simonandschuster.com.

Preface

Men's and women's health encompasses many of life's essentials—not just disorders affecting the sex organs, but topics such as sexuality, fertility, family planning, pregnancy, and giving birth. Information about these topics can be found on the web, in magazines, and in many books. So why do we need this book? What makes it different from other sources?

One difference is in the quality of information. *The Merck Manual of Women's and Men's Health* is adapted from the bestselling *The Merck Manual of Medical Information—Second Home Edition*. This book, written in everyday language, is a translation of *The Merck Manual of Diagnosis and Therapy*, commonly referred to as *The Merck Manual*. *The Merck Manual* is the oldest continuously published general medical textbook in the English language and the most widely used medical textbook in the world. Building on that tradition, *The Merck Manual of Women's and Men's Health* has been reviewed extensively and includes contributions from more than 15 experts. The material reflects the most widely accepted medical knowledge and practice.

The Merck Manual of Women's and Men's Health is comprehensive and detailed. All major aspects of sexual and reproductive health are discussed, with topics ranging from how to be an active and informed patient to the biology of the sex organs, breast disorders, pelvic floor disorders, sexual dysfunction, prostate disorders, family planning, infertility, sexually transmitted diseases, and much more. This book explains what a disorder is, who is likely to get it, what its symptoms are, how it is diagnosed, what its prognosis is, and how it can be prevented and treated. Normal pregnancy and delivery, as well as complications of pregnancy and delivery, are covered. Medical terms are defined so that readers can more easily understand their doctors. Also included are bullet points that summarize topics and "Did You Know" boxes that describe particularly interesting, important, or surprising facts. The many illustrations, sidebars, and tables and the comprehensive index aid in locating and understanding the material.

No book can replace the expertise of an experienced health care practitioner. This book is meant to supplement that relationship, not replace it. As a source of reliable information, *The Merck Manual of Women's and Men's Health* can help readers communicate better with their health care practitioners.

The strength of this book ultimately derives from the efforts of the contributors, whose names are included following the table of contents, and the consulting editors. They deserve a degree of thanks that cannot be adequately expressed here.

We welcome all comments and suggestions.

Justin L. Kaplan, MD
Robert S. Porter, MD

Special Note to Readers

The contributors, reviewers, editors, and publisher have made extensive efforts to ensure that the information is accurate and conforms to the standards accepted at the time of publication. However, constant changes in information resulting from continuing research and clinical experience, reasonable differences in opinions among authorities, unique aspects of individual situations, and the possibility of human error in preparing such an extensive text require that the reader exercise judgment when making decisions and consult and compare information from other sources. In particular, the reader is advised to discuss information obtained in this book with a doctor, pharmacist, nurse, or other health care practitioner.

Contents

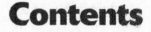

Part III   Men's Health

Contributors

David B. Acker, MD
Associate Professor of Obstetrics, Gynecology, and Reproductive Biology, Harvard Medical School; Director of Obstetrics, Brigham and Women's Hospital

Hervy E. Averette, MD (Deceased)
Professor of Clinical Oncology, University of Miami; American Cancer Society Professor and Sylvester Professor of Gynecologic Oncology

George R. Brown, MD
Professor and Associate Chairman, Department of Psychiatry, East Tennessee State University; Chief of Psychiatry, Mountain Home VAMC

Ralph E. Cutler, MD
Professor of Medicine (Emeritus), Department of Medicine, Loma Linda University School of Medicine; Consultant, Nephrology Section, VA Loma Linda Healthcare System

Sherman Elias, MD
John J. Sciarra Professor and Chair, Department of Obstetrics and Gynecology, Feinberg School of Medicine, Northwestern University; Chairman, Obstetrics and Gynecology, Prentice Women's Hospital of Northwestern Memorial Hospital

Norah C. Feeny, PhD
Associate Professor, Department of Psychology, Case Western Reserve University

Michael R. Foley, MD
Clinical Professor of Obstetrics & Gynecology, University of Arizona at the Health Sciences Center

Michael F. Greene, MD
Professor of Obstetrics, Gynecology, and Reproductive Biology, Harvard Medical School; Director of Obstetrics, Massachusetts General Hospital

Susan L. Hendrix, DO

Professor, Department of Obstetrics and Gynecology, Wayne State University School of Medicine, Hutzel Women's Hospital

Pamela J. Adams Hillard, MD

Professor, Dept. of Obstetrics/Gynecology and of Pediatrics, University of Cincinnati College of Medicine; Director, Obstetrics and Gynecology, Cincinnati Children's Hospital Medical Center

Fran E. Kaiser, MD

Executive Medical Director, Merck & Co., Inc.; Clinical Professor of Medicine, University of Texas Southwestern Medical Center, Adjunct Professor of Medicine, Saint Louis University

Paul Lui, MD

Associate Professor of Surgery, Division of Urology, Loma Linda University School of Medicine

J. Allen McCutchan, MD, MSc

Professor of Medicine, Division of Infectious Diseases, University of California at San Diego School of Medicine

Daniel R. Mishell, Jr., MD

The Lyle G. McNeile Professor and Chairman, Department of Obstetrics and Gynecology, Keck School of Medicine, University of Southern California

Pamela A. Moalli, MD, PhD

Assistant Professor, University of Pittsburgh School of Medicine; Assistant Professor, Magee-Womens Hospital

Robert W. Rebar, MD

Executive Director, American Society for Reproductive Medicine; Volunteer Clinical Professor, Department of Obstetrics and Gynecology, University of Alabama

Victor G. Vogel, MD

Professor of Medicine and Epidemiology, University of Pittsburgh School of Medicine; Director, Breast Cancer Prevention Program, University of Pittsburgh Cancer Institute/Magee-Womens Hospital

Committed to Providing Medical Information: Merck and The Merck Manuals

In 1899, the American drug manufacturer Merck & Co. first published a small book titled *Merck's Manual of the Materia Medica*. It was meant as an aid to physicians and pharmacists, reminding doctors that "Memory is treacherous." Compact in size, easy to use, and comprehensive, *The Merck Manual* (as it was later known) became a favorite of those involved in medical care and others in need of a medical reference. Even Albert Schweitzer carried a copy to Africa in 1913, and Admiral Byrd carried a copy to the South Pole in 1929.

By the 1980s, the book had become the world's largest selling medical text and was translated into more than a dozen languages. While the name of the parent company has changed somewhat over the years, the book's name has remained constant, known officially as *The Merck Manual of Diagnosis and Therapy* but usually referred to as *The Merck Manual* and sometimes "The Merck."

In 1990, the editors of *The Merck Manual* introduced *The Merck Manual of Geriatrics*. This new book quickly became the best-selling textbook of geriatric medicine, providing specific and comprehensive information on the care of older people. The 3rd edition was published in five languages. The creation of this book reflects Merck's commitment to the world's aging population and the company's desire to improve geriatric care globally.

In 1997, *The Merck Manual of Medical Information—Home Edition* was published. In this revolutionary book, the editors translated the complex medical information in *The Merck Manual* into plain language, producing a book meant for all those people interested in medical care who did not have a medical degree. The book received critical acclaim and sold over 2 million copies. *The Second Home Edition* was released in 2003 and continued Merck's commitment to providing comprehensive, understandable medical information to all people.

The Merck Manual of Health & Aging, published in 2004, continued Merck's commitment to education and geriatric care, providing information on aging and the care of older people in words understandable by the lay public.

As part of its commitment to ensuring that all who need and want medical information can get it, Merck provides the content of these Merck Manuals on the web (visit www.merckmanuals. com) for free. Registration is not required, and use is unlimited. The web publications are continuously updated to ensure that the information is as up-to-date as possible.

Merck also supports the community of chemists and others with the need to know about chemical compounds with *The Merck Index*. First published in 1889, this publication actually predates *The Merck Manual* and is the most widely used text of its kind. *The Merck Veterinary Manual* was first published in 1955. It provides information on the health care of animals and is the preeminent text in its field.

The Merck Manual of Women's and Men's Health, published in 2007, is the latest book in the venerable tradition of The Merck Manuals. Adapted from *The Second Home Edition, The Merck Manual of Women's and Men's Health* is a reliable resource for information about sexual health, pregnancy, and disorders that affect the reproductive organs.

Merck & Co., Inc. is one of the world's largest pharmaceutical companies. Merck is committed to providing excellent medical information and, as part of that effort, continues to proudly provide all of The Merck Manuals as a service to the community.

Part I

General Issues

CHAPTER 1

Women's and Men's Health—An Overview

For men and women, the health of the entire body, including the function of all organs—heart, lungs, gastrointestinal tract, muscles, nerves, eyes, ears, and other organs—is important. However, discussions of men's and women's health usually focus on sexuality and the healthy functioning of the reproductive organs. Nevertheless, maintaining the best possible overall health care involves taking part in preventive self-care measures, being an active and informed patient, as well as recognizing the importance of genital and sexual health.

What Does Women's Health Involve?

Women's health focuses on the breasts and female reproductive system—vulva, vagina, cervix, uterus, ovaries, and fallopian tubes. Inflammation, infection, cancer, and many other disorders may affect these organs. Problems related to reproduction and sexual function can develop.

Doctors who specialize in the female reproductive system are called gynecologists. Some gynecologists specialize in obstetrics, the care of women throughout pregnancy and delivery. Physicians who handle obstetrics are called obstetricians or obstetrician-gynecologists. Some gynecologists specialize in the care of older women, women going through menopause, and women who have urinary problems. Some women see their gynecologist for primary care. Some gynecologic care can be provided by another health care practitioner such as an internist, a nurse-midwife, a physician's assistant, or a general, family, or nurse practitioner. Which type of practitioner women see for care sometimes depends on what the problem is, what the health care practitioner's experience and training are, and how medicine is practiced in the geographic region. A woman should choose a practitioner with whom she can comfortably discuss sensitive topics, such as sex, birth control, pregnancy, and problems related to menopause.

Aside from certain obvious differences, how are men and women different? In the past, research studies tended to use only men as subjects. Over time, people began to question whether the results of such studies could be applied to women. They also wondered whether prevention and treatment of disorders common among or unique to women had been researched adequately. To answer some of these questions, a long-term major research study, funded by the United States government, was begun in 1991. It is called the Women's Health Initiative (WHI).

The WHI aimed to study major causes of death, disability, and frailty in postmenopausal women. These disorders include heart disorders, stroke, blood clots in the legs and lungs, osteoporosis, dementia, and certain cancers. Heart disease (usually coronary artery disease) is the leading cause of death in postmenopausal women, and about half of all deaths related to heart disease occur in women. Osteoporosis is a common cause of fractures, which contribute to increased disability, lessen the quality of life, and may shorten life. The WHI included the highest quality long-term research studies on hormone therapy and the risks of disorders among women. Also, the WHI studied the effects of calcium and vitamin D on the risk of fractures and colorectal cancer and the relationship between dietary fat intake and breast cancer.

The WHI is ongoing, but some important data have already been collected. The WHI and other studies have provided information about the risks and benefits of long-term postmeno-

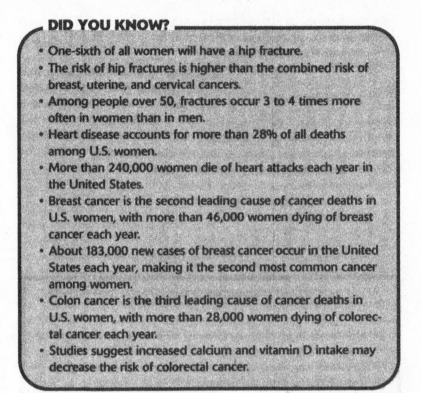

DID YOU KNOW?

- One-sixth of all women will have a hip fracture.
- The risk of hip fractures is higher than the combined risk of breast, uterine, and cervical cancers.
- Among people over 50, fractures occur 3 to 4 times more often in women than in men.
- Heart disease accounts for more than 28% of all deaths among U.S. women.
- More than 240,000 women die of heart attacks each year in the United States.
- Breast cancer is the second leading cause of cancer deaths in U.S. women, with more than 46,000 women dying of breast cancer each year.
- About 183,000 new cases of breast cancer occur in the United States each year, making it the second most common cancer among women.
- Colon cancer is the third leading cause of cancer deaths in U.S. women, with more than 28,000 women dying of colorectal cancer each year.
- Studies suggest increased calcium and vitamin D intake may decrease the risk of colorectal cancer.

pausal hormone therapy. This information provides women with some guidance about hormone use. Choosing whether or not to use hormone therapy is an important health decision.

What Does Men's Health Involve?

Men's health usually focuses on the male reproductive system—the penis, testes, scrotum, and prostate. Inflammation, infection, cancer, and many other disorders may affect these organs. Problems related to reproduction and sexual function can also develop.

Doctors who specialize in the male reproductive system are called urologists. Urologists also treat urinary tract problems in men and women. Care for some men's health problems can be provided by a primary care practitioner (physician, nurse practitioner, or physician's assistant) or a urologist, depending on what the problem is, what the primary care practitioner's experience and training are, and how medicine is practiced in the geographic region. When possible, a man should choose a practitioner with whom he is comfortable and can discuss sensitive topics such as sex.

Men have certain health challenges other than those that involve the reproductive system. For example, men tend to smoke (1 of every 4 men over age 20) and drink more than women and generally lead less healthy lives. About 7 of every 10 men over the age of 20 are overweight, and more than one quarter of them have high blood pressure. Men do not seek medical help as often as women. Young men tend to join in fearless, risky behaviors more than women. Men are significantly less likely than women to recognize the health benefits of fruits and vegetables, such as their role in reducing the risk of many cancers, heart disease, high blood pressure, and diabetes. Many of the major health risks for men can be prevented and treated if they are identified early.

SOME IMPORTANT DISPARITIES BETWEEN MEN AND WOMEN

- Men have a shorter life expectancy (74.5 years for men versus 79.9 years for women).
- The death rate from cardiovascular disease is 1.5 times higher (men: 297.4 per 100,000; women: 197.2).
- The HIV/AIDS death rate is 3 times higher (men: 7.4 per 100,000; women: 2.5).
- The total cancer death rate is 1.5 times higher (men: 238.9 per 100,000; women: 163.1).
- Men are 4.4 times more likely to die from suicide (men: 18.4 per 100,000; women: 4.2).
- Men are 2.2 times more likely to die from unintentional injuries (men: 51.6 per 100,000; women: 23.5).
- Men are 2.3 times more likely to die from motor vehicle injuries (men: 22.1 per 100,000; women: 9.6).

Source: National Center for Health Statistics, Centers for Disease Control and Prevention, 2004.

Some experts are calling for more research on how disorders that can affect both sexes affect men specifically. Men's shorter life expectancy cannot be explained by differences in the severity of disorders that affect only men and those that affect only women.

Rather, certain disorders that affect both sexes may somehow be more severe in men. Also, although many research studies in the past tended to include mostly men, most such studies did not exclude women completely. Past studies focused on a particular disorder, not on how the disorder affected men.

Preventive Health Care for Women and Men

Preventive medicine aims to prevent disorders from occurring in the first place or to diagnose a disorder early, ideally when there are no symptoms. There are four major components:

1. Vaccinations to prevent infectious diseases
2. Screening programs, such as those for high blood pressure, diabetes, and cancer
3. Chemoprevention (drug therapy), such as cholesterol-lowering drugs to prevent atherosclerosis, aspirin to prevent heart attacks or strokes, and antihypertensive drugs to reduce blood pressure and prevent strokes
4. Counseling to help people make healthy lifestyle choices, such as not smoking, wearing seat belts, exercising, brushing and flossing their teeth, and eating a healthy diet

What a specific person needs to prevent a disorder is based on the person's risk of developing a disorder. That risk depends on such factors as age, sex, family history, lifestyle, and physical and social environment.

Prevention in Young to Middle-Aged Adults

For young and middle-aged adults, the risk of major health problems is established by periodically measuring blood pressure, weight, and cholesterol levels. Some experts recommend also measuring blood sugar levels. A health care practitioner may check for depression and stress by asking questions about mood and sleep patterns. A person may be asked questions about the work environment to determine any health hazards.

Papanicolaou (Pap) tests (for cervical cancer) and mammograms (depending on the woman's age or family history of breast cancer) are recommended for women, and breast self-examination is encouraged. For men older than 50 (or younger if there is a family history suggesting increased risk), some experts recommend an

Preventing Major Health Problems

HEALTH PROBLEM	PREVENTIVE MEASURES
Heart disease	Maintain the best possible cholesterol levels through diet, exercise, and drugs (if necessary)
	Maintain the best possible blood pressure through diet, exercise, stress reduction, and drugs (if necessary)
	Eat a balanced diet high in fiber and limited in fat and cholesterol
	Do not smoke
Cancer*	Do not smoke (lung cancer)
	Eat a balanced diet high in fiber and limited in fat and cholesterol (breast cancer, colorectal cancer, and possibly other cancers)
	Regularly examine the breasts (for women aged 20 and over) or testes (for men aged 12 to about 40)
	Avoid too much exposure to the sun, and use sunscreens with a high sun-protection factor (skin cancer)
	Check the skin for growths that change or bleed and perhaps ask another person (such as a spouse) to look at locations that are difficult to see, such as the back or behind the ears (skin cancer)
	Check for bleeding from the rectum (colorectal cancer)
Stroke	Do not smoke
	Maintain the best possible blood pressure through diet, exercise, stress reduction, and drugs (if necessary)
	Maintain the best possible cholesterol levels through diet, exercise, and drugs (if necessary)
	Avoid stress and fatigue
Chronic obstructive pulmonary disease	Do not smoke
	Avoid exposure to toxic substances (especially in industrial settings)
Injuries	Wear a seat belt in motor vehicles
	When possible, use a car with the best safety equipment (such as multiple air bags, anti-lock brakes, and electronic stability control)

Preventing Major Health Problems (Continued)

Injuries (*continued*)	Wear a helmet when riding a bicycle or motorcycle
	Store firearms safely
	Install smoke and carbon monoxide detectors in the home and make sure they are working
	Never swim alone
	Learn cardiopulmonary resuscitation (CPR) and other methods to relieve airway obstruction, such as the Heimlich maneuver
	Remove or secure throw rugs, make sure lighting is adequate, and install handrails or grab bars where needed to prevent falls
	Exercise regularly
	Drink alcohol in moderation if at all
Diabetes	Exercise regularly
	Eat a balanced diet
	Measure weight intermittently and attempt to maintain an ideal body weight
Pneumonia	Get a pneumonia (pneumococcal) vaccine once, then once again after 5 years if older than 65 or at high risk
Influenza	Get an influenza vaccine every year
Tooth loss	Brush the teeth and use dental floss regularly
	Do not eat sweets frequently
	Visit a dentist regularly
Sexually transmitted diseases	Practice abstinence or limit the number of sex partners
	Use condoms and follow safe sex practices
	Get the vaccine against human papillomavirus to prevent cervical cancer and genital warts
Liver disease	Drink alcohol in moderation if at all
	Get a vaccination against hepatitis B if at high risk
Stress	Check mental health—for example, for unusual irritability, anxiety, symptoms of depression, thoughts of suicide or violence, excessive consumption of alcohol, or substance abuse

*In addition to these preventive measures, screening programs are available for breast, cervical, colorectal, and prostate cancer.

annual rectal examination to screen for prostate cancer. A blood test for prostate-specific antigen (PSA) is sometimes recommended in addition. Men, especially adolescents to men aged 40, may be advised to examine their testes to help detect testicular cancer. An annual test for hidden (occult) blood in the stool and periodic colonoscopy or another colon cancer screening method are recommended for men and women over 50.

Depending on the person's risk profile, the health care practitioner may offer counseling on stopping smoking, avoiding alcohol or certain drugs (illicit drugs and drugs that cause drowsiness) while driving, wearing seat belts, using motorcycle or bicycle helmets, having working smoke and carbon monoxide detectors in the home, having heating systems and fireplaces cleaned and inspected periodically, and making sure all firearms are safely stored. People who spend a lot of time outdoors in areas where Lyme disease is common are advised to take precautions.

The health care practitioner usually emphasizes the importance of eating a balanced diet that includes whole grains, fresh fruits and vegetables, and adequate calcium and that is limited in fat and cholesterol. The need for regular exercise is also emphasized. Sexual behavior is discussed. Depending on the person's risk profile, the discussion may focus on preventing sexually transmitted diseases and unintended pregnancies. Women who are planning on becoming pregnant are advised to take a multivitamin with folic acid, to stop smoking, and to eliminate or limit alcohol.

Vaccinations are not a focus in this age group, although tetanus/diphtheria (Td) boosters are recommended every 10 years, and people at high risk of complications of the flu or pneumonia would benefit from getting the influenza vaccine every year and the pneumonia (pneumococcal) vaccine. The pneumonia vaccine may need to be repeated once, at least 5 years after the first immunization with the vaccine. Hepatitis B vaccine (HBV) is recommended for all young adults.

Chemoprevention sometimes includes aspirin for people at risk of heart attacks, cholesterol-lowering drugs for people with high cholesterol levels that have not responded to diet and exercise, and drugs that improve or preserve bone density for people with or at risk of osteoporosis.

Prevention in Older Adults

Many screening measures are important for people over age 65. For example, blood pressure, height, weight, blood sugar level,

A Partial Screening Schedule for Adults[*]

TEST	AGE (YEARS)	HOW OFTEN
Blood pressure	18 and older	Every office visit or annually
Height	18 and older	Periodically
Weight	18 and older	Every office visit or annually
Rectal examination for occult (hidden) blood in stool and, in men, for prostate cancer	50 and older	Annually
Cholesterol	Men 35 and older Women 45 and older	Every 5 years if levels are within normal limits
Hearing	65 and older	Periodically
Mammography (for women)	50 and older (some experts say age 40 and older)	Annually
Papanicolaou (Pap) test (for women)	18 and older	Every 1 to 3 years
Colonoscopy	50 and older	Every 3 to 10 years
Prostate-specific antigen (PSA) level (for men)	50 and older	Annually
Dental and oral health examination	18 and older	Annually
Breast examination	40 and older	Annually
Bone density	65 and older	Periodically

[*]Based on recommendations by most major experts in the United States. However, differences exist among the recommendations of the various experts.

and cholesterol level are measured regularly. Rectal examinations, vision and hearing tests, stool tests for hidden blood, colon cancer screening, mammograms, Pap tests, bone density tests for women, and PSA tests for men are often useful.

Counseling may include smoking cessation, alcohol curtailment, prevention of sexually transmitted diseases, and the need for regular dental visits. Preventing injuries is discussed. Older people may be advised to remove throw rugs and install bathtub rails and grab bars to prevent falls, to install large-numbered telephones, and to set the hot water heater at not more than 130°F (to prevent burns).

A balanced diet limited in fat and cholesterol is emphasized, as is adequate calcium and vitamin D, especially for women to prevent osteoporosis. Regular exercise is still beneficial for this age group. It helps prevent heart disease, diabetes, stroke, osteoporosis, cancer, and frailty, among other health problems.

Three vaccinations are recommended for people over 65. The pneumonia (pneumococcal) vaccine is recommended for every person once after reaching 65 years of age, unless the person had the same vaccine before age 65 and within the last 5 years. The vaccine may need to be repeated once, at least 5 years after the first immunization with the vaccine. This vaccination prevents the most common types of pneumonia that develop among people living in the community. The influenza vaccine is recommended every year, and a tetanus/diphtheria (Td) booster is recommended every 10 years.

Chemoprevention can include cholesterol-lowering drugs to prevent atherosclerosis, antihypertensive drugs to control blood pressure and prevent stroke, and drugs that improve or preserve bone density to prevent osteoporosis or broken bones in people who have osteoporosis.

Being an Active and Informed Patient

Having a Primary Care Practitioner

A primary care practitioner provides most preventive care and, when possible, is the first practitioner involved when a person needs care for a problem. The primary care practitioner can also coordinate testing and any referrals to specialists. In addition, if a person needs advice about what to do about a new problem (for example, an injury or a new symptom) or is not sure whether a problem requires a visit to an emergency department, the primary care practitioner's office can often be called.

Talking With the Practitioner

Communication is often better and medical decisions are more easily made when people have established a relationship with a primary care practitioner. People who do not have a primary care practitioner are more likely to be seen by a doctor they do not know. The primary care practitioner usually knows the person well. Thus, important information about the person is less likely to be ignored because the person forgets to tell the doctor, does not know about it, or cannot fully explain it. People are more likely to trust practitioners they know and tend to experience less anxiety when a medical problem arises. Also, practitioners who are familiar with their patients can often avoid unnecessary testing. Primary care practitioners often have long-standing relationships with their patients and are familiar with what their patients want, how they best receive information, how they cope with adversity, whether they are able to purchase prescribed drugs, and which family members they rely on.

Making the Most of a Health Care Visit

Preparing for the health care visit enables a person to get the most out of the time spent. During a first visit, the person may wish to tell the practitioner any personal, religious, or ethnic considerations that may affect health care decisions. If the person already has an advance directive such as a living will or a durable power of attorney agreement, a copy should be given to the practitioner. A person who does not already have an advance directive may wish to discuss why one is needed or how to prepare one. Also, the person should ask questions about office practices, such as whether to expect other practitioners (such as other doctors, nurse practitioners, or physician assistants) to participate in care from time to time and how to handle sudden urgent health problems that occur at night or during weekends.

The person should describe any previous hospitalizations, use of home health services, and care from specialists or other health care practitioners. Providing the names, addresses, and phone numbers of other practitioners helps the primary care practitioner communicate with these sources and obtain copies of medical records (with the person's written permission). The person should tell the practitioner about any plans for diagnostic tests or new treatments.

Before any visit, the person should collect all drugs currently being taken, including medicinal herbs, vitamins, and other over-the-counter drugs, to bring to the practitioner. Any forms that need to be completed by office personnel should also be brought. Any significant medical symptoms or questions about medical issues should be written down. Questions are easily forgotten during a busy office visit. Because there may not be time to discuss all questions, the most important questions should be asked first.

The person should listen carefully to the practitioner and respond as honestly and completely as possible. A common topic that requires clear and honest communication is the use of prescribed drugs. For example, a person who has not been taking a drug as prescribed needs to say so and to provide an explanation (for example, "I seem to get stomach cramps from the medicine" or "I cannot afford the medicine" or, if true, "I often forget"). Other common topics requiring honest discussion include exercise, sleep, diet, mental health issues, sexual practices, and use of caffeine, tobacco, drugs (including illicit), and alcohol.

Symptoms should be described as honestly and openly as possible. Exaggerating the severity of symptoms may make their cause difficult to determine and may also detract from a person's long-term credibility with the practitioner. Similarly, minimizing the severity of symptoms may cause important disorders to be overlooked or pain or other symptoms to be ineffectively treated. All symptoms should be described, no matter how embarrassing.

If tests are ordered, the person should ask how and when results will be communicated. Knowing who is responsible (the practitioner or the person) for initiating follow-up of results is particularly important. For example, some practitioners or their office personnel telephone the person promptly about abnormal results but mail normal results or discuss them at the next visit. New technology means some people can access their laboratory results through the Internet at a secure web site.

If an invasive diagnostic procedure or treatment is proposed, its effectiveness and possible side effects, as well as possible alternatives, should be discussed. Also, the person should ask what the specific goals for the treatment are and how the response to treatment will be followed or monitored. Before certain diagnostic procedures, the person may be asked to sign an informed consent form, which describes the pertinent risks, benefits, and alternatives. In such cases, the person should ask as many questions as needed to feel comfortable with making a decision.

The person should request an explanation of anything that is not understood and ask for a patient education sheet or handout on the subject if one is available. Asking the practitioner to write out instructions and reading the instructions back to the doctor at the end of the visit is one way to help clarify communication. It offers the practitioner the opportunity to correct any miscommunication. If a person cannot read or has impaired vision, speech, or hearing, other approaches may be needed to keep track of the information. For example, instructions may be recorded or a family member or friend may be asked to read the instructions. All of these strategies can also help when a person goes to the pharmacy for drugs.

Before leaving the office, a person should check the list of questions made before the visit and ask the practitioner about anything not covered. If many questions remain, another appointment may be necessary, or the person may need to be referred to another health care practitioner, such as a nurse, pharmacist, or dietitian, for further information.

After the visit, a follow-up appointment should be scheduled if needed. Prescriptions should be filled, and any material included by the pharmacist about the drug should be reviewed. Keeping a diary of important aspects of care may be useful. For example, a person with constant headaches may want to record when headaches occur, what activities or other factors are associated with them, and how they respond to drugs.

Getting a Second Opinion
Despite similar training, doctors have their own opinions, experiences, and thoughts on how to practice, including diagnosing and treating disorders. Some doctors are conservative

and may order fewer tests or pursue fewer or less invasive treatments. Others are more aggressive. Also, doctors differ in how they analyze and weigh risks and benefits of treatment alternatives. Health care is highly specialized and constantly changing, and becoming skilled in all the latest technologies is difficult. For these reasons, getting a second opinion from a different doctor can give a person additional insight and more information about how to treat a disorder. A second opinion should be considered when contemplating an invasive diagnostic test or deciding between different courses of treatment. Options can be weighed, and the result is a more informed choice about what to do. Whether the second opinion is similar to or different from the first, a person can also get a third opinion.

HOW TO GET A SECOND OPINION

- Check with the health insurance company to see if the cost of a second opinion is covered. If it is not covered, consider whether a second opinion would be worth the cost of paying for it. Ask about and follow any special procedures for getting a second opinion.

- Ask the doctor to recommend a second doctor. Most doctors welcome another opinion. Alternatively, contact another trusted doctor for a recommendation. University teaching hospitals and medical societies can also provide names of expert doctors.

- Arrange to have medical records sent to the second doctor before the visit. The new doctor then has time to look at the records, and repeat diagnostic tests will be avoided. Because of HIPAA (Health Insurance and Portability and Accountability Act) regulations, written permission is required before any records or test results can be forwarded.

- Learn as much as possible about the disorder. Write questions and concerns down, and bring the list to discuss with the doctor.

- Visit the doctor to get the second opinion. Do not rely on the telephone or Internet. For a second opinion to be meaningful, the doctor should thoroughly review medical records and perform any relevant parts of the physical examination.

Keeping Medical Records

Keeping a personal record that includes hospitalizations (dates, location, attending doctor's name, and diagnoses), family medical history, allergic reactions to drugs, and significant medical problems is important. Memory alone is not always accurate, and records may not be available when needed. For example, institutions may be unable to provide medical records from long ago.

Immunization records, which are traditionally kept for children, are important to keep and to keep up-to-date throughout life. The person's drug regimen should be written out on one sheet of paper or kept on a computer. The regimen can be updated as new events occur and the information changes. Copies of laboratory results are also useful to keep for future reference.

State laws vary regarding which parts of the medical record in the doctor's office are available to patients. Doctors often own the records but can be required by the courts to submit copies or summaries of the records for specific legal situations. At the patient's request, a doctor's office usually copies and releases the records to the patient or creates a summary of portions or all of the record to send to other health care practitioners. The Health Insurance and Portability and Accountability Act of 1996 (HIPAA) dictates that a person's medical records are confidential and that disclosing information about a person's medical conditions generally requires the person's consent. Patients who want a copy of all of their medical records for personal use may or may not be entitled to these records, depending on state law. Generally, a complete record is not needed. Rather, a file should be maintained of the most important items, including the information needed for the personal record.

Medical records are increasingly being recorded and stored electronically. This practice may enable different practitioners who care for a person to share information about the person more easily and with fewer errors.

Researching a Disorder

When a disorder is first diagnosed, the practitioner may supply an information sheet or pamphlet that summarizes key points. The person may have some general knowledge of the disorder based on newspaper or magazine articles or television or radio shows.

Additional sources of information are available for people who want to learn more. Many books provide helpful, general information. Some local, university, or hospital libraries have useful resources, sometimes including a research librarian. The Internet provides information too. However, judging the reliability of printed and online materials is not always easy. When asked, doctors and registered nurses may help people determine what sources are reliable and may also be a source of additional reliable information. Some online government medical sources are authoritative. Examples are the National Institutes of Health (NIH; www.nih.gov), the Agency for Healthcare Research and Quality (AHRQ; www.ahrq.gov), and the Centers for Disease Control and Prevention (CDC; www.cdc.gov). Many disorder-specific, patient-oriented Internet sites (such as the National Multiple Sclerosis Society) provide reliable information for people with a particular disorder. Sites designed to sell products or services may provide biased or inaccurate information.

Support groups may provide helpful information as well as psychologic support. Such groups can be located through local newspapers, phone directories, hospitals, doctors' offices, other health care practitioners' offices, and the Internet. Many cities have support groups, sometimes for specific disorders. For example, Gilda's Club, which supports people living with cancer, is located in several cities. In support groups, people who have the same disorder can share practical and useful suggestions for day-to-day living, such as where to find pieces of specialized equipment, what equipment works best, and how to interact with or care for someone with a disorder. In addition, chat rooms on the Internet enable people with a specific disorder to communicate with one another, to learn more about their disorder, and to share resources.

Talking to a Partner About Sex

Sexuality is natural and healthy. Emotional, spiritual, psychologic, social, and ethical factors are involved. Most older people remain interested in sex and report quite satisfying sex lives well into old age. Talking honestly and thoughtfully with one's partner about sex throughout a relationship tends to improve satisfaction with sex as well as the relationship.

Some people hide their sexuality because they think doing so is expected of them based on their sex or age. Some people deny their sexual fantasies or repress their desires. People may feel that their partner does not understand how to satisfy them sexually. People respond so differently in what they find sexually arousing that the only way partners get to know each other's preferences is by communicating.

Initiating talk about sex might be difficult. Partners should choose a time when both are free of distractions. A book or magazine article might help break the ice. A relaxing environment in a public location (so that there is no expectation of sexual activity), such as a park or a coffee bar, may take some of the pressure off. Open-ended questions (for example, "What do you want from…?") might focus on relationship expectations and on desired sexual practices. Partners new to a sexual relationship should discuss contraceptive use and testing for sexually transmitted diseases, including HIV (human immunodeficiency virus) infection. Good communication involves the following:

- Being open to discussion
- Listening attentively, without interruption and without judging
- Recognizing when a topic is uncomfortable for one's partner
- Communicating one's own preferences honestly and respectfully.

At one time or another, most people have a problem with their sex lives. Common problems include difficulty getting aroused, difficulty reaching orgasm, having sex end too quickly, and differences between partners in the frequency and type of sexual activity they desire. A problem may arise when a physical change, such as a mastectomy, alters a person's body image and affects sexuality. Some sexual problems go away eventually or can be treated by a primary care practitioner, gynecologist, or urologist. Another option is sex therapy. Sex therapists are trained counselors or health care practitioners who help people with sexual problems.

They have training in the physical and emotional issues linked to sexuality and sex. A sex therapist can help a couple see their situation from a completely different viewpoint. The therapist asks questions to help discover any emotional or physical reasons for the problem. Ideally, sex therapists work with both partners when the problem affects the couple. Exercises and tasks to be done at home may be prescribed. As with visits to any health care practitioner, sessions with a sex therapist are strictly confidential.

CHAPTER 2

Sexuality

Sexuality is a normal part of the human experience. However, the types of sexual behavior that are considered normal vary greatly within and among different cultures. In fact, it may be impossible to define "normal" sexuality. There are wide variations not only in "normal" sexual behavior but also in the frequency of or need for sexual release. Some people desire sexual activity several times a day, whereas others are satisfied with infrequent activity (for example, a few times a year).

Although younger people are often reluctant to view older people as sexually interested, most older people remain interested in sex and report quite satisfying sex lives well into old age. Problems with sexual function, such as erectile dysfunction in men (see page 419) and dyspareunia, vaginismus, or anorgasmia in women (see page 193), affect people of all ages, although such problems tend to be more common in older people.

Societal attitudes about sexuality change with time. Examples of such changes can be seen regarding masturbation, homosexuality, and frequent sexual activity with different sex partners.

Masturbation

Masturbation, which was once regarded as a perversion and even a cause of mental disease, is now recognized as a normal sexual activity throughout life. It is estimated that more than 97% of males and 80% of females have masturbated. In general, males masturbate more frequently than females, even if

DID YOU KNOW?

- The types of sexual activity that people engage in and how often they engage in these activities vary so much that it is almost impossible to define "normal" sexual activity.
- Most older people have satisfying sex lives.
- Masturbation is extremely common, even among people involved in sexually gratifying relationships.
- Homosexuality is widely regarded as a sexual orientation that is present from childhood and is thus not a "choice."
- Homosexuality is not considered a disorder.

involved in a sexually gratifying relationship. Although masturbation is normal and is often recommended as a "safe sex" option, it may cause guilt and psychologic suffering that stems from the disapproving attitudes of others. This can result in considerable distress and can even affect sexual performance.

Homosexuality

As with masturbation, homosexuality, once considered abnormal by the medical profession, is no longer considered a disorder; it is widely recognized as a sexual orientation that is present from childhood. An estimated 4 to 5% of adults are involved exclusively in homosexual relationships throughout their lives, with an additional 2 to 5% of people periodically engaging in sex with someone of the same sex (bisexuality). Adolescents may experiment with same-sex play, but this does not necessarily indicate an enduring interest in homosexual or bisexual activity as adults.

Homosexuals discover that they are attracted to people of the same sex, just as heterosexuals discover that they are attracted to people of the opposite sex. The attraction appears to be the end result of biologic and environmental influences and is not a matter of choice. Therefore, the popular term "sexual preference" makes little sense in matters of sexual orientation.

Most homosexuals adjust well to their sexual orientation, although they must overcome widespread societal disapproval and prejudice. This adjustment may take a long time and may be associated with substantial psychologic stress. Many homosexual men and women experience bigotry in social situations and in the workplace, adding to their stress. Discrimination based on sexual orientation (or perceived sexual orientation) remains widespread.

Frequent Sexual Activity With Different Partners

For some heterosexuals and homosexuals, frequent sexual activity with different partners is a common practice throughout life. This behavior may serve as a reason to seek professional counseling, because the transmission of certain diseases (for example, HIV infection, hepatitis, syphilis, gonorrhea, cervical cancer) is linked to having many sex partners and because having many sex partners may signify difficulty in forming meaningful, lasting relationships.

Gender Identity

- How a person sees himself or herself, whether masculine or feminine (gender identity) is well established by 18 to 24 months of age.
- Gender identity disorder is a discrepancy between a person's sexual anatomy and gender identity.
- Transsexualism is an extreme form of gender identity disorder.

Gender identity is how a person sees himself or herself, whether masculine, feminine, or somewhere in-between. Gender role is the objective, public presentation in our culture as masculine, feminine, or mixed. For most people, gender identity is consistent with gender role (as when a man has an inner sense of his masculinity and publicly acts in ways that support this feeling).

Gender identity is well established by early childhood (18 to 24 months of age). During childhood, boys come to know they are boys, and girls come to know they are girls. Children sometimes prefer activities considered to be more appropriate for the other sex. However, this does not mean that a young girl who likes to play baseball and wrestle, for example, has a gender identity problem, as long as she sees herself as, and is content with being, female.

Similarly, a boy who plays with dolls and prefers cooking to sports or to rough types of play does not have a gender identity problem as long as he identifies himself as, and is comfortable with being, male.

Children born with genitals that are not clearly male or female usually do not have a gender identity problem if they are decisively reared as one sex or the other, even if they are raised in the gender role that is opposite their biologic sex pattern. There have been some highly publicized cases, however, in which this approach has failed.

Gender Identity Disorder and Transsexualism

People who experience a significant discrepancy between their anatomy and their inner sense of self as masculine, feminine, mixed, or neutral often have a gender identity disorder. The extreme form of gender identity disorder is called transsexualism.

People who are transsexuals believe that they are victims of a biologic accident and that they are cruelly imprisoned within a body incompatible with their gender identity. Most transsexuals are biologic males who identify themselves as females, usually early in childhood, and regard their genitals and masculine features with repugnance. Transsexualism appears to occur in about 1 of 30,000 males and 1 of 100,000 females.

Transsexuals may seek psychologic help, either to assist them in coping with the difficulties of living in a body that they do not feel comfortable with or to help them through a gender transition. Many transsexuals appear to be helped most by a combination of counseling, hormone therapy, electrolysis, and genital surgery.

Some transsexuals are satisfied with changing their gender role by working, living, and dressing in society as a member of the opposite sex, which may include obtaining identification (such as a driver's license) that reinforces their change in gender role. They may never seek to actually alter their anatomy in any way. Many of these people, who are sometimes referred to as "transgenderists," meet no criteria for a mental health disorder.

Other transsexuals, in addition to adopting the behavior, dress, and mannerisms of the opposite sex, also receive hormone treatments to change their secondary sex characteristics. In biologic males, use of the female hormone estrogen causes breast growth and other body changes, such as wasting of the genitals (genital atrophy) and the inability to maintain an erection. In biologic females, use of the male hormone testosterone causes such changes as the growth of facial hair, deepening of the voice, and changes in body odor.

Still other transsexuals seek to undergo sex reassignment surgery. For biologic males, this involves removal of the penis and testes and the creation of an artificial vagina. For biologic females, this involves removal of the breasts and the internal reproductive organs (uterus and ovaries), closure of the vagina, and creation of an artificial penis. For both sexes, surgery is preceded by use of the appropriate sex hormone (estrogen in male-to-female transformation, testosterone in female-to-male transformation).

Although transsexuals who undergo sex reassignment surgery are unable to have children, many are able to have quite satisfactory sexual relations. The ability to achieve orgasm is often retained after surgery, and some people report feeling comfortable sexually for the first time. However, few transsexuals endure the sex reassignment process for the sole purpose of being able to function sexually in the opposite sex. Confirmation of gender identity is the usual motivator.

Paraphilias

Paraphilias are attractions that in extreme forms are socially unacceptable deviations from the traditionally held norms of sexual relationships and attractions.

- Paraphilias may take the form of fetishism, transvestic fetishism, pedophilia, exhibitionism, voyeurism, masochism, or sadism, among others.
- The difference between paraphilias and unusual sexual behaviors is that paraphilias are extreme and seriously impair the capacity for affectionate, reciprocal sexual activity.

The key features of a paraphilia include repetitive, intense, sexually arousing fantasies or behaviors that usually involve objects (for example, shoes, underwear, leather or rubber products), the infliction of suffering or pain on oneself or one's partner, or having sex with nonconsenting people (for example, with children, with helpless people, or in rape situations). Once these arousal patterns are established, usually in late childhood or near puberty, they are often lifelong.

Some degree of variety is very common in healthy adult sexual relationships and fantasies. When people mutually agree to engage in them, noninjurious sexual behaviors of an unusual nature may be an intrinsic part of a loving and caring relationship. When taken to the extreme, however, such sexual behaviors are paraphilias, psychosexual disorders that seriously impair the capacity for affectionate, reciprocal sexual activity. Partners of people with a paraphilia may feel like an object or as if they are unimportant or unnecessary in the sexual relationship.

Paraphilias may take the form of fetishism, transvestic fetishism, pedophilia, exhibitionism, voyeurism, masochism, or sadism, among others. Most people with paraphilias are men, and many have more than one type of paraphilia.

DID YOU KNOW?

- Most people with paraphilias are men, and many have more than one type of paraphilia.
- Cross-dressing is not always considered a mental health disorder and may not adversely affect a couple's sexual relationship.
- Exhibitionists rarely commit rape.
- Partial asphyxiation (for example, by tying a noose or cloth around the neck) as a way to enhance orgasm may result in accidental death.

Fetishism

In fetishism, sexual activity makes use of physical objects (the fetish), sometimes in preference to contact with humans. People with fetishes may become sexually stimulated and gratified by wearing another person's undergarments, wearing rubber or leather, or holding, rubbing, or smelling objects, such as high-heeled shoes. People with this disorder may not be able to function sexually without their fetish.

Transvestic Fetishism

In transvestic fetishism, a man prefers to wear women's clothing, or, far less commonly, a woman prefers to wear men's clothing (cross-dressing). In neither case, however, does the person wish to change his or her sex, as transsexuals do. Cross-dressing is not always considered a mental health disorder and may not adversely affect a couple's sexual relationship.

Transvestic fetishism is a disorder only if it causes distress, results in impairment of some type, or involves "daredevil" behavior likely to lead to injury, loss of a job, or imprisonment. Transvestites also cross-dress for reasons other than sexual stimulation, for example, to reduce anxiety, to relax, or, in the case of male transvestites, to experiment with the feminine side of their otherwise male personalities.

Pedophilia

Pedophilia is a preference for sexual activity with young children. In Western societies, pedophilia is defined as sexual fantasy about or sexual relations with a child younger than 13 by a person 16 or older. Some pedophiles are attracted only to children, often of a specific age range or developmental stage, whereas others are attracted to both children and adults.

Although state laws vary, the law generally considers a person older than 18 to be committing statutory rape if the victim is 16 or younger. Statutory rape cases often do not meet the definition of pedophilia, highlighting the somewhat arbitrary nature of selecting a specific age cutoff point in a medical or legal definition.

Pedophilia is much more common among men than among women. Both boys and girls can be victims, although more reported cases involve girls. Pedophiles may focus only on children within their families (incest), or they may prey on children in the community. Force or coercion may be used to engage children sexually, and threats may be invoked to prevent disclosure by the victim.

Pedophilia can be treated with psychotherapy and drugs that alter the sex drive, with varying results. Such treatment may be sought voluntarily or only after criminal apprehension and legal action. Incarceration, even long-term, does not change pedophilic desires or fantasies.

Exhibitionism

In exhibitionism, a person (usually male) exposes his genitals to unsuspecting strangers and becomes sexually excited when doing so. Further sexual contact is almost never sought, so exhibitionists rarely commit rape. Most exhibitionists are younger than 40 and may or may not be married. Exposure of genitals to unsuspecting strangers for sexual excitement is rare among women. Provocative dressing by women is increasingly accepted by society as normal. In addition, social venues in which women can expose themselves are not uncommon, and such behavior may not constitute a mental health disorder.

Voyeurism

In voyeurism, a person becomes sexually aroused by watching someone who is disrobing, naked, or engaged in sexual activity. It is the act of observing (peeping) that is arousing, not sexual activity with the observed person. Some degree of voyeurism is particularly common, more among boys and men but increasingly among women. Society often regards mild forms of this behavior as normal. As a disorder, voyeurism is much more common among men; it may become the preferred method of sexual activity and consume countless hours of watching. The amount and variety of sexually explicit materials and shows available to men and women have increased significantly, but engaging in these activities lacks the element of secret observation that is the hallmark of voyeurism. The Internet has made voyeurism easier to engage in without the neighborhood prowling traditionally associated with this behavior.

Sexual Masochism and Sadism

Sexual masochism involves acts in which a person derives sexual excitement from being humiliated, beaten, bound, or otherwise abused. Sexual sadism involves acts in which a person derives sexual pleasure from inflicting physical or psychologic suffering on another person. Some people act out their sadistic urges with a consenting partner (who may have sexual masochism); rarely, some act them out on nonconsenting victims. Fantasies of total control and dominance are often important, and the sadist may bind and gag the partner in elaborate ways.

Some amount of sadism and masochism is commonly play-acted in healthy sexual relationships, and mutually compatible partners often seek one another out. For example, the use of silk handkerchiefs for simulated bondage and mild spanking during sexual activity are common practices between consenting partners and are not considered sadomasochistic.

In contrast, the disorder of sexual masochism or of sexual sadism takes these acts to an extreme and can result in severe bodily or psychologic harm and even death. For example, masochistic sexual activity may involve asphyxiophilia, whereby the person is partially choked or strangled (either by a partner or by the self-application of a noose around the neck). A temporary decrease in oxygen to the brain at the point of orgasm is sought as an enhancement to sexual release, but the practice may accidentally result in death.

CHAPTER 3

Family Planning

Family planning involves using various methods to control the number and timing of pregnancies. A couple may use contraception to avoid pregnancy temporarily or sterilization to avoid pregnancy permanently. Abortion may be used to end an unwanted pregnancy when contraception has failed or not been used.

DID YOU KNOW?

- The effectiveness of certain contraceptive measures, such as the pill or rhythm methods, depends a great deal on how well instructions are followed.
- Contraceptive hormones can be taken by mouth, inserted into the vagina, applied to the skin, or injected into muscle.
- Contraceptive hormones, which have serious side effects in some women, may also have health benefits.
- Latex condoms are the only contraceptive method that helps protect against all common sexually transmitted diseases, including HIV infection.
- Intrauterine devices (IUDs) provide effective contraception and have few serious side effects.

Contraception

Contraception is prevention of the fertilization of an egg by a sperm (conception) or the attachment of the fertilized egg to the lining of the uterus (implantation).

There are several methods of contraception. None is completely effective, but some methods are far more reliable than others. Each contraceptive method has advantages and disadvantages. Choice of method depends on a person's lifestyle and preferences and on the degree of reliability needed.

How Effective Is Contraception?

METHOD	PERCENTAGE OF WOMEN WHO BECOME PREGNANT DURING THE FIRST YEAR OF USE
Oral contraceptives:	
Combination estrogen-progestin tablets	0.1–5
Progestin-only tablets	0.5–5
Implants	0.1
Injections of medroxypro-gesterone	0.3
Condom:	
Male	3–14
Female	5–21
Diaphragm with spermicide	6–20
Cervical cap with spermicide	9–40
Intrauterine device (IUD)	0.1–0.6
Natural family planning (rhythm) method	1–25
Withdrawal method	4–19

HORMONAL METHODS

The hormones used to prevent conception include estrogen and progestins (drugs similar to the hormone progesterone). Hormonal methods prevent pregnancy mainly by stopping the ovaries from releasing eggs or by keeping the mucus in the cervix thick so that sperm cannot pass through the cervix into the uterus. Thus, hormonal methods prevent the egg from being fertilized.

Oral Contraceptives

Oral contraceptives, commonly known as the pill, contain hormones—either a combination of a progestin and estrogen or a progestin alone.

Combination tablets are typically taken once a day for 3 weeks, not taken for a week (allowing the menstrual period to occur), then started again. Inactive tablets may be included for the week when combination tablets are not taken to establish a routine of taking one tablet a day. Fewer than 0.2% of women who take combination tablets as instructed become pregnant during the first year of use. However, the chances of becoming pregnant increase if a woman skips or forgets to take a tablet, especially the first ones in a monthly cycle.

The dose of estrogen in combination tablets varies. Usually, combination tablets with a low dose of estrogen (20 to 35 micrograms) are used because they have fewer serious side effects than those with a high dose (50 micrograms). Healthy women who do not smoke can take low-dose estrogen combination contraceptives without interruption until menopause.

Progestin-only tablets are taken every day of the month. They often cause irregular bleeding. About 0.5 to 5% of women who take these tablets become pregnant. Progestin-only tablets are usually prescribed only when taking estrogen may be harmful. For example, these tablets may be prescribed for women who are breastfeeding because estrogen reduces the amount and quality of breast milk produced. Progestin-only tablets do not affect breast milk production.

Before starting oral contraceptives, a woman should have a physical examination, including measurement of blood pressure, to make sure she has no health problems that would make taking the contraceptives risky for her. If she or a close relative has had diabetes or heart disease, a blood test is usually performed to measure levels of cholesterol, other fats (lipids), and sugar (glucose). If the cholesterol or sugar level is high or other lipid levels are abnormal, doctors may still prescribe a low-dose estrogen combination contraceptive. However, they periodically perform blood tests to monitor the woman's lipid and sugar levels. Three months after starting oral contraceptives, the woman should have another examination to be sure her blood pressure has not changed. After that, she should have an examination at least once a year.

Also before starting oral contraceptives, a woman should discuss with her doctor the advantages and disadvantages of oral contraceptives for her situation.

Advantages: The main advantage is reliable, continuous contraception if oral contraceptives are taken as instructed. Also, taking oral contraceptives reduces the occurrence of menstrual cramps, premenstrual syndrome, irregular bleeding, anemia, breast cysts, ovarian cysts, mislocated (ectopic) pregnancies (almost always in the fallopian tubes), and infections of the fallopian tubes. Also, women who have taken oral contraceptives are less likely to develop rheumatoid arthritis or osteoporosis.

Taking oral contraceptives reduces the risk of developing several types of cancer, including uterine (endometrial) cancer, ovarian, colon, and rectal cancers. The risk is reduced for many years after the contraceptives are discontinued. Breast cancer is slightly more likely to be diagnosed in women while they are taking oral contraceptives but not after the contraceptives are discontinued, even in women who have a family history of breast cancer.

Oral contraceptives taken early in a pregnancy do not harm the fetus. However, they should be discontinued as soon as the woman realizes she is pregnant. Oral contraceptives do not have any long-term effects on fertility, although a woman may not release an egg (ovulate) for a few months after discontinuing the drugs.

Disadvantages: The disadvantages of oral contraceptives may include bothersome side effects. Irregular bleeding is common during the first few months of oral contraceptive use but usually stops as the body adjusts to the hormones. Also, taking oral contraceptives every day, without any breaks, for several months can reduce the number of bleeding episodes.

Some side effects are related to the estrogen in the tablet. They may include nausea, bloating, fluid retention, an increase in blood pressure, breast tenderness, and migraine headaches. Others are related mostly to the type or dose of the progestin. They may include mood disorders, weight gain, acne, and nervousness.

Some women who take oral contraceptives gain 3 to 5 pounds because of fluid retention. They may gain even more because appetite also increases. Some women have headaches and difficulty sleeping. Many of these side effects are uncommon with the low-dose tablets.

In some women, oral contraceptives cause dark patches (melasma) on the face, similar to those that may occur during pregnancy (see page 279). Exposure to the sun darkens the patches even more. If the woman discontinues oral contraceptives, the dark patches slowly fade.

Taking oral contraceptives increases the risk of developing some disorders. The risk of developing blood clots in the veins is higher for women who take combination oral contraceptives than for those who do not. The risk is 7 times higher with tablets containing a high dose of estrogen. However, the risk is 2 to 4 times higher with tablets containing a low dose of estrogen: This risk is half of that during pregnancy. Because surgery also increases the risk of developing blood clots, a woman must discontinue oral contraceptives a month before major elective surgery and not take them again until a month afterward. Because the risk of developing blood clots in leg veins is high during pregnancy and for a few weeks after delivery, doctors recommend that women wait 2 weeks after delivery before they take oral contraceptives. For healthy women who do not smoke, taking low-dose estrogen combination tablets does not increase the risk of having a stroke or heart attack.

Use of oral contraceptives, particularly for more than 5 years, may increase the risk of developing cervical cancer. Women who are taking oral contraceptives should have a Papanicolaou (Pap) test at least once a year. Such tests can detect precancerous changes in the cervix early—before they lead to cancer.

The likelihood of developing gallstones increases during the first few years of oral contraceptive use, then decreases.

For women in certain situations, the risk of developing certain disorders is substantially increased if they take oral contraceptives. For example, women who are older than 35 and who smoke should not use oral contraceptives because the risk of heart attack is increased. For women who have certain disorders, risks are increased if they take oral contraceptives. But if closely monitored by a health care practitioner, such women may be able to take oral contraceptives.

Some sedatives, antibiotics, and antifungals can reduce the effectiveness of oral contraceptives. Women taking oral contraceptives may become pregnant if they simultaneously take one of these drugs.

WHEN TAKING ORAL CONTRACEPTIVES IS RESTRICTED*

A woman must not take oral contraceptives if any of the following situations apply:

- She smokes and is older than 35
- She has an active liver disorder or liver tumors
- She has very high triglyceride levels (250 mg/dL or higher)
- She has untreated high blood pressure
- She has diabetes with blocked arteries
- She has a kidney disorder
- She has had blood clots
- She has a leg immobilized (as in a cast)
- She has coronary artery disease
- She has had a stroke
- She has had cholestasis (jaundice) of pregnancy or jaundice while she was previously taking oral contraceptives
- She has breast or uterine (endometrial) cancer
- She has had a heart attack

A woman may take oral contraceptives with a doctor's supervision if any of the following situations apply:

- She is depressed
- She has premenstrual syndrome
- She frequently has migraine headaches (but no numbness in the limbs)
- She smokes cigarettes but is younger than 35
- She has had hepatitis or another liver disorder and has fully recovered
- She has high blood pressure that is controlled with treatment

(*Continued*)

WHEN TAKING ORAL CONTRACEPTIVES IS RESTRICTED*
(Continued)

- She has varicose veins
- She has a seizure disorder that is being treated with drugs
- She has fibroids in the uterus
- She has been treated for precancerous abnormalities or cancer of the cervix
- She is obese
- She has close relatives who have had blood clots

*These restrictions apply only when estrogen and a progestin are used together.
mg/dL = milligrams per deciliter of blood.

Skin Patches and Vaginal Rings

Skin patches and vaginal rings that contain estrogen and a progestin are used for 3 of 4 weeks. In the fourth week, no contraception is used to allow the menstrual period to occur.

A contraceptive skin patch is placed on the skin once a week for 3 weeks. The patch is left in place for 1 week, then removed, and a new patch is placed on a different area of the skin. During the fourth week, no patch is used. Exercise and use of saunas or hot tubs do not displace the patches.

A vaginal ring is a small plastic device that is placed in the vagina and left there for 3 weeks. Then it is removed for 1 week. A woman can place and remove the vaginal ring herself. The ring comes in one size and can be placed anywhere in the vagina. Usually, the ring is not felt by the woman's partner during intercourse. A new ring is used each month.

With either method, a woman has a regular menstrual period. Spotting or bleeding between periods (breakthrough bleeding) is uncommon. Side effects and restrictions on use are similar to those of combination oral contraceptives.

Contraceptive Implants

Contraceptive implants are plastic capsules or rods containing a progestin. After numbing the skin with an anesthetic, a doctor makes a small incision or uses a needle to place the implants under the skin of the inner arm above the elbow. No stitches are necessary. The implants release the progestin slowly into the bloodstream. No implants are currently available in the United States. A single plastic implant, which is inserted through a needle and is effective for 3 years (but must be removed through an incision), will soon be available.

The most common side effects are irregular or no menstrual periods during the first year of use. After that, periods frequently become regular. Headaches and weight gain may also occur. These side effects prompt some women to have the implants removed. Because the implants do not dissolve in the body, a doctor has to remove them. Removal is more difficult than insertion because tissue under the skin thickens around the implants. Removal may result in a minor scar. As soon as the implants are removed, the ovaries return to their normal functioning, and the woman becomes fertile again.

Contraceptive Injections

Two contraceptive formulations are available as injections. Each is injected by a health care practitioner into a muscle of the arm or buttocks, and each is very effective as a contraceptive.

Medroxyprogesterone acetate, a progestin, is injected once every 3 months. Medroxyprogesterone acetate can completely disrupt the menstrual cycle. About one third of women using this contraceptive have no menstrual bleeding during the 3 months after the first injection, and another third have irregular bleeding and spotting for more than 11 days each month. After this contraceptive is used for a while, irregular bleeding occurs less often. After 2 years, about 70% of the women have no bleeding at all. When the injections are discontinued, a regular menstrual cycle resumes in about half of the women within 6 months and in about three fourths within 1 year. Fertility may not return for up to a year after injections are discontinued.

Side effects include a slight weight gain and a temporary decrease in bone density. Bones usually return to their previous density after the injections are discontinued. Medroxyprogesterone acetate does not increase the risk of developing any cancer, including breast cancer. It greatly reduces the risk of developing uterine (endometrial) cancer. Interactions with other drugs are uncommon.

The other formulation is a once-a-month injection. It contains estrogen and a much smaller amount of medroxyprogesterone acetate than the injections given every 3 months. Consequently, bleeding usually occurs regularly about 2 weeks after each injection is given, and bone density does not decrease. Because the dose of medroxyprogesterone acetate is lower, fertility returns much more rapidly after the injections are discontinued.

Emergency Contraception

Emergency contraception, the so-called morning-after pill, involves the use of hormones within 72 hours after one act of unprotected sexual intercourse or after one occasion when a contraceptive method fails (for example, if a condom breaks).

Two regimens are available. The more effective regimen consists of one dose of levonorgestrel, a progestin, followed by another dose 12 hours later. With this regimen, about 1% of women become pregnant, and fewer side effects occur than with the other regimen. Alternatively, two tablets of a combination oral contraceptive are taken within 72 hours of the unprotected intercourse. Then two more tablets are taken 12 hours later. With this regimen, only about 2% of women become pregnant, but as many as 50% have nausea and 20% vomit. Antiemetic drugs, such as hydroxyzine taken by mouth, are given to prevent nausea and vomiting.

BARRIER CONTRACEPTIVES

Barrier contraceptives physically block the sperm's access to a woman's uterus. They include the condom (male or female), diaphragm, and cervical cap.

Condoms made of latex are the only contraceptives that provide protection against sexually transmitted diseases, including those due to bacteria (such as gonorrhea and syphilis) as well as those due to viruses (such as HIV—human immunodeficiency virus—infection). However, this protection, though considerable, is not complete. Male condoms made of polyurethane also provide protection, but they are thinner and more likely to tear. Male condoms made of lambskin do not protect against viral infections such as HIV infection and thus are not recommended.

Blocking Access: Barrier Contraceptives

Barrier contraceptives prevent sperm from entering a woman's uterus. They include condoms, diaphragms, and cervical caps. Some condoms contain spermicides. Spermicides should be used with condoms and other barrier contraceptives that do not already contain them.

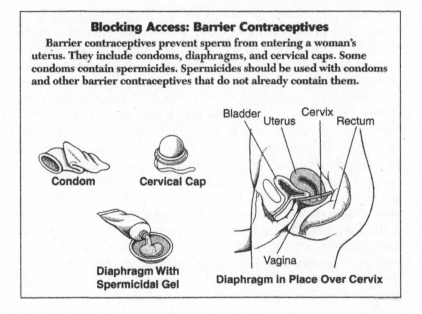

Condom

Cervical Cap

Diaphragm With Spermicidal Gel

Bladder Uterus Cervix Rectum

Vagina

Diaphragm in Place Over Cervix

Condoms must be used correctly to be effective. With some male condoms, the tip needs to be positioned so that it extends about ½ inch beyond the penis to provide a space to collect semen. Other male condoms have a reservoir at the tip for this purpose. Immediately after ejaculation, the penis should be withdrawn while the condom's rim is held firmly against the base of the penis to prevent the condom from slipping off and spilling semen. The condom should then be removed carefully. If semen is spilled, sperm could enter the vagina, resulting in pregnancy. A new condom should be used after each ejaculation, and the condom should be discarded if its integrity is in doubt. A spermicide, which may be included in the condom's lubricant or inserted separately into the vagina, increases the effectiveness of condoms.

The female condom is held in the vagina by a ring. It resembles a male condom but is larger and is not as effective.

The **diaphragm**, a dome-shaped rubber cup with a flexible rim, is inserted into the vagina and positioned over the cervix. A diaphragm prevents sperm from entering the uterus.

Diaphragms come in various sizes and must be fitted by a health care practitioner, who also teaches the woman how to insert it. A diaphragm should cover the entire cervix without causing discomfort. Neither the woman nor her partner should notice its presence. A contraceptive cream or jelly should always be used with a diaphragm, in case the diaphragm is displaced during intercourse. The diaphragm is inserted before intercourse and should remain in place for at least 8 hours but no more than 24 hours afterward. If sexual intercourse is repeated while the diaphragm is in place, additional spermicide should be inserted into the vagina to continue protection. If a woman has gained or lost more than 10 pounds, has had a diaphragm for more than a year, or has had a baby or an abortion, she must be refitted for a diaphragm because the vagina's size and shape may have changed. During the first year of diaphragm use, the percentage of women who become pregnant varies from about 3% when the diaphragm is used correctly to about 14% when it is used the way most people use it.

The **cervical cap** resembles the diaphragm but is smaller and more rigid. It fits snugly over the cervix. Cervical caps must be fitted by a health care practitioner. A contraceptive cream or jelly should always be used with a cervical cap. The cap is inserted before intercourse and left in place for at least 8 hours after intercourse, up to 48 hours at a time.

SPERMICIDES

Spermicides are preparations that kill sperm on contact. They are available as vaginal foams, creams, gels, and suppositories and are placed in the vagina before sexual intercourse. These contraceptives also provide a physical barrier to sperm. No single type of preparation seems to be more effective than another. They are best used in combination with a barrier contraceptive, such as a male condom, female condom, or diaphragm.

INTRAUTERINE DEVICES

Intrauterine devices (IUDs) are small, flexible plastic devices that are inserted into the uterus. An IUD is left in place for 5 or 10 years, depending on the type, or until the woman wants the device removed. IUDs must be inserted and removed by a doctor or other health care practitioner. Insertion takes only a few minutes. Removal is also quick and usually causes minimal discomfort. IUDs kill or immobilize sperm and prevent fertilization of the egg.

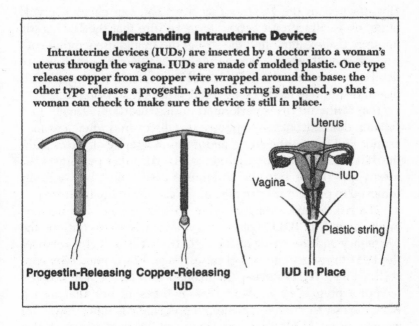

Understanding Intrauterine Devices

Intrauterine devices (IUDs) are inserted by a doctor into a woman's uterus through the vagina. IUDs are made of molded plastic. One type releases copper from a copper wire wrapped around the base; the other type releases a progestin. A plastic string is attached, so that a woman can check to make sure the device is still in place.

Uterus

IUD

Vagina

Plastic string

Progestin-Releasing IUD   **Copper-Releasing IUD**   **IUD in Place**

Two types of IUDs are currently available in the United States. One type, which releases a progestin, is effective for 5 years. The other, which releases copper, is effective for at least 10 years. One year after removal of an IUD, 80 to 90% of women who try to conceive do so.

An IUD inserted up to 1 week after one act of unprotected sexual intercourse is nearly 100% effective as a method of emergency contraception.

The uterus is briefly contaminated with bacteria at the time of insertion, but an infection rarely results. After the first month of use, an IUD does not increase the risk of a pelvic infection.

Bleeding and pain are the main reasons that women have IUDs removed, accounting for more than half of all removals before the usual replacement time. The copper-releasing IUD increases the amount of menstrual bleeding. In contrast, the progestin-releasing IUD reduces or, after 6 months of use, completely prevents menstrual bleeding.

About 10% of IUDs are expelled during the first year after insertion, often during the first few months. A plastic string is usually attached to the IUD so that a woman can check every so often, especially after a period, to make sure that the IUD is still in place. If she cannot find the string, she should use another contraceptive method until she can see her health care practitioner to determine whether the IUD is still in place. If another IUD is inserted after one has been expelled, it usually stays in place.

Rarely, the uterus is perforated during insertion. Usually, perforation does not cause symptoms. It is discovered when a woman cannot find the plastic string and ultrasonography or x-rays show the IUD located outside the uterus. An IUD that perforates the uterus and passes into the abdominal cavity must be surgically removed to prevent it from injuring and scarring the intestine.

The risk of miscarriage is about 55% in women who become pregnant with an IUD in place. If a woman wishes to continue the pregnancy and the string of the IUD is visible, a doctor removes the IUD to reduce the risk of miscarriage. For women who conceive with an IUD in place, the likelihood of having a mislocated (ectopic) pregnancy is about 5%—5 times higher than usual. Nonetheless, the risk of an ectopic pregnancy is much lower for women using IUDs than for those not using a contraceptive method, because IUDs prevent pregnancy effectively.

TIMING METHODS

Some contraceptive methods depend on timing rather than on drugs or devices.

Natural Family Planning Methods

Natural family planning (rhythm) methods depend on abstinence from sexual intercourse during the woman's fertile time of the month. In most women, the ovary releases an egg about 14 days before the start of a menstrual period. Although the unfertilized egg survives only about 12 hours, sperm can survive for as long as 6 days after intercourse. Consequently, fertilization can result from intercourse that occurred up to 6 days before the release of the egg.

The calendar method is the least effective natural family planning method, even for women who have regular menstrual cycles. To calculate when to abstain from intercourse, women subtract 18 days from the shortest and 11 days from the longest of their previous 12 menstrual cycles. For example, if a woman's cycles last from 26 to 29 days, she must avoid intercourse from day 8 through day 18 of each cycle.

Other, more effective natural family planning methods include the temperature, mucus, and symptothermal methods.

For the temperature method, a woman determines the temperature of the body at rest (basal body temperature) by taking her temperature each morning before she gets out of bed. This temperature decreases before the egg is released and increases slightly after the egg is released. The couple avoids intercourse from the beginning of the woman's menstrual period until at least 48 hours after the day her basal body temperature increased.

For the mucus method, the woman's fertile period is established by observing cervical mucus, which is usually secreted in larger amounts and becomes more watery shortly before the egg is released. The woman can have intercourse with a low risk of conception after her menstrual period ends until she observes an increase in the amount of cervical mucus. She then avoids intercourse until 4 days after the largest amount of mucus has been observed.

The symptothermal method involves observing changes in both cervical mucus and basal body temperature as well as other symptoms that may be associated with the release of the egg, such as slight cramping pain. Of the natural family planning methods, this one is the most reliable.

Withdrawal Before Ejaculation

To prevent sperm from entering the vagina, a man can withdraw the penis from the vagina before ejaculation, when sperm are released during orgasm. This method, also called coitus interruptus, is not reliable because sperm may be released before orgasm. It also requires that the man have a high degree of self-control and precise timing.

Abortion

Induced abortion is the intentional ending of a pregnancy by medical means.

- When surgical evacuation is used to end pregnancy, a suction tube or forceps is used to remove the contents of the uterus.
- Drugs used to induce abortions include mifepristone followed by misoprostol.
- Complications are uncommon when an abortion is done by a trained health care practitioner in a hospital or clinic.

Worldwide, the status of abortion varies from being legally banned to being available on request. About two thirds of the women in the world have access to legal abortion. In the United States, laws regarding how late in the pregnancy elective abortion can be performed vary from state to state. In the United States, about 25% of all pregnancies are ended by elective abortion, making it one of the most common surgical procedures performed.

Abortion methods include use of surgery (surgical evacuation) and use of drugs. The method used depends in part on how long a woman has been pregnant. The length of the pregnancy may be hard to estimate if any bleeding has occurred after conception, if the woman is overweight, or if the uterus points backward rather than forward. In these situations, ultrasonography is usually performed to estimate the length of the pregnancy.

Surgical evacuation involves removing the contents of the uterus through the vagina. It is used for about 95% of abortions. Different techniques are used depending on the length of the pregnancy.

A technique called suction curettage is almost always used for pregnancies of less than 12 weeks. Typically, doctors use a small, flexible tube attached to a vacuum source, usually a machine suction pump or hand pump but occasionally a vacuum syringe. The tube is inserted through the opening of the cervix into the interior of the uterus, which is then gently and thoroughly emptied.

Sometimes this procedure does not terminate the pregnancy, especially in the first week after the menstrual period is missed.

For pregnancies of 4 to 6 weeks, suction curettage can be performed with little or no dilation of the cervix, because a small suction tube can be used. For pregnancies of 7 to 12 weeks, the cervix is usually dilated because a larger suction tube is used. To reduce the possibility of injuring the cervix, a doctor can use natural substances that absorb fluids, such as dried seaweed stems (laminaria), rather than mechanical devices. Laminaria are inserted into the opening of the cervix and left in place for at least 4 to 5 hours, usually overnight. As the laminaria absorb large amounts of fluid from the body, they expand and stretch the opening of the cervix. Drugs such as prostaglandins can also be used to dilate the cervix.

DID YOU KNOW?

- Abortion is one of the most common surgical procedures done in the United States.
- The cervix may be dilated using dried seaweed, which absorbs fluids from the body and stretches the opening of the cervix.

For pregnancies of more than 12 weeks, a technique called dilation and evacuation is most commonly used. After the cervix is dilated, suction and forceps are used to remove the fetus and placenta. Then the uterus may be gently scraped to make sure everything has been removed. This technique results in fewer minor complications than do the drugs used to induce abortion. However, for pregnancies of more than 18 weeks, dilation and evacuation can cause serious complications, such as damage to the uterus or intestine.

Drugs used to induce abortions include mifepristone (RU-486) and prostaglandins, such as misoprostol. Mifepristone, given by mouth, blocks the action of the hormone progesterone, which prepares the lining of the uterus to support the fetus. Mifepristone is approved only for pregnancies of 7 weeks or less. Prostaglandins are hormonelike substances that stimulate the uterus to contract.

They are given by mouth, placed in the vagina, or given by injection. After mifepristone is given, a prostaglandin is given. The regimen now used involves taking 1 to 3 tablets of mifepristone and, 2 days later, taking a prostaglandin (misoprostol) by mouth or vaginally. This regimen causes abortion in about 95% of cases. If abortion does not occur, surgical evacuation is performed.

Complications

In general, abortion has a higher risk of complications than contraception or sterilization, especially for young women. The risk of complications from an abortion is related to the length of the pregnancy and the abortion method used. The longer a woman has been pregnant, the greater the risk. However, complications are uncommon when an abortion is performed by a trained health care practitioner in a hospital or clinic.

The uterus is perforated by a surgical instrument in 1 of 1,000 abortions. Sometimes the intestine or another organ is also injured. Severe bleeding occurs during or immediately after the procedure in 6 of 10,000 abortions. Some techniques can tear the cervix, especially during the 2nd trimester of pregnancy.

Later, infections or blood clots in the legs may develop. Bleeding can occur if part of the placenta is left in the uterus. Very rarely, sterility results from scarring of the uterine lining due to the procedure or a subsequent infection—a disorder called Asherman's syndrome. If the fetus has Rh-positive blood, a woman who has Rh-negative blood may produce Rh antibodies— as in any pregnancy, miscarriage, or delivery. Such antibodies may endanger subsequent pregnancies unless the woman is given injections of Rh0(D) immune globulin (see page 322).

Sterilization

Sterilization involves making a person incapable of reproduction.

- Disrupting the tubes that carry sperm or the egg ends the ability to reproduce.
- Vasectomy is a short procedure for men, done in the doctor's office.
- The traditional procedure for women, tubal ligation, is more complicated, requiring an abdominal incision.

- In a new procedure for women called Essure, small inserts are placed in the fallopian tubes without making an incision.
- The procedures, although considered permanent, can sometimes be reversed in many men and women.

About one third of all married couples in the United States who use family planning methods choose sterilization. Sterilization should always be considered permanent. However, an operation that reconnects the appropriate tubes (reanastomosis) can be performed to restore fertility. Reanastomosis is less likely to be effective in men than in women. For couples, pregnancy rates are 45 to 60% after reanastomosis in men and 50 to 80% after reanastomosis in women.

Vasectomy is performed to sterilize men. It involves cutting and sealing the vasa deferentia (the tubes that carry sperm from the testes). A vasectomy, which is performed by a urologist in the office, takes about 20 minutes and requires only a local anesthetic. Through a small incision on each side of the scrotum, a section of each vas deferens is removed and the open ends of the tubes are sealed off. A man who has had a vasectomy should continue contraception for a while. Usually, he does not become sterile until about 15 to 20 ejaculations after the operation, because many sperm are stored in the seminal vesicles. A laboratory test can be performed to be sure that ejaculates are free of sperm.

Complications of vasectomy include bleeding (in fewer than 5% of men), an inflammatory response to sperm leakage, and spontaneous reopening (in fewer than 1%), usually shortly after the procedure. Sexual activity, with contraception, may resume as soon after the procedure as the man desires. Fewer than 1% of women become pregnant after their partner is sterilized.

DID YOU KNOW?

- Contraception should be continued for a while after a vasectomy, until the sperm stored in the body are ejaculated.
- A pregnancy that occurs after tubal ligation is often mislocated—in the fallopian tubes rather than the uterus.

Tubal ligation is used to sterilize women. It involves cutting and tying or blocking the fallopian tubes, which carry the egg from the ovaries to the uterus. More complicated than vasectomy, tubal ligation requires an abdominal incision and a general or regional anesthetic. Women who have just delivered a child can be sterilized immediately after childbirth or on the following day, without staying in the hospital any longer than usual. Sterilization also may be planned in advance and performed as elective surgery.

Sterilization for women is often performed by laparoscopy. Working through a thin tube inserted through a small incision in the woman's abdomen, a doctor cuts the fallopian tubes and ties off the cut ends. Or a doctor may use electrocautery (a device that produces an electrical current to cut through tissue) to seal off about 1 inch of each tube. The woman usually goes home the same day. After laparoscopy, up to 6% of women have minor complications, such as a skin infection at the incision site or constipation. Fewer than 1% have major complications, such as bleeding or punctures of the bladder or intestine. About 2% of women become pregnant during the first 10 years after they are sterilized. About one third of these pregnancies are mislocated (ectopic) pregnancies that develop in the fallopian tubes.

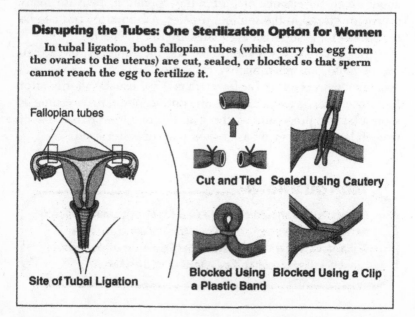

Disrupting the Tubes: One Sterilization Option for Women

In tubal ligation, both fallopian tubes (which carry the egg from the ovaries to the uterus) are cut, sealed, or blocked so that sperm cannot reach the egg to fertilize it.

Fallopian tubes

Cut and Tied   Sealed Using Cautery

Blocked Using   Blocked Using a Clip
a Plastic Band

Site of Tubal Ligation

Various mechanical devices, such as plastic bands and spring-loaded clips, can be used to block the fallopian tubes instead of cutting or sealing them. Sterilization is easier to reverse when these devices are used because they cause less tissue damage. However, reversal is successful in only about three fourths of the women.

Essure, another sterilization procedure for women, involves no incisions. A flexible viewing tube (hysteroscope) is passed through the vagina, cervix, and uterus and used to place microinserts in the fallopian tubes. The inserts are made of polyester fibers and metals (nickel titanium and stainless steel). During the first 3 months, the woman's body and the microinserts work together to form a tissue barrier to permanently prevent sperm from reaching an egg. During this 3-month period, another form of birth control is needed. After 3 months, an x-ray procedure using a radiopaque dye injected into the cervix (hysterosalpingography) is done to make sure the fallopian tubes are completely blocked.

Surgical removal of the uterus (hysterectomy) results in sterility. This procedure is usually performed to treat a disorder rather than as a sterilization technique.

CHAPTER 4

Infertility

Infertility is the inability of a couple to achieve a pregnancy after repeated intercourse without contraception for 1 year.

Infertility affects about one of five couples in the United States. It is becoming increasingly common because people are waiting longer to marry and to have a child. Nevertheless, up to 60% of the couples who have not conceived after a year of trying do conceive eventually, with or without treatment. The goal of treatment is to reduce the time needed to conceive or to provide couples who might not otherwise conceive the opportunity to do so. Before treatment is begun, counseling that provides information about the treatment process (including its duration) and the chances of success is beneficial.

The cause of infertility may be due to problems in the man, the woman, or both. Problems with sperm, ovulation, or the fallopian tubes each account for almost one third of infertility cases. In a small percentage of cases, infertility is caused by problems with mucus in the cervix or by unidentified factors. Thus, the diagnosis of infertility problems requires a thorough assessment of both partners.

Age is a factor, primarily for women. As women age, becoming pregnant becomes more difficult and the risk of complications during pregnancy increases. Also, women, particularly after age 35, have a limited time to resolve infertility problems before menopause.

Even when no cause of infertility can be identified, the couple may still be treated. In such cases, the woman may be given drugs to stimulate several eggs to mature and be released—so-called fertility drugs (see page 57). Examples are clomiphene and human gonadotropins. A woman's chances of becoming pregnant are about 10 to 15% with each month of treatment. Alternatively, an artificial insemination technique that selects only the most active sperm may be tried.

DID YOU KNOW?

- About one of five couples in the United States is infertile.
- Many drugs can impair fertility by affecting sperm production or ovulation.
- Infertility may result from problems in the man, woman, or both.
- A couple can be treated for infertility even when the cause cannot be diagnosed.
- Treatment for infertility, which may be stressful and expensive, is sometimes ultimately unsuccessful.

While a couple is undergoing treatment for infertility, one or both partners may experience frustration, emotional stress, feelings of inadequacy, and guilt. They may alternate between hope and despair. Feeling isolated and unable to communicate, they may become angry at or resentful toward each other, family members, friends, or the doctor. The emotional stress can lead to fatigue, anxiety, sleep or eating disturbances, and an inability to concentrate. In addition, the financial burden and time commitment involved in diagnosis and treatment can cause marital strife.

These problems can be lessened if both partners are involved in and are given information about the treatment process, regardless of which one has the diagnosed problem. Knowing what the chances of success are, as well as realizing that treatment may not be successful and cannot continue indefinitely, can help a couple cope with the stress. Information about when to end treatment, when to seek a second opinion, and when to consider adoption is also helpful. Counseling and psychologic support, including support groups such as RESOLVE and the American Infertility Association, can help.

Problems With Sperm

- Sperm may be abnormal, too few in number, absent, or unable to reach the penis for ejaculation.
- Heat, hormonal or genetic disorders, injuries, mumps, some drugs and toxins, and blockages in the ejaculatory ducts can cause problems with sperm.
- Doctors base the diagnosis on the medical history and results of the physical examination, semen analysis, and sperm function tests.
- In vitro fertilization and gamete intrafallopian tube transfer are the treatments most likely to result in pregnancy.

To be fertile, a man must be able to deliver an adequate quantity of normal sperm to a woman's vagina, and sperm must be able to fertilize the egg. Conditions that interfere with this process can make a man less fertile.

Conditions that increase the temperature of the testes (where sperm are produced) can greatly reduce the number of sperm and the vigor of sperm movement and can increase the number of abnormal sperm. Temperature may be increased by exposure to excessive heat, disorders that produce a prolonged fever, undescended testes (a rare abnormality present at birth), and varicose veins in the testes (varicocele).

Certain hormonal or genetic disorders may interfere with sperm production. Hormonal disorders include hyperprolactinemia, hypothyroidism, hypogonadism, and disorders of the adrenal gland (which produces testosterone and other hormones) or pituitary gland (which controls testosterone production). Genetic disorders involve an abnormality of the sex chromosomes, as occurs in Klinefelter syndrome.

Other causes of reduced sperm production include mumps that affect the testes (mumps orchitis), injury to the testes, exposure to industrial or environmental toxins, and drugs. Drugs include androgens (such as testosterone), aspirin when taken for a long time, chlorambucil, cimetidine, colchicine, corticosteroids (such as prednisone), cotrimoxazole, cyclophosphamide, drugs used to treat malaria, estrogens taken to treat prostate cancer, marijuana, medroxyprogesterone, methotrexate, monoamine oxidase inhibitors (MAOIs—a type of antidepressant), nicotine, nitrofurantoin, opioids (narcotics), spironolactone, and sulfasalazine. Use of anabolic steroids may affect hormone levels and thus also interfere with sperm production. Excessive consumption of alcohol may reduce sperm production.

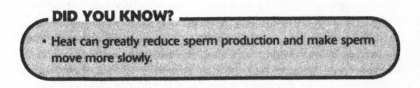

DID YOU KNOW?

- Heat can greatly reduce sperm production and make sperm move more slowly.

Some disorders result in the complete absence of sperm (azoospermia) in semen. They include serious disorders of the testes and blocked or missing vasa deferentia, missing seminal vesicles, and blockage of both ejaculatory ducts.

Occasionally, semen, which contains the sperm, moves in the wrong direction (into the bladder instead of down the penis). This disorder, called retrograde ejaculation (see page 427), is more common among men who have diabetes or who have had pelvic surgery, such as prostate removal. Infertility may result.

Diagnosis

Doctors ask the man about his medical history and perform a physical examination to try to identify the cause. Doctors check for physical abnormalities, such as undescended testes, and for signs of hormonal or genetic disorders that can cause infertility. Levels of hormones (including testosterone) may be measured in the blood.

Often, a semen analysis, the main screening procedure for male infertility, is needed. For this procedure, the man is asked not to ejaculate for 2 to 3 days before the analysis. Then he is asked to ejaculate, usually by masturbation, into a clean glass jar, preferably at the laboratory site. For men who have difficulty producing a semen sample this way, special condoms that have no lubricants or chemicals toxic to sperm can be used to collect semen during intercourse. An analysis based on two or three samples, obtained at least 2 weeks apart, is more reliable than an analysis based on a single sample.

The volume of the semen sample is measured. Whether the color and consistency of semen are normal is determined. The sperm are examined under a microscope to determine whether they are abnormal in shape, size, movement, or number.

If the semen sample is abnormal, the analysis may be repeated because samples from the same man normally vary greatly. If the semen still seems to be abnormal, the doctor tries to identify the cause. However, a low sperm count may indicate only that too little time had elapsed since the last ejaculation or that only some of the semen was deposited in the collection jar. Furthermore, a low sperm count does not mean that fertility is reduced, and a normal sperm count does not guarantee fertility.

Tests of sperm function and quality can be performed. One test detects antibodies to sperm. Another determines whether sperm membranes are intact. Still others can determine the sperm's ability to bind to an egg and penetrate it. Sometimes a biopsy of the testes is performed to obtain more detailed information about sperm production and the function of the testes.

Treatment

Clomiphene, a drug used to trigger (induce) ovulation in women, may be used to try to increase sperm counts in men. However, clomiphene does not improve the sperm's ability to move or reduce the number of abnormal sperm, and it has not been proved to increase fertility.

For men who have a low sperm count with normal sperm, artificial insemination may slightly increase their partner's chances of pregnancy. This technique uses the first portion of the ejaculated semen, which has the greatest concentration of sperm. A technique that selects only the most active sperm (washed sperm) is somewhat more successful. In vitro fertilization, often with intracytoplasmic sperm injection (the injection of a single sperm into a single egg), and gamete intrafallopian tube transfer (GIFT) are much more complex and costly procedures. They are successful in treating many types of male infertility.

For men who produce no sperm, inseminating the woman with sperm from another man (a donor) may be considered. Because of the danger of contracting sexually transmitted diseases, including infection with human immunodeficiency virus (HIV), fresh semen samples from donors are no longer used. Instead, frozen sperm samples are obtained from a certified sperm bank, which has tested the donors for sexually transmitted diseases.

Varicoceles can be treated with surgery. Sometimes fertility improves as a result.

The partner of a man who has fertility problems may be treated with human gonadotropins, to stimulate several eggs to mature and be released (see page 58).

Problems With Ovulation

- Women may be infertile because their ovaries do not release an egg each month.
- Such problems occur when the system that controls reproductive function malfunctions.
- Ultrasonography, ovulation predictor kits (used at home), blood or urine tests, or endometrial biopsy can identify problems with ovulation.
- Clomiphene, human gonadotropins plus human chorionic gonadotropin, or sometimes gonadorelin may be used to trigger ovulation.

In women, a common cause of infertility is an ovulation problem—that is, the ovaries do not release an egg each month (see page 111). Ovulation problems result when one part of the system that controls reproductive function malfunctions. This system includes the hypothalamus (an area of the brain), pituitary gland, adrenal glands, thyroid gland, and genital organs. For example, the ovaries may not produce enough progesterone, the female hormone that causes the lining of the uterus to thicken in preparation for a potential fetus. Ovulation may not occur because the hypothalamus does not secrete gonadotropin-releasing hormone, which stimulates the pituitary gland to produce the hormones that trigger ovulation (luteinizing hormone and follicle-stimulating hormone). High levels of prolactin (hyperprolactinemia), a hormone that stimulates milk production, may result in low levels of the hormones that trigger ovulation. Prolactin levels may be high because of a pituitary gland tumor (prolactinoma), which is almost always noncancerous. Ovulation problems may be due to polycystic ovary syndrome, thyroid gland disorders, adrenal gland disorders, excessive exercise, diabetes, weight loss, obesity, or psychologic stress. Sometimes the cause is early menopause—when the supply of eggs has run out early.

Ovulation is often the problem in women who have irregular periods or no periods (amenorrhea—see page 155). It is sometimes the problem in women who have regular menstrual periods but do not have premenstrual symptoms, such as breast tenderness, lower abdominal swelling, and mood changes.

Diagnosis

To determine if or when ovulation is occurring, doctors may ask a woman to take her temperature at rest (basal body temperature) each day. Usually, the best time is immediately after awakening. A low point in basal body temperature suggests that ovulation is about to occur. An increase of more than 0.9°F (0.5°C) in temperature usually indicates that ovulation has occurred. However, basal body temperature does not reliably or precisely indicate when ovulation occurs. At best, it predicts ovulation only within 2 days. More accurate techniques include ultrasonography and ovulation predictor kits (which detect an increase in luteinizing hormone in the urine 24 to 36 hours before ovulation). These kits are used at home to test urine on several consecutive days. Also, the level of progesterone in the blood or saliva or the level of one of its by-products in the urine may be measured. A marked increase in these levels indicates that ovulation has occurred.

To determine whether ovulation is occurring normally, doctors may perform an endometrial biopsy. A small sample of tissue is removed from the lining of the uterus 10 to 12 days after ovulation is thought to have occurred. The sample is examined under a microscope. If changes that normally occur after ovulation are seen, ovulation has occurred normally. If the normal changes appear

DID YOU KNOW?

- Irregular or absent periods may indicate a problem with ovulation.
- Drugs used to trigger ovulation sometimes overstimulate the ovaries and may have to be stopped.

delayed, the problem may be inadequate production or inactivity of progesterone.

Treatment

A drug to trigger ovulation may be used. The particular drug is selected based on the specific problem. If ovulation has not occurred for a long time, clomiphene with medroxyprogesterone is usually preferred. First, the woman takes medroxyprogesterone, usually by mouth, to trigger a menstrual period. Then she takes clomiphene by mouth. Usually, she ovulates 5 to 10 days after clomiphene is discontinued and has a period 14 to 16 days after ovulation. Clomiphene is not effective for all causes of ovulation problems. It is most effective when the cause is polycystic ovary syndrome.

If a woman does not have a period after treatment with clomiphene, she takes a pregnancy test. If she is not pregnant, the treatment cycle is repeated. A higher dose of clomiphene is used in each cycle until ovulation occurs or the maximum dose is reached. When the dose that triggers ovulation is determined, the woman takes that dose for at least three to four more treatment cycles. Most women who become pregnant do so by the fourth cycle in which ovulation occurs. About 75 to 80% of women treated with clomiphene ovulate, but only about 40 to 50% become pregnant. About 5% of pregnancies in women treated with clomiphene involve more than one fetus, primarily twins.

Side effects of clomiphene include hot flashes, abdominal bloating, breast tenderness, nausea, vision problems, and headaches. About 5% of women treated with clomiphene develop ovarian hyperstimulation syndrome. In this syndrome, the ovaries enlarge greatly and a large amount of fluid moves out of the bloodstream into the abdomen. This syndrome may be life threatening. To try to prevent it, doctors prescribe the lowest effective dose of clomiphene, and if the ovaries enlarge, they discontinue the drug.

If a woman does not ovulate or become pregnant during treatment with clomiphene, hormonal therapy with human gonadotropins, injected into a muscle or under the skin, can be tried. Human gonadotropins stimulate the follicles of the ovaries to mature. Follicles are fluid-filled cavities, each of which contain an egg (see page 108). Blood tests to measure estrogen levels and ultrasonography can detect when the follicles are mature. Then, the woman is given an injection of a different hormone, human chorionic gonadotropin, to trigger ovulation. When human gonadotropins are used appropriately, more than 95% of women treated with them ovulate, but only 50 to 75% become pregnant. About 10 to 30% of pregnancies in women treated with human gonadotropins involve more than one fetus, primarily twins.

Human gonadotropins can have severe side effects, so doctors closely monitor the woman during treatment. About 10 to 20% of women treated with human gonadotropins develop ovarian hyperstimulation syndrome (which can also occur with clomiphene). If hyperstimulation occurs (if the ovaries enlarge markedly or if estrogen levels increase too much), doctors do not give the woman human chorionic gonadotropin to trigger ovulation. Human gonadotropins are also expensive.

If the cause of infertility is early menopause, neither clomiphene nor human gonadotropins can stimulate ovulation.

If the hypothalamus does not secrete gonadotropin-releasing hormone, a synthetic version of this hormone, called gonadorelin, may be useful. This drug, like the natural hormone, stimulates the pituitary gland to produce the hormones that trigger ovulation. The risk of ovarian hyperstimulation is low with this treatment, so close monitoring is not needed. However, this drug is not available in the United States.

When the cause of infertility is high levels of the hormone prolactin, the best drug is one that acts like dopamine, called a dopamine agonist, such as bromocriptine or cabergoline. (Dopamine is a chemical messenger that generally inhibits the production of prolactin.)

Problems With the Fallopian Tubes

- If the fallopian tubes are blocked or malfunction, the egg cannot reach the uterus or the sperm cannot reach the egg.
- Hysterosalpingography or laparoscopy with a tubal dye study is done to detect blockages.
- Abnormalities may be removed or dislodged using a hysteroscope or surgery.
- In vitro fertilization is recommended for most couples.

The fallopian tubes may be abnormal in structure or function. If they are blocked, the egg cannot move from the ovary to the uterus. Causes of fallopian tube problems include previous infections (such as pelvic inflammatory disease), endometriosis, a ruptured appendix, and surgery in the pelvis. A mislocated (ectopic) pregnancy in the fallopian tubes can also cause damage. Structural disorders can block the fallopian tubes. These disorders include birth defects of the uterus and fallopian tubes, fibroids in the uterus, and bands of scar tissue between normally unconnected structures (adhesions) in the uterus or pelvis.

Diagnosis and Treatment

To determine whether the fallopian tubes are blocked, doctors can use hysterosalpingography. In this procedure, x-rays are taken after a radiopaque dye is injected through the cervix. The dye outlines the interior of the uterus and fallopian tubes. This procedure is performed shortly after a woman's menstrual period ends. This procedure can detect structural disorders that can block the fallopian tubes. However, in about 15% of cases, hysterosalpingography indicates that the fallopian tubes are blocked when they are not—called a false-positive result. After hysterosalpingography with normal results, fertility appears to be slightly improved, possibly because the procedure temporarily widens (dilates) the tubes or clears the tubes of mucus. Therefore, doctors may wait to see if a woman becomes pregnant after this procedure before additional tests of fallopian tube function are performed.

Another procedure (called sonohysterography) is sometimes used to evaluate the uterus. A salt (saline) solution is injected into the interior of the uterus through the cervix during ultrasonography so that the interior is distended and abnormalities can be seen. This procedure is quick and does not require an anesthetic.

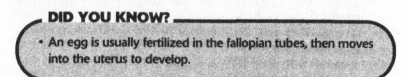

DID YOU KNOW?

• An egg is usually fertilized in the fallopian tubes, then moves into the uterus to develop.

If an abnormality within the uterus is detected, doctors examine the uterus with a viewing tube called a hysteroscope, which is inserted through the cervix into the uterus. If adhesions, a polyp, or a small fibroid is detected, the hysteroscope may be used to dislodge or remove the abnormal tissue, increasing the chances that the woman will become pregnant.

If evidence suggests that the fallopian tubes are blocked or that a woman may have endometriosis, a small viewing tube called a laparoscope is inserted in the pelvic cavity through a small incision just below the navel. Usually, a general anesthetic is used. This procedure enables doctors to directly view the uterus, fallopian tubes, and ovaries. The laparoscope may also be used to dislodge or remove abnormal tissue in the pelvis.

Treatment depends on the cause. Surgery can be performed to repair a damaged fallopian tube caused by an ectopic pregnancy or an infection. However, after such surgery, the chances of a normal pregnancy are small, and those of an ectopic pregnancy are great. Consequently, surgery is not often recommended. In vitro fertilization is recommended for most couples.

Problems With Mucus in the Cervix

• Mucus may remain thick at ovulation or contain antibodies to sperm, preventing fertilization.

Normally, mucus in the cervix (the lower part of the uterus that opens into the vagina) is thick and impenetrable to sperm until just before release of an egg (ovulation). Then, just before ovulation, the mucus becomes clear and elastic (because the level of the hormone estrogen increases). As a result, sperm can move through the mucus into the uterus to the fallopian tubes, where fertilization can take place. If the mucus does not change at ovulation (usually because of an infection), pregnancy is unlikely. Pregnancy is also unlikely if the mucus contains antibodies to sperm, which kill sperm before they can reach the egg.

Diagnosis and Treatment

A postcoital test, performed between 2 and 8 hours after sexual intercourse, involves evaluating cervical mucus and determining whether sperm can survive in the mucus. The test is scheduled for the midpoint of the menstrual cycle, when the estrogen level is highest and the woman is ovulating. A sample of mucus is taken with forceps or a syringe. The thickness and elasticity of the mucus and the number of sperm in the mucus are determined. Abnormal results include overly thick mucus, no sperm, and sperm clumping together because the mucus contains antibodies to the sperm. However, abnormal results do not always indicate that there is a problem with the mucus or that pregnancy cannot occur. Sperm may be absent only because they were not deposited into the vagina during intercourse, and the mucus may be overly thick only because the test was not performed at the proper time in the menstrual cycle.

Treatment may include intrauterine insemination, in which semen is placed directly in the uterus to bypass the mucus. Drugs to thin the mucus, such as guaifenesin, may be used. However, there is no proof that either treatment increases the chances of pregnancy.

Fertilization Techniques

- For in vitro fertilization, the ovaries are stimulated, eggs are retrieved and fertilized in a laboratory, and some of the resulting embryos are transferred back to the woman's uterus.
- If the man has a low sperm count, one sperm may be injected into one egg.
- When the fallopian tubes are normal, active sperm and eggs may be retrieved, then placed in the far end of the fallopian tube for fertilization.

If treatment has not resulted in pregnancy after four to six menstrual cycles, fertilization techniques, such as in vitro fertilization or gamete intrafallopian tube transfer, may be considered.

In vitro (test tube) fertilization involves stimulating the ovaries, retrieving released eggs, fertilizing the eggs, growing the resulting embryos in a laboratory, and then implanting the embryos in the woman's uterus.

Typically, a woman's ovaries are stimulated with human gonadotropins and a gonadotropin-releasing hormone agonist or antagonist (drugs that prevent ovulation from occurring until after several eggs have matured). As a result, many eggs usually mature. Guided by ultrasonography, a doctor inserts a needle through the woman's vagina into the ovary and removes several eggs from the follicles. The eggs are placed in a culture dish and fertilized with sperm selected as the most active. After about 3 to 5 days, two or three of the resulting embryos are transferred from the culture dish into the woman's uterus through the vagina. Additional embryos can be frozen in liquid nitrogen to be used later if pregnancy does not occur. Despite the transfer of several embryos, the chances of producing one full-term baby are only about 18 to 25% each time eggs are placed in the uterus.

DID YOU KNOW?

- The chances of having a full-term baby after using fertilization techniques (such as in vitro fertilization) vary by age but are generally less than 25%.
- Women take drugs to stimulate the ovaries before fertilization techniques are used.

Intracytoplasmic sperm injection may be used with in vitro fertilization to improve the chances that the woman will become pregnant, particularly when the man has a very low sperm count. In this procedure, a single sperm is injected into a single egg. With this procedure, the chances of producing a full-term baby are about the same as those with in vitro fertilization alone.

Gamete intrafallopian tube transfer (GIFT) can be performed if the fallopian tubes are functioning normally. Eggs and selected active sperm are obtained as for in vitro fertilization, but the eggs are not fertilized with the sperm in the laboratory. Instead, the eggs and sperm are transferred to the far end of the woman's fallopian tube through the abdomen (using a laparoscope) or the vagina (guided by ultrasonography), so that the egg can be fertilized in the fallopian tube. Thus, this procedure is more invasive than in vitro fertilization. For each transfer, the chances of producing a full-term baby are about the same as those with in vitro fertilization.

Variations of in vitro fertilization and GIFT include the transfer of a more mature embryo (blastocyst transfer), use of eggs from another woman (donor), and transfer of frozen embryos to a surrogate mother. These techniques raise moral and ethical issues, including questions about the disposal of stored embryos (especially in cases of death or divorce), legal parentage if a surrogate mother is involved, and selective reduction of the number of implanted embryos (similar to abortion) when more than three develop.

CHAPTER 5

Sexually Transmitted Diseases

Sexually transmitted (venereal) diseases are infections that are passed from person to person through sexual contact.

Because sexual activity includes intimate contact, it provides an easy opportunity for organisms to spread from one person to another. A variety of infectious microorganisms can be spread by sexual contact. Bacterial sexually transmitted diseases (STDs) include syphilis, gonorrhea, nongonococcal urethritis and chlamydial cervicitis, lymphogranuloma venereum, chancroid, granuloma inguinale, and trichomoniasis. Viral STDs include genital warts, genital herpes, molluscum contagiosum, and HIV infection or AIDS (see page 84). Some infections that are spread by skin-to-skin contact or by ingestion of the microorganism can be transmitted during sex, even though they are not considered classical STDs.

DID YOU KNOW?

- Successful treatment of sexually transmitted diseases usually requires treatment of all sex partners.
- Sometimes, sexually transmitted diseases do not cause symptoms, particularly in women.
- Many sexually transmitted diseases can be treated and cured with a single dose of an antibiotic.

STDs are among the most common infectious diseases. It is estimated that over 3 million people contract gonorrhea and chlamydia every year in the United States—making these the two most common STDs in the country.

Although STDs usually result from having vaginal, oral, or anal sex with an infected partner, genital penetration is not necessary to spread an infection. Some diseases may also be transmitted by kissing or by close body contact. Also, the organisms responsible for some STDs (for example, HIV and hepatitis viruses) can be transmitted through nonsexual means, such as from mother to child at birth or through breastfeeding or exposure to contaminated food, water, blood, medical instruments, or needles.

Effective drugs are available for most STDs caused by bacteria, although a number of new antibiotic-resistant strains of bacteria

PROPER CONDOM USE

- Use a new condom for each act of sexual intercourse.
- Use the correct size condom.
- Carefully handle the condom to avoid damaging it with fingernails, teeth, or other sharp objects.
- Put the condom on after the penis is erect and before any genital contact with the partner.
- Place the rolled condom over the tip of the erect penis.
- Leave $1/2$ inch at the tip of the condom to collect semen.
- With one hand, squeeze trapped air out of the tip of the condom.
- If uncircumcised, pull the foreskin back before rolling the condom down.
- With the other hand, roll the condom over the penis to its base and smooth out any air bubbles.
- Make sure that lubrication is adequate during intercourse.
- With latex condoms, use only water-based lubricants. Oil-based lubricants (such as petroleum jelly, shortening, mineral oil, massage oils, body lotions, and cooking oil) can weaken latex and cause the condom to break.
- Hold the condom firmly against the base of the penis during withdrawal, and withdraw the penis while it is still erect to prevent slippage.

OTHER DISEASES THAT MAY BE TRANSMITTED SEXUALLY

- Amebiasis
- Campylobacteriosis
- Pediculosis pubis (crabs, lice)
- Cytomegalovirus infection
- Giardiasis
- Hepatitis A, B, and C
- Salmonellosis
- Scabies
- Shigellosis

---

have become widespread. Viral STDs, especially herpes and HIV, persist for life and have effective treatment but no known cure.

Preventing or controlling STDs depends on practicing safe sex and getting prompt diagnosis and treatment. Knowing how to prevent the spread of STDs—in particular, knowing the proper method for using a condom—is crucial.

One strategy health care workers use to help control the spread of some STDs is contact tracing. Health care workers try to trace and treat (if treatment is available) all of an infected person's sexual contacts. People who have been treated are reexamined to make sure they are cured.

Syphilis

Syphilis is a sexually transmitted disease caused by the bacterium Treponema pallidum.

- Symptoms progress through stages, usually starting with a painless sore at the infection site (usually the penis, vulva, or vagina), then a rash (which may occur on the palms or soles) as well as mouth sores and general symptoms, then a stage without symptoms.
- Tertiary syphilis, the final stage, can severely damage the cardiovascular and nervous systems.
- To make the diagnosis, doctors use different tests depending on the stage of the infection.

- Penicillin, given by injection, is the best antibiotic for all stages of infection.
- Infected people must avoid sexual contact until they and their partner have completed treatment.

Syphilis is highly contagious during the primary and secondary stages: a single sexual encounter with a person who has syphilis results in infection about one third of the time. The bacterium enters the body through mucous membranes, such as those in the vagina or mouth, or through the skin. Within hours, the bacterium reaches nearby lymph nodes, then spreads throughout the body by way of the bloodstream. Syphilis can infect a fetus during pregnancy, causing birth defects and other problems.

The annual number of people with newly diagnosed symptomatic syphilis last peaked in 1990 with 50,000 cases in the United States. Since then—largely because of focused public health measures—numbers dropped to 6,000 in 1999 and have since increased, reaching nearly 8,000 in 2004. Most cases are detected by blood tests in people without symptoms.

DID YOU KNOW?

- A single unprotected sexual encounter with someone who has syphilis results in infection about one third of the time.

Symptoms

Symptoms of syphilis usually begin 3 to 4 weeks after infection, although they may start as early as 1 week or as late as 13 weeks after infection. Syphilis progresses through several stages (primary, secondary, latent, and tertiary) if not treated. Infection can persist for many years and may cause heart damage, brain damage, and death.

In the **primary stage,** a painless sore or ulcer (chancre) appears at the infection site—typically the penis, vulva, or vagina. The chancre may also appear on the anus, rectum, lips, tongue, throat, cervix, fingers, or, rarely, other parts of the body. Usually, a person has only one chancre, but occasionally several develop.

The chancre begins as a small red raised area, which soon turns into a painless open sore. The chancre does not bleed and is hard to the touch. Nearby lymph nodes usually swell and are also painless. About half of infected women and one third of infected men are unaware of it. Others ignore the chancre because it causes few symptoms. The chancre usually heals in 3 to 12 weeks, after which the person appears to be completely healthy.

The **secondary stage** usually begins with a skin rash, which typically appears 6 to 12 weeks after infection. About 25% of infected people still have a healing chancre at this time. The rash usually does not itch or hurt and can have many different appearances. Unlike rashes from most other diseases, the rash of secondary syphilis commonly appears on the palms or soles. The skin rash may be short-lived or may last for months. Even if a person is not treated, the rash eventually clears up. New rashes, however, may appear weeks or months later.

Secondary-stage syphilis is a generalized disease that can cause fever, fatigue, loss of appetite, and weight loss. Mouth sores develop in more than 80% of people. About 50% have enlarged lymph nodes throughout the body, and about 10% develop inflammation of the eyes. The eye inflammation usually causes no symptoms, although occasionally the optic nerve swells, which may cause some blurring of vision. About 10% of people have inflamed bones and joints that ache. Jaundice may result from inflammation of the liver. A small number of people develop acute syphilitic meningitis, which causes headaches, neck stiffness, and sometimes deafness.

Raised areas (condylomata lata) may develop where the skin adjoins mucous membrane (for example, at the inner edges of the lips and vulva) and in moist areas of the skin. These extremely infectious areas may flatten and turn a dull pink or gray. The hair often falls out in patches, leaving a moth-eaten appearance.

After the person has recovered from the secondary stage, the disease enters a **latent stage,** in which the infection persists but no symptoms occur. This stage may last for years to decades—or for the rest of the person's life. Syphilis is generally not contagious in the latent stage.

During the **tertiary (third) stage,** syphilis is also not contagious but produces symptoms that range from mild to devastating.

Three main types of tertiary syphilis may occur: benign tertiary syphilis, cardiovascular syphilis, and neurosyphilis.

Benign tertiary syphilis is rare today. Lumps called gummas appear on the skin or in various organs. These lumps grow slowly, heal gradually, and leave scars. The lumps can develop almost anywhere in the body but are most common on the scalp, face, upper trunk, and leg (just below the knee). The bones may be affected, resulting in a deep, penetrating pain that is usually worse at night.

Cardiovascular syphilis usually appears 10 to 25 years after the initial infection. A person may develop an aneurysm (weakening and dilation) of the aorta (the main artery leaving the heart) or leakage of the aortic valve. These changes may lead to chest pain, heart failure, or death.

Neurosyphilis (syphilis of the nervous system) affects about 5% of all people with untreated syphilis, although it is rare in developed countries. It can cause many serious problems in the brain and spinal cord, interfering with thinking, walking, talking, and many other activities of daily life.

Neurosyphilis occurs in three forms: meningovascular, paretic (also called general paralysis of the insane), and tabetic (tabes dorsalis). Meningovascular neurosyphilis is a chronic form of meningitis that affects the brain and spinal cord. Paretic neurosyphilis usually does not start until the person is 40 or 50. It begins with gradual behavioral changes, such as deterioration in personal hygiene, mood swings, and progressive confusion. Tabetic neurosyphilis is a progressive disease of the spinal cord that begins gradually, typically with an intense, stabbing pain in the legs that comes and goes irregularly. Later, the person becomes unsteady while walking.

Diagnosis

A chancre or a typical rash on the palms and soles usually leads a doctor to suspect syphilis. A definitive diagnosis is based on the results of laboratory tests.

Two types of blood test are used. The first is a screening test, such as the Venereal Disease Research Laboratory (VDRL) or the rapid plasma reagin (RPR) test. Screening tests are inexpensive and easy to perform, but they may need to be repeated because the results can be falsely negative in the first few weeks of primary syphilis. Screening tests sometimes come back falsely positive because of diseases other than syphilis. Therefore, a positive screening test result usually must be confirmed with a second, specialized blood test that measures antibodies to syphilis bacteria. Screening test results become negative after successful treatment, but the second, confirmatory test stays positive indefinitely.

In the primary or secondary stages, syphilis may also be diagnosed by obtaining fluid from a skin or mouth sore and identifying the bacteria under a microscope. For neurosyphilis, a spinal tap (lumbar puncture) is needed to obtain spinal fluid for antibody testing. In the latent stage, syphilis is diagnosed only by antibody tests of the blood and spinal fluid. In the tertiary stage, syphilis is diagnosed from the symptoms and an antibody test.

Treatment and Prognosis

Because people with primary and secondary syphilis can pass the disease to others, they must avoid sexual contact or take careful precautions until they and their sex partners have completed treatment. With primary-stage syphilis, all sex partners for the previous 3 months are at risk of being infected. With secondary-stage syphilis, all sex partners for the previous year are at risk. Sex partners in these categories need to be screened with an antibody test performed on a blood sample. If the test is positive, they need to be treated. Some doctors simply treat all sex partners without waiting for test results.

Penicillin given by injection is the best antibiotic for all stages of syphilis. For primary-stage syphilis, a one-time treatment with penicillin is adequate, although some doctors repeat the dose in one week. For secondary-stage syphilis, the second dose is always given. Penicillin is also given for latent-stage syphilis and for all forms of tertiary-stage syphilis, although more frequent or longer treatment given intravenously may be needed. People who are allergic to penicillin may receive azithromycin once by mouth, ceftriaxone by injection daily for 10 days, or doxycycline by mouth for 14 days.

More than half of the people with syphilis in its early stages, especially those with secondary-stage syphilis, develop a reaction 2 to 12 hours after the first treatment. This reaction is called the

Jarisch-Herxheimer reaction and is believed to result from the sudden death of millions of bacteria. Symptoms of the reaction include a feeling of overall illness, fever, headache, sweating, shaking chills, and temporary worsening of the syphilitic sores. Rarely, people with neurosyphilis may experience seizures or paralysis. The symptoms of this reaction are temporary and rarely cause permanent harm.

After treatment, the prognosis for primary-, secondary-, and latent-stage syphilis is excellent. The prognosis is poor for tertiary-stage syphilis of the brain or heart, because existing damage usually cannot be reversed. A person who has been cured of syphilis does not become immune to it and can acquire the infection again.

Gonorrhea

Gonorrhea is a sexually transmitted disease caused by the bacterium Neisseria gonorrhoeae *that infects the inner lining of the urethra, cervix, rectum, and throat, or the membranes (conjunctivae) of the eyes.*

- Symptoms of gonorrhea may be absent or may include discharge from the penis or vagina, pain while urinating, a frequent need to urinate, and, in women, lower abdominal pain.
- A sample of the discharge is used to make the diagnosis.
- Antibiotics are given to kill the bacterium that causes gonorrhea; treatment against *Chlamydia* is often given at the same time because people with gonorrhea often also have chlamydia.

While the rate of gonorrhea has declined by 75% since 1985, there were still 330,000 reported cases in the United States in 2004. Gonorrhea usually causes problems only at the site of infection, although the disease can spread through the bloodstream to other parts of the body, especially the skin and joints. In women, the disease may ascend the genital tract and infect the membranes inside the pelvis, causing pelvic pain and reproductive problems.

Symptoms

In men, the first symptoms usually appear 2 to 7 days after infection. Symptoms start with mild discomfort in the urethra, followed a few hours later by mild to severe pain during urination, discharge of pus from the penis, and a frequent and urgent need to urinate, which worsens as the disease spreads to the upper part of the urethra. The penile opening may become red and swollen.

Infected women often have no symptoms for weeks or months, and the disease may be discovered only after the woman's male partner is diagnosed and she is examined as a contact. If symptoms do occur, they usually appear 7 to 21 days after infection and are usually mild. However, some women have severe symptoms, such as a frequent need to urinate, pain while urinating, a discharge from the vagina, and fever. The cervix, uterus, fallopian tubes, ovaries, urethra, and rectum may be infected, causing tenderness or severe deep pelvic pain, especially during intercourse. Pus, which appears to come from the vagina, may be coming from the cervix, urethra, or glands near the vaginal opening.

Anal sex with an infected partner may result in gonorrhea of the rectum. The disease may cause discomfort around the anus and a discharge from the rectum. The area around the anus may become red and raw, and the stool may be coated with mucus and pus. When a doctor examines the rectum with a viewing tube (anoscope), mucus and pus may be visible on the wall of the rectum.

Oral sex with an infected partner may result in gonorrhea of the throat (gonococcal pharyngitis). Usually, the infection produces no symptoms, but sometimes it causes a sore throat and discomfort during swallowing.

If infected fluids come into contact with the eyes, gonococcal conjunctivitis may develop, causing swelling of the eyelids and a discharge of pus from the eyes. A pregnant woman with gonorrhea can infect the eyes of her baby during birth. In adults, often only one eye is affected. Newborns usually have infection in both eyes. Blindness may result if the infection is not treated early.

Gonorrhea in infant and young girls is usually the result of sexual abuse by adults or teens. Symptoms may include irritation, redness, and swelling of the vulva, with a discharge of pus from the vagina. The girl may be sore in the vaginal area or have pain during urination. The rectum also may be inflamed. The underpants may be stained with discharge.

In some people, gonorrhea spreads through the bloodstream to one or more joints, causing them to become swollen, tender, and extremely painful and limiting movement. A bloodstream infection may also cause fever, a general feeling of illness, pain that moves from joint to joint, and the formation of red pus-filled spots on the skin (arthritis-dermatitis syndrome).

The interior of the heart may become infected (endocarditis). Infection of the covering of the liver (perihepatitis) causes pain in the upper right part of the abdomen similar to that of gallbladder disease. These infections are treatable and rarely fatal, but recovery from arthritis or endocarditis may be slow.

Diagnosis

A doctor can make a diagnosis almost immediately by identifying the bacterium (gonococcus) under a microscope. In more than 90% of infected men, this diagnosis can be made using a sample of discharge from the penis. The sample is usually obtained by passing a small swab a few centimeters into the urethra. Microscopic examination of a sample of the discharge from the cervix is less reliable; gonococci can be seen in only about 60% of infected women. The sample of discharge is also sent to the laboratory for culture, which is very reliable in both sexes but takes longer than a microscopic examination. If a doctor suspects an infection of the throat or rectum, samples from these areas are sent for culture.

Highly sensitive methods for detecting the DNA of the two bacteria that cause gonorrheal and chlamydial infections enable laboratories to test for both infections in a single specimen. Because these tests can be performed on urine samples from both sexes, they are convenient for screening people who have no symptoms or who are unwilling to have specimens taken from their penis or vagina.

Because a person may have more than one STD, a doctor should take a sample of blood to determine whether the person with gonorrhea also has syphilis or human immunodeficiency virus (HIV) infection.

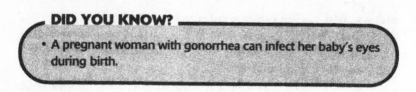

DID YOU KNOW?

• A pregnant woman with gonorrhea can infect her baby's eyes during birth.

Treatment

People with gonorrhea are usually given antibiotics to kill both *Chlamydia* and gonococci, because people with gonorrhea are often infected with *Chlamydia* at the same time. A single injection of ceftriaxone into a muscle or a single dose of cefixime, levofloxacin, ciprofloxacin, or ofloxacin by mouth is usually adequate to cure gonorrhea but a week-long course of another oral antibiotic (doxycycline or levofloxacin) is routinely given to cure chlamydia. Alternatively, a single large dose of azithromycin can be used to cure chlamydial infections. If gonorrhea has spread through the bloodstream, the person usually is treated in the hospital with intravenous antibiotics.

If symptoms recur or persist at the end of treatment, the doctor may obtain specimens for culture to make sure the person is cured. Symptoms of urethritis may recur in men (postgonococcal urethritis) and are most commonly caused by *Chlamydia* and other organisms that do not respond to treatment with ceftriaxone.

Nongonococcal Urethritis and Chlamydial Cervicitis

Nongonococcal urethritis and chlamydial cervicitis are sexually transmitted diseases caused by the bacterium Chlamydia trachomatis *and various other microorganisms that produce inflammation of the urethra and cervix.*

- Several different microorganisms cause gonorrhea-like diseases; the most common is that caused by *Chlamydia trachomatis*.
- The most common symptoms are pain or burning while urinating, a discharge from the penis or vagina, and the urge to urinate frequently; however, in many people infected with these organisms, symptoms do not develop.
- Chlamydia can be diagnosed from a sample of discharge.

- Infections with *Ureaplasma* and *Mycoplasma* can be diagnosed with expensive tests, but the diagnosis is usually based on symptoms in a person with no evidence of gonorrhea.
- Infection is usually treated with an antibiotic for at least 7 days.

Several different microorganisms cause diseases that resemble gonorrhea. These microorganisms include *Chlamydia trachomatis*, *Trichomonas vaginalis*, and several different types of *Mycoplasma*. In the past, these microorganisms were difficult for laboratories to identify, so the infections they caused were simply called "nongonococcal" to indicate that they were not caused by *Neisseria gonorrhoeae*, the bacterium that causes gonorrhea.

Chlamydia trachomatis infection (chlamydia) is very common, with 929,000 reported cases in the United States in 2004. Because the infection sometimes produces no symptoms, even more people may be affected. In men, chlamydia causes about half of the urethral infections not caused by gonorrhea. Most of the remaining male urethral infections are caused by *Ureaplasma urealyticum*. In women, chlamydia accounts for virtually all of the pus-forming cervical infections not caused by gonorrhea. Both sexes may acquire gonorrhea and chlamydia at the same time.

Symptoms and Diagnosis

Between 4 and 28 days after intercourse with an infected person, an infected man typically has a mild burning sensation in his urethra while urinating. A clear or cloudy discharge from the penis may be evident. The discharge is usually less thick than the discharge that occurs in gonorrhea. Early in the morning, the opening of the penis is often red and stuck together with dried secretions. Occasionally, the disease begins more dramatically. The man needs to urinate frequently, finds urinating painful, and has discharge of pus from the urethra.

Although most women infected with *Chlamydia* have few or no symptoms, some experience frequent urges to urinate and pain while urinating, pain in the lower abdomen, pain during sexual intercourse, and secretions of yellow mucus and pus from the vagina.

Anal infections may cause pain and a yellow discharge of pus and mucus.

In most cases, a doctor can diagnose chlamydia by examining discharge from the penis or cervix in a laboratory. Newer tests that amplify DNA or RNA, such as the polymerase chain reaction (PCR), enable a doctor to diagnose chlamydia or gonorrhea from a urine sample. These tests are recommended for screening of sexually active women between the ages of 15 and 25. Genital infections with *Ureaplasma* and *Mycoplasma* are not diagnosed specifically in routine medical settings, because culturing of these microorganisms is difficult and other techniques for diagnosis are expensive. The diagnosis of nongonococcal infections is often presumed if the person has characteristic symptoms and no evidence of gonorrhea.

If chlamydia is not treated, symptoms usually disappear in 4 weeks. However, an untreated infection can cause a number of complications. Untreated chlamydial cervicitis often ascends to the fallopian tubes (tubes that connect the ovaries to the uterus), where inflammation may cause pain and scarring. The scarring can cause infertility and ectopic pregnancy (see page 318). These complications can occur in women without symptoms and result in considerable suffering and medical costs. In men, chlamydia may cause epididymitis, which produces painful swelling of the scrotum on one or both sides (see page 398). Whether *Ureaplasma* has a role in these complications is unclear.

COMPLICATIONS OF CHLAMYDIAL AND UREAPLASMAL INFECTIONS

In men
- Infection of the epididymis
- Narrowing (stricture) of the urethra

In women
- Infection of the fallopian tubes and linings of the pelvic cavity
- Infection of the surface of the liver

In men and women
- Infection of the membranes of the eyes (conjunctivitis)

In newborns
- Conjunctivitis
- Pneumonia

Treatment

Chlamydial and ureaplasmal infections are usually treated with tetracycline, doxycycline, or levofloxacin taken by mouth for at least 7 days or with a single dose of azithromycin taken by mouth. Because the symptoms are so similar to those of gonorrhea, doctors usually give an antibiotic such as ceftriaxone to treat gonorrhea at the same time. Pregnant women are given erythromycin instead of tetracycline or doxycycline. If symptoms persist or return, treatment is then repeated for a longer period.

Infected people who have sexual intercourse before completing treatment may infect their partners. Also, partners who are infected may re-infect the treated person. Thus, sex partners are treated simultaneously if possible. The risk of a repeat infection of chlamydia or another STD within 3 to 4 months is high enough that screening may be repeated at that time.

Lymphogranuloma Venereum

Lymphogranuloma venereum is a sexually transmitted disease caused by Chlamydia trachomatis *that produces painful swellings in the groin.*

Lymphogranuloma venereum is caused by a subtype of *Chlamydia trachomatis* other than those that cause nongonococcal urethritis and chlamydial cervicitis. The disease occurs mostly in tropical and subtropical areas and is uncommon in the United States, with only 27 reported cases in 2004.

Symptoms begin 3 or more days after infection. A small, painless, fluid-filled blister develops usually on the penis or in the vagina. Typically, the blister becomes a sore that quickly heals—often going unnoticed. Next, lymph nodes in the groin on one or both sides may swell and become tender. With prolonged or repeated episodes of infection, the lymphatic vessels may become obstructed, causing tissue to swell. Rectal infection may cause scarring, which can result in a narrowing of the rectum.

A doctor suspects lymphogranuloma venereum based on its characteristic symptoms. The diagnosis can be confirmed by a blood test that identifies antibodies against *Chlamydia trachomatis*. If given early in the disease, treatment with oral doxycycline, erythromycin, or tetracycline for 3 weeks results in rapid healing.

Chancroid

Chancroid is a sexually transmitted disease caused by the bacterium Haemophilus ducreyi *that produces painful genital sores.*

While quite common in other parts of the world, chancroid is rare in the United States, with only 30 cases reported in 2004.

Symptoms begin 3 to 7 days after infection. Small, painful blisters form on the genitals or around the anus and rapidly rupture to form shallow sores. These sores may enlarge and connect. The lymph nodes in the groin may become tender, enlarged, and matted together, forming an abscess (a collection of pus). The skin over the abscess may become red and shiny and may break down and discharge pus onto the skin.

Several antibiotics are effective for chancroid. A single injection of ceftriaxone is effective, as is a single oral dose of azithromycin, 3 days of oral ciprofloxacin, or 7 days of oral erythromycin.

Granuloma Inguinale

Granuloma inguinale is a rare sexually transmitted disease caused by the bacterium Calymmatobacterium granulomatis *that leads to chronic inflammation of the genitals.*

Granuloma inguinale is rare in developed countries, with only eight cases reported in the United States in 1999. It is more common in people living under primitive conditions in Papua New Guinea, Australia, and South Africa.

Symptoms usually begin 1 to 12 weeks after infection. The first symptom is a painless, red nodule that slowly grows into one or more round, raised lumps that then break down to form a sore. Sites of infection include the penis, scrotum, groin, and thighs in men and the vulva, vagina, and surrounding skin areas in women. Either trimethoprim-sulfamethoxazole or doxycycline taken by mouth for at least 3 weeks is effective.

Trichomoniasis

Trichomoniasis is a sexually transmitted disease of the vagina or urethra caused by Trichomonas vaginalis, *a single-celled organism.*

- Women usually have a discharge from the vagina, sore vulva, pain while urinating, or frequency of urination; men may have no symptoms or discharge from the penis, pain while urinating, or frequency of urination.
- A sample of the discharge is used to make the diagnosis.
- A single dose of metronidazole in women and a 7-day course in men usually cures the infection.

Trichomonas vaginalis commonly infects the genitals and urinary tract of men and women. However, women are more likely to develop symptoms. About 20% of women develop trichomoniasis of the vagina during their reproductive years.

In men, urethral infection with no or minimal symptoms is common, although rarely the epididymis and prostate are infected. In some populations, *Trichomonas* may account for 5 to 10% of all cases of nongonococcal urethritis.

Symptoms and Diagnosis

In women, the disease usually starts with a greenish yellow, frothy vaginal discharge. In some women the discharge is slight. The vulva may be irritated and sore, and sexual intercourse may be painful. In severe cases, the vulva and surrounding skin may be inflamed and the labia swollen. Pain on urination or frequency of urination, such as occurs in a bladder infection, may occur alone or with the other symptoms.

Men with trichomoniasis may have no symptoms but still infect their sex partners. Many men have nongonococcal urethritis with symptoms of discharge from the urethra, pain during urination, and a need to urinate frequently. The role of *Trichomonas* in prostate infections is unclear.

The organism is more difficult to detect in men than in women. In women, the diagnosis can usually be made quickly by seeing the organism in a sample of vaginal secretions under a microscope or after several days by culture. Tests for other STDs are usually performed as well, because *Trichomonas* is common in people with gonorrhea or chlamydia. In men, secretions from the end of the penis (obtained in the morning, before urination) may be examined under a microscope and sent to the laboratory for culture. Microscopic examination of the urine may also detect *Trichomonas*.

DID YOU KNOW?

- Although women more often develop symptoms and thus more often seek treatment, cure requires treating her and her male sex partner.
- A person should avoid drinking alcohol while being treated.

Treatment

A single dose of metronidazole taken by mouth cures up to 95% of infected women; however, they may become reinfected unless their sex partners are treated simultaneously. It is not known whether a single-dose treatment is effective in men, but men are usually cured after 7 days of treatment.

If taken with alcohol, metronidazole may cause nausea and flushing of the skin. The drug also may cause a metallic taste in the mouth, nausea, or a decrease in the number of white blood cells and, in women, an increased susceptibility to vaginal yeast infections (genital candidiasis). Metronidazole is best avoided during pregnancy, at least during the first 3 months. Infected people who have sexual intercourse before the infection is cured are likely to infect their partners.

Genital Warts

Genital warts (condylomata acuminata) *are growths in or around the vagina, penis, or rectum caused by sexually transmitted papillomaviruses.*

- Papillomaviruses cause genital warts as well as cervical cancer in women.
- Many people have no symptoms, but some may experience burning pain.
- Genital warts can usually be diagnosed from their appearance.
- Treatment methods include laser, freezing therapy, and surgery; however, treatment is not always successful, as warts tend to come back.

Genital warts are common; in the United States an estimated 500,000 people per year develop genital warts. About 22% of sexually active young women have been infected with one of the viruses that causes these warts. Because of the location of these warts, condoms may not protect against infection.

Genital warts are caused by certain types of papillomavirus, other types of which cause the common warts that appear on other parts of the body. Several types of papillomavirus infect the genitals, but not all of them cause plainly visible external genital warts. Some types cause tiny raised areas on the cervix that may only be visible with a magnifying instrument called a culposcope. Although these less-visible spots generally do not cause symptoms, the papillomaviruses causing them increase the risk of developing cervical cancer and therefore should be treated (see page 247). Vaccination against the papillomaviruses that cause genital warts and cervical cancer is available in the United States for girls and women 9 to 26 years old. The vaccine should be administered before the onset of sexual activity, but girls and women who are sexually active should still be vaccinated.

Symptoms and Diagnosis

Genital warts occur most often on warm, moist surfaces. In men, the usual areas are on the penis, especially below the foreskin (if the penis is uncircumcised). In women, genital warts occur on the vulva, vaginal wall, cervix, and skin surrounding the vaginal area. Genital warts may develop in the area around the anus and in the rectum, especially in people who engage in anal sex. Many people have no symptoms from the warts, but some feel occasional burning pain.

The warts usually appear 1 to 6 months after infection with papillomavirus, beginning as tiny, soft, moist, pink or red swellings. They grow rapidly and appear as rough, irregular bumps, which sometimes grow out from the skin on narrow stalks. Groups of warts often grow in the same area, and their rough surfaces give them the appearance of a small cauliflower. The warts may grow very rapidly in pregnant women, in people with an impaired immune system (for example, people with AIDS or those who are taking immunosuppressive drugs), and in people who have inflammation of the skin.

Genital warts usually can be diagnosed from their appearance. Unusual-looking or persistent warts may be removed surgically and examined under a microscope to make sure that they are not cancerous. Regular Papanicolaou (Pap) tests to detect the early stages of cancer are very important in women who have warts on the cervix.

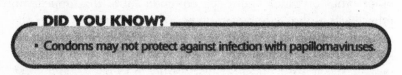

DID YOU KNOW?

• Condoms may not protect against infection with papillomaviruses.

Treatment

In many people, the immune system eventually controls the papillomavirus. Half the time, the infection is gone after 8 months; less than 10% of people are infected longer than 2 years.

No treatment is completely satisfactory, and some treatments are uncomfortable and leave scars. External genital warts may be removed by laser, freezing (cryotherapy), or surgery using local anesthetics. Podophyllin toxin, imiquimod, or trichloroacetic acid can be applied directly to the warts. This approach, however, requires many applications over weeks to months, may burn the surrounding skin, and frequently fails. Imiquimod cream produces less burning but may be less effective. The warts may return after apparently successful treatment.

Warts in the urethra may be removed by endoscopic surgery (a procedure in which a flexible viewing tube with surgical attachments is used). This is sometimes followed by injection of the wart with a chemotherapy drug, 5-fluorouracil. Interferon-alpha injections into the wart are somewhat effective, but they must be administered several times a week for many weeks and are very expensive.

In uncircumcised men, circumcision may help prevent recurrence. All sex partners should be examined for warts and other STDs and treated, if necessary.

Other Sexually Transmitted Diseases

Some bacteria (*Shigella, Campylobacter,* and *Salmonella*), viruses (hepatitis A, B, and C), and parasites (*Giardia* and other amebas) that are usually transmitted nonsexually can sometimes be transmitted during sex. Infection by these organisms, with the exception of hepatitis B and C, is usually acquired by mouth. Thus, activities in which the mouth comes into contact with the anus of an infected person can transmit these infections. Symptoms are typically those of the specific organism transmitted and may involve diarrhea, fever, abdominal pain or bloating, nausea and vomiting, and jaundice. Infections recur frequently, especially in homosexual men with many sex partners. Some infections cause no symptoms but may lead to serious long-term complications, such as chronic hepatitis B or C.

CHAPTER 6

Human Immunodeficiency Virus Infection

- HIV is transmitted through contact with body fluids that contain the virus or infected cells.
- A few weeks after the infection is transmitted, fever, rashes, swollen lymph nodes, and fatigue may develop, then usually disappear.
- Blood tests can detect HIV infection within weeks of infection.
- Over years, HIV destroys white blood cells called CD4+ lymphocytes, which help to defend the body against other infections.
- When levels of CD4+ lymphocytes in the blood are low, AIDS develops with symptoms that may include weight loss, recurring fever, diarrhea, anemia, and thrush (fungal infection of the mouth or vagina); opportunistic infections (those caused by microorganisms that do not harm people with normal immune systems); and cancers.
- The CD4+ lymphocyte count indicates how severely the immune system is damaged, what infections may occur, and how a person is responding to treatment.
- Antiretroviral drugs of four types (nucleoside reverse transcriptase inhibitors, non-nucleoside reverse transcriptase inhibitors, protease inhibitors, and fusion inhibitors) are given

in 3-drug combinations to increase their potency and prevent resistance to individual drugs.

- These drug combinations prevent HIV from replicating and help restore the immune system but do not eliminate HIV, so they must be taken indefinitely.

Human immunodeficiency virus (HIV) infection is an infection by one of two viruses, HIV-1 and HIV-2. The HIV viruses progressively destroy some types of white blood cells called lymphocytes. Lymphocytes are an important part of the body's immune defenses. When lymphocytes are destroyed, the body becomes susceptible to attack by many other infectious organisms. Many of the complications of HIV infection, including death, are usually the result of these other infections and not of the HIV infection itself.

WHAT IS A RETROVIRUS?

The human immunodeficiency virus (HIV) is a retrovirus, which like many other viruses stores its genetic information as RNA rather than as DNA. When the virus enters a targeted host cell, it releases its RNA and an enzyme (reverse transcriptase), and then makes DNA using the viral RNA as a pattern. The viral DNA is then incorporated into the host cell DNA. This reverses the usual process of copying information in human cells, which make RNA copies from the pattern of human DNA (thus, the term "retro" for "backward"). Other RNA viruses, such as polio or measles, do not make DNA copies to reproduce but simply copy their own RNA.

Each time a host cell divides, it makes a new copy of the integrated viral DNA along with its own genes.

HIV DNA can either lie latent (hidden) and do no damage or activate to produce thousands of copies of the HIV RNA by taking over the functions of the cell and killing it. These new HIV copies are released from the infected cell to invade other cells and repeat the cycle.

Acquired immunodeficiency syndrome (AIDS) is the most severe form of HIV infection. A person with HIV infection is considered to have AIDS when at least one complicating illness develops or his ability to defend against infection significantly declines as measured by a low CD4+ lymphocyte count.

HIV infection and AIDS have reached epidemic proportions. About 40 million people are infected worldwide. In parts of Africa, AIDS threatens to destroy large numbers of adults between the ages of 15 and 45, leaving millions of orphans.

Infections with HIV-1 and HIV-2 are serious and tend to occur in different regions. HIV-1 is most common in the Western Hemisphere; Europe; Asia; and Central, South, and East Africa. HIV-2 is common in West Africa, although many people there are infected with HIV-1.

Transmission of Infection

The transmission of HIV requires contact with a body fluid that contains either the virus or infected cells. HIV can appear in nearly any body fluid, but transmission mainly comes from blood, semen, vaginal secretions, and breast milk. Although low concentrations of HIV are also present in tears, urine, and saliva, transmission from these fluids is extremely rare.

HIV is transmitted in the following ways:

* Sexual contact with an infected person, during which the mucous membrane lining the mouth, vagina, penis, or rectum is exposed to contaminated body fluids (unprotected sex)
* Injection or infusion of contaminated blood, as occurs with blood transfusions, the sharing of needles, or an accidental prick from an HIV-contaminated needle
* Transfer of the virus from an infected mother to a child before birth, during birth, or after birth through the mother's milk.

Susceptibility to HIV infection increases when the skin or a mucous membrane is torn or damaged—even minimally—as can happen during vigorous vaginal or anal intercourse. Sexual transmission of HIV is more likely if either partner has herpes, syphilis, or another sexually transmitted disease (STD) that produces breaks in the skin or inflammation of the genitals. However, HIV can be transmitted even if neither partner has other STDs or obvious breaks in the skin. HIV transmission also can occur during oral sex, although it is far less common than during vaginal or anal intercourse.

In the United States, Europe, and Australia, HIV has mainly been transmitted through male homosexual contact and the sharing of needles among injecting drug users, but transmission through heterosexual contact has been rapidly increasing.

A health care worker who is pricked with an HIV-contaminated needle or other sharp object has about a 1 in 300 chance of contracting HIV. The risk increases if the object penetrates deeply or if contaminated blood is injected. Infected fluid splashing into the mouth or eyes has less than a 1 in 1,000 chance of causing

DID YOU KNOW?

- Many people die of another infection rather than HIV infection itself.
- HIV can be transmitted from mother to child in breast milk.
- HIV infection is more easily transmitted when skin or mucous membranes are damaged by traumatic sexual activity or inflamed by other sexually transmitted diseases such as herpes or syphilis.
- HIV is not transmitted by casual contact at work, school, or home; coughing or sneezing; or insects such as mosquito bites.
- Infected people can spread HIV immediately after becoming infected even if they have no symptoms.
- Some blood tests for HIV may be negative during the first several weeks of infection.
- HIV infection is almost completely preventable—through sexual abstinence or condom use and access to clean needles.
- Even without treatment, some infected people remain well for over a decade, but others become severely ill within a few years of infection. Blood tests can determine who needs and who can safely defer treatment.
- Taking anti-HIV drugs irregularly may enable the virus to become resistant, begin to replicate, and resume its ill effects on immune function.
- If antiviral drugs are used correctly, most people can live productive, active lives for years.

infection. Taking a combination of antiretroviral drugs soon after exposure appears to reduce, but not eliminate, the risk of becoming infected and is recommended.

People with hemophilia require frequent infusions of whole blood or other blood products. Before 1985, many people with hemophilia in the United States became infected with HIV

THE HIV TRANSMISSION RISK OF SEVERAL SEXUAL ACTIVITIES

No risk (unless sores are present)

- Dry kissing
- Body-to-body rubbing and massage
- Using unshared inserted sexual devices
- Being masturbated by a partner, without semen or vaginal fluids
- Bathing and showering together
- Contact of intact skin with feces or urine

Theoretical risk (extremely low risk unless sores are present)

- Wet kissing
- Oral sex performed on male (no ejaculation, with or without a condom)
- Oral sex performed on female (with barrier)
- Oral-anal contact
- Digital vaginal or anal penetration, with or without a glove
- Using shared but disinfected inserted sexual devices

Low risk

- Oral sex performed on male (with ejaculation, with or without ingestion of semen)
- Oral sex performed on female (no barrier)
- Vaginal or anal intercourse (with proper use of a condom)
- Using shared but not disinfected inserted sexual devices

High risk

- Vaginal or anal intercourse (with or without ejaculation, condom not used or used improperly)

because the blood products they received were contaminated with HIV. AIDS became the leading cause of death among these people. Since 1985, all blood collected for transfusion has been tested for HIV, and when possible, some blood products are treated with heat to eliminate the risk of HIV infection. The current risk of HIV infection from a single blood transfusion is estimated to be less than 1 in 500,000.

HIV infection in a large number of women of childbearing age has led to HIV infection in children. In about 25 to 35% of the pregnancies involving women infected with HIV, the virus is transmitted to the fetus through the placenta or, more commonly, at birth during passage through the birth canal. Infants who are breast-fed can contract HIV infection through breast milk. A few children contract HIV infection through sexual abuse.

HIV is not transmitted by casual contact or even by close, nonsexual contact at work, school, or home. No case of HIV transmission has been traced to the coughing or sneezing of an infected person or to a mosquito bite. Transmission from an infected doctor or dentist to a patient is extremely rare.

Mechanism of Infection

Once in the body, HIV attaches to several types of white blood cells, the most important being the helper T lymphocyte. Helper T lymphocytes activate and coordinate other cells of the immune system. These lymphocytes have a receptor protein called CD4 in their outer membrane (and are therefore designated as CD4+). HIV has its genetic material encoded in RNA. Once inside a CD4+ lymphocyte, the virus turns its RNA into DNA by means of an enzyme called reverse transcriptase. The viral DNA is incorporated into the DNA of the infected lymphocyte. The lymphocyte's own machinery then reproduces (replicates) the virus inside the cell, eventually destroying the cell. The thousands of new viruses produced by each infected cell infect other lymphocytes and can destroy them as well. Within a few days or weeks, enough HIV may be produced to reduce numbers of lymphocytes substantially and enable the person to spread the HIV infection to others.

Simplified Life Cycle of the Human Immunodeficiency Virus

Like all viruses, human immunodeficiency virus (HIV) reproduces (replicates) using the genetic machinery of its host cell, usually a CD4+ lymphocyte. Currently licensed drugs inhibit two critical enzymes (reverse transcriptase and protease) that the virus uses to replicate. Drugs targeted at a third enzyme, integrase, are being developed.

1. HIV first attaches to and penetrates its target cell.
2. HIV releases RNA, the genetic code of the virus, into the cell. For the virus to replicate, its RNA must be converted into DNA; the enzyme that performs the conversion is called reverse transcriptase. HIV mutates easily at this point, because reverse transcriptase is prone to errors during the conversion of viral RNA to DNA.
3. The viral DNA enters the cell's nucleus.
4. With the help of an enzyme called integrase, the viral DNA becomes integrated with the cell's DNA.
5. The DNA now replicates and reproduces RNA and proteins. The proteins are in the form of a long chain that must be cut into pieces after the virus leaves the cell.
6. A new virus is assembled from RNA and short pieces of protein.
7. The virus buds through the membrane of the cell, wrapping itself in a fragment of the cell membrane (envelope).
8. To be able to infect other cells, the budded virus must mature. It becomes mature when another viral enzyme (HIV protease) cuts structural proteins within the virus, causing them to rearrange.

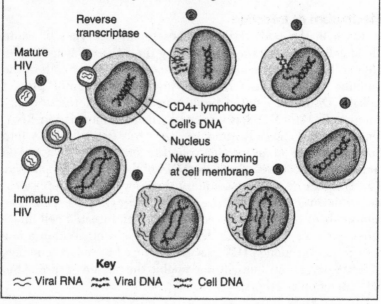

Reverse transcriptase

Mature HIV

CD4+ lymphocyte

Cell's DNA

Nucleus

New virus forming at cell membrane

Immature HIV

Key

≈ Viral RNA   ≋ Viral DNA   ≈ Cell DNA

Because HIV infection destroys CD4+ lymphocytes, it weakens the body's system for protecting itself against certain infections and cancers. This weakening of the immune system is part of the reason that the body is unable to eliminate HIV infection once it has started. However, the immune system is able to mount some response. Within a month or two of infection, the body produces lymphocytes and antibodies that help to lower the amount of HIV in the blood and keep the infection under control. For this reason, HIV infection can continue for a long time in some people before it causes serious problems.

Because the number of CD4+ lymphocytes in the blood helps determine the ability of the immune system to protect the body from infections, it is a good measure of the severity of the damage done by HIV infection. A healthy person has a CD4+ lymphocyte count of roughly 800 to 1,300 cells per microliter of blood. Typically, blood levels of CD4+ lymphocytes are reduced 40 to 60% in the first few months of infection. After about 6 months, the CD4+ count stops falling so quickly, but it continues to decline.

If the CD4+ count falls below about 200 cells per microliter of blood, the immune system becomes less able to fight certain infections (for example, the fungal infection that causes *Pneumocystis carinii* pneumonia [PCP]). These infections do not usually appear in people with a healthy immune system and are called opportunistic infections. A count below about 50 cells per microliter of blood is particularly dangerous, because additional opportunistic infections that can rapidly cause severe weight loss, blindness, or death commonly occur.

The amount of HIV in the blood is called the **viral load**. In the first few months after infection, a large number of virus particles circulate in the blood. The infection is very contagious at this stage. Later, the viral load drops to a lower level that remains constant for some time. This level is an important indicator of how contagious a person's infection is and how fast the disease is likely to progress. Doctors measure the viral load during treatment, because a decreasing or very low level indicates that treatment is working. The goal of treatment is to lower the viral load to the point where it is undetectable (suppressed) in the blood, although some virus is probably still present. A rise in the viral load may indicate the development of drug resistance or failure to take the drugs.

Symptoms

Most people experience no noticeable symptoms upon initial infection. However, fever, rashes, swollen lymph nodes, fatigue, and a variety of less common symptoms may develop within a few weeks of HIV infection and last a few weeks. The symptoms disappear, although the lymph nodes may stay enlarged. An infected person is able to spread the virus soon after becoming infected; this is true even if there are no symptoms.

A person can have HIV infection for years—even a decade or longer—before developing AIDS. Before AIDS develops, many people feel well, although some develop a variety of nonspecific symptoms. These symptoms include swollen lymph nodes, weight loss, fatigue, recurring fever or diarrhea, anemia, and thrush (a fungal infection of the mouth).

The main symptoms of AIDS are those of the specific opportunistic infections and cancers that develop. HIV can also directly infect the brain, causing memory loss, weakness, difficulty walking, and difficulty in thinking and concentrating (dementia). In some people, HIV is probably directly responsible for AIDS wasting, which is a significant loss of weight with or without an obvious cause. Wasting in people with AIDS may also be caused by a series of infections or an untreated infection (such as tuberculosis) that persists. Kidney failure, which may be a direct effect of HIV, is more common in blacks than in whites.

Kaposi's sarcoma, a cancer that appears as painless, red to purple, raised patches on the skin, affects many people with AIDS, especially homosexual men. Cancers of the immune system (lymphomas, typically non-Hodgkin's lymphoma) may develop, sometimes first appearing in the brain, where they can cause confusion, personality changes, and memory loss. Women are prone to developing cancer of the cervix. Homosexual men are prone to developing cancer of the rectum.

Usually, death is caused by the cumulative effects of wasting, dementia, opportunistic infections, or cancers.

Diagnosis

A relatively simple, accurate blood test that detects antibodies to HIV (ELISA test) is used to screen people for HIV infection. If the ELISA result is positive, it is confirmed with a more accurate

Common Opportunistic Infections Associated With AIDS

INFECTION	DESCRIPTION	SYMPTOMS
Candida esophagitis	A yeast infection of the esophagus	Painful swallowing, burning in chest
Pneumocystis carinii pneumonia	An infection of the lungs with *Pneumocystis* fungus	Difficulty breathing, cough, fever
Toxoplasmosis	Infection with the parasite *Toxoplasma,* which usually affects the brain	Headache, confusion, lethargy, seizures
Tuberculosis	Infection of the lungs and sometimes other organs with tuberculosis bacteria	Cough, fevers, night sweats, weight loss, chest pain
Mycobacterium avium complex	Infection of the intestines or lungs with a type of bacteria that resembles tuberculosis bacteria	Fever, weight loss, diarrhea, cough
Cryptosporidiosis	Infection of the intestines with the parasite *Cryptosporidium*	Diarrhea, abdominal pain, weight loss
Cryptococcal meningitis	Infection of the lining of the brain with the yeast *Cryptococcus*	Headache, fever, confusion
Cytomegalovirus infection	Infection of the eyes or intestinal tract with cytomegalovirus	Eye: blindness Intestinal tract: diarrhea, weight loss
Progressive multifocal leukoencephalopathy	Infection of the brain with a polyomavirus	Weakness on one side of the body, loss of coordination or balance

test, usually the Western Blot. Both tests often are not positive in the first month or two after HIV infection because it takes the body that long to produce antibodies against the virus. Other tests (for example, viral load tests or P24 antigen) detect HIV in the blood much sooner after infection. P24 antigen is currently used along with other tests to screen blood donated for transfusions.

People diagnosed with HIV infection have their blood tested regularly to measure the CD4+ count and viral load. CD4+ counts indicate the health of a person's immune system and, when low, their chances of becoming ill from an infection. Viral load is a predictor of how fast the CD4+ count is likely to drop over the next year. Doctors use these two measurements to decide when to start drugs for both the treatment of HIV and the prevention of the complicating infections. Doctors also use these tests to monitor the effects of treatment. With successful treatment, the viral load falls to low levels within weeks and the CD4+ count begins a long, slow recovery toward normal levels. AIDS is diagnosed when the CD4+ count falls below 200 cells per microliter of blood, there is extreme wasting, or certain opportunistic infections and cancers develop.

Prevention

Because HIV is nearly always transmitted by sexual contact or the sharing of needles, infection is almost completely preventable. Unfortunately, the measures required for prevention—sexual abstinence or condom use (see page 65) and access to clean needles—are sometimes personally or socially unpopular. Many people have difficulty changing their addictive or sexual behaviors, so they continue to engage in behavior that puts them at risk for HIV infection. Additionally, safe sex practices are not foolproof: condoms can leak or break.

Vaccines for preventing HIV infection or slowing the progression of AIDS in people who are already infected have so far proved elusive.

Because HIV is not transmitted through the air or by casual contact (such as touching, holding, or dry kissing), hospitals and clinics do not isolate HIV-infected people unless they have another contagious infection. HIV-contaminated surfaces can easily be cleaned and disinfected because HIV is inactivated by heat and by common disinfectants such as hydrogen peroxide and alcohol. People who are likely to come into contact with blood or other body fluids at their job should wear protective gear, including latex gloves, masks, and eye shields. These universal precautions apply to body fluids from all people, not just those from someone with HIV, for two reasons: people with HIV may not know that they are infected, and other viruses can be transmitted by body fluids.

People who have been exposed to HIV from a blood splash, needlestick, or sexual contact may reduce the chance of infection by taking a brief course of anti-HIV drugs. These drugs must be started as soon as possible after the exposure. Four weeks of preventive treatment with two or three drugs is currently recommended. Because the risk of infection varies, doctors and infected people make treatment decisions individually based on the type of exposure.

STRATEGIES FOR PREVENTING THE TRANSMISSION OF HIV

- Abstain from sexual activity.
- Use a condom (preferably made of latex) for each act of intercourse with an infected partner or a partner whose HIV status is unknown (vaginal spermicides and sponges do not protect against HIV infection).
- If engaging in oral sex, withdraw before ejaculation; avoid brushing teeth for several hours before and after oral sex.
- Newly monogamous couples should get tested for HIV and other sexually transmitted diseases (STDs) before engaging in unprotected sexual intercourse.
- Never share needles or syringes.
- Wear rubber gloves (preferably latex) when touching body fluids of a person who might be infected with HIV.
- If exposed to HIV by needlestick, seek treatment to prevent infection.

Treatment

Four classes of drugs are available to treat HIV infection: nucleoside reverse transcriptase inhibitors, non-nucleoside reverse transcriptase inhibitors, protease inhibitors, and fusion inhibitors. Both types of reverse transcriptase inhibitors work by interfering with the HIV enzyme reverse transcriptase, which converts viral RNA into DNA. Protease inhibitors interfere with the HIV enzyme protease, which is needed to activate certain proteins inside newly produced viruses. Failure to activate these proteins results in immature, defective HIV that does not infect new cells. None of these drugs kill HIV; they prevent the virus from replicating. If replication is sufficiently slowed, the destruction of CD4 cells by HIV is decreased dramatically and CD4+ counts begin to rise. The result can be reversal of much of the damage to the immune system caused by HIV.

HIV usually develops resistance to any of these drugs when they are used alone and even in combinations of two drugs. Resistance can develop after a few days to several months of use, depending on the drug and the person. Therefore, treatment is most effective when at least two or preferably three of the drugs are given in combination—usually one or two reverse transcriptase inhibitors plus a protease inhibitor. This combination of drugs is sometimes referred to as a "drug cocktail." Combinations of drugs are used for three reasons. First, combinations are more powerful than single drugs in reducing levels of HIV in the blood. Second, combinations help prevent the development of drug resistance. Third, some HIV drugs (like ritonavir) boost the blood levels of other HIV drugs (including most protease inhibitors) by slowing their removal from the body. Drug combinations have delayed the onset of AIDS in HIV-infected people, thus extending their lives.

Combinations of HIV drugs have both unpleasant and serious side effects. Disturbances in the metabolism of fats appear to be caused primarily by the protease inhibitors. Symptoms are the slow migration of body fat from the face, arms, and legs to the abdomen ("protease paunch") and sometimes to the breasts of women. Blood levels of cholesterol and triglycerides, two forms of fat in the blood, are increased—probably increasing the risk of future heart attacks and strokes.

Nucleoside reverse transcriptase inhibitors damage mitochondria, a critical site of energy generation in human cells. Their side effects include anemia, painful feet caused by nerve damage, and liver damage that rarely progresses to liver failure. Individual drugs differ in their tendency to cause these problems. Careful monitoring and changes of drugs can usually prevent serious problems.

Drug treatment is beneficial only when the drugs are taken on schedule. Missed doses allow the virus to replicate and develop resistance. The goal of combination therapy is to reduce the viral load so it is below detectable levels. No treatments have proven able to eliminate the virus from the body, although levels often fall below what can be measured; if treatment is stopped, viral load increases and CD4+ counts begin to fall.

It is not yet clear for which infected people drug treatment should be started, but people with low CD4+ counts or high viral loads require treatment, even if they have no symptoms. Because of the many significant and unpleasant side effects and because the drugs are very expensive, it is not easy for people with HIV infection to take the drugs for many years without fail. Because taking HIV drugs irregularly often leads to drug resistance, doctors try to ensure that anyone prescribed these drugs is both willing and able to adhere to the treatment schedule.

People with low CD4+ counts are routinely prescribed drugs to prevent opportunistic infections. To prevent *Pneumocystis* pneumonia, the combination of sulfamethoxazole and trimethoprim is given when the CD4+ count drops below 200 cells per microliter of blood. This combination of drugs also prevents toxoplasmosis, which can damage the brain of a person with AIDS. For people with CD4+ counts below 50 cells per microliter of blood, azithromycin taken weekly or clarithromycin or rifabutin taken daily may prevent *Mycobacterium avium* infections. People recovering from cryptococcal meningitis or those experiencing repeated infections of the mouth, esophagus, or vagina with the fungus *Candida* may be given the antifungal drug fluconazole for prolonged periods. People with recurring episodes of herpes simplex infections of the mouth, lips, genitals, or rectum may require prolonged treatment with an antiviral drug (such as acyclovir) to prevent relapses.

Other drugs may help with the weakness and weight loss associated with AIDS. Megestrol and dronabinol (a marijuana derivative) stimulate appetite. Many people with AIDS claim that natural marijuana is even more effective. Anabolic steroids (such as testosterone) can also significantly reverse the loss of muscle tissue. Testosterone levels are reduced in some men and can be replaced by use of injections or patches on the skin.

Drugs for HIV Infection

DRUG	SIDE EFFECTS
Fusion inhibitor	
Fuseon	Inflammation at injection sites
Non-nucleoside reverse transcriptase inhibitors	
Delavirdine	Rash, headaches
Efavirenz	Dizziness, sleepiness, nightmares, confusion, agitation, forgetfulness, euphoria, rash
Nevirapine	Rash (occasionally severe or life threatening), liver dysfunction
Nucleoside and nucleotide reverse transcriptase inhibitors	
	All may cause lactic acidosis and liver damage
Abacavir	Fever, rash (occasionally severe or life threatening), nausea and vomiting, low white blood count
Didanosine (ddI)	Peripheral nerve damage, pancreas inflammation, nausea, diarrhea
Emtricibine	
Lamivudine (3TC)	Headache, fatigue
Stavudine (d4T)	Peripheral nerve damage, loss of facial fat
Tenofovir	Mild to moderate diarrhea, nausea and vomiting, flatulence
Zalcitabine (ddC)	Peripheral nerve damage, pancreas inflammation, mouth sores
Zidovudine (AZT)	Anemia and susceptibility to infection (resulting from bone marrow toxicity), headache, insomnia, weakness, muscle aches

Drugs for HIV Infection (Continued)

Protease inhibitors	
	All produce nausea, vomiting, diarrhea, and abdominal discomfort; high blood sugar and cholesterol are common; increased abdominal fat ("protease paunch") may occur; bleeding in hemophilia; liver dysfunction
Amprenavir	
Darunavir	
Indinavir	Kidney stones
Lopinavir	Mouth tingling, altered taste
Nelfinavir	
Ritonavir	Mouth tingling, altered taste
Saquinavir	
Tipranavir	Brain hemorrhage is a rare complication

Prognosis

Exposure to HIV does not always lead to infection, and some people who have had repeated exposures over many years remain uninfected. Moreover, many HIV-infected people remain well for more than a decade before becoming ill. Why some people become ill so much sooner than others is not fully understood, but a number of human genetic factors influence both susceptibility to infection and progression to AIDS after infection.

Of the people infected with HIV who do not receive drug treatment, each year 1 to 2% develop AIDS for the first several years after infection. Every year thereafter, about 5% of the people with untreated HIV infection develop AIDS. Within 10 to 11 years of contracting HIV infection, half of the people who have not received treatment develop AIDS. Eventually, more than 95% of untreated infected people develop AIDS, and it is possible that they all will if they live long enough, although a few people have remained well for more than 15 years.

Before effective therapy was developed in the mid 1990s, many people with AIDS experienced a rapid decline in their quality of life after first being hospitalized for the infection—often spending much of their remaining time in the hospital. Most people died within 2 years of developing AIDS. However, current therapy has changed AIDS into a more stable, manageable disease. Many people have lived for years with AIDS, continuing to lead productive and active lives. Nevertheless, illness from infections and the expense and side effects of drugs may reduce quality of life. For people unable to tolerate or take drugs consistently, the natural progression of the disease resumes. Cure is not yet possible, although intensive research continues.

Part II

Women's Health

CHAPTER 7

Female Reproductive System

The female reproductive system consists of the external and internal genital organs. (The breasts are sometimes considered part of the reproductive system—see page 206.) However, other parts of the body also affect the development and functioning of the reproductive system. They include the hypothalamus (an area of the brain), the pituitary gland (located directly below the hypothalamus), and the adrenal glands (located on top of the kidneys). The hypothalamus orchestrates the interactions among the genital organs, pituitary gland, and adrenal glands. These parts of the body interact with each other by releasing hormones. Hormones are chemical messengers that control and coordinate activities in the body. The hypothalamus produces gonadotropin-releasing hormone, which stimulates the pituitary gland to produce luteinizing hormone and follicle-stimulating hormone. These hormones stimulate the ovaries to produce the female sex hormones, estrogen and progesterone, and some male sex hormones (androgens). (Male sex hormones stimulate the growth of pubic and underarm hair at puberty and maintain muscle mass in girls as well as boys.) After childbirth, the hypothalamus signals the pituitary gland to produce prolactin, a hormone that stimulates milk production. The adrenal glands produce small amounts of female and male sex hormones.

External Genital Organs

The external genital organs consist of the mons pubis, labia majora, labia minora, Bartholin's glands, and clitoris. The area containing these organs is called the vulva. The external genital organs have three main functions: enabling sperm to enter the body, protecting the internal genital organs from infectious organisms, and providing sexual pleasure.

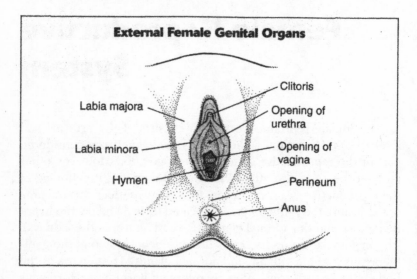

External Female Genital Organs

The mons pubis is a rounded mound of fatty tissue that covers the pubic bone. During puberty, it becomes covered with hair. The mons pubis contains oil-secreting (sebaceous) glands that release pheromones, which are involved in sexual attraction. The labia majora (literally, large lips) are relatively large, fleshy folds of tissue that enclose and protect the other external genital organs. They are comparable to the scrotum in males. The labia majora contain sweat and sebaceous glands, which produce lubricating secretions. After puberty, hair appears on the labia majora.

The labia minora (literally, small lips) can be very small or up to 2 inches wide. The labia minora lie just inside the labia majora and surround the openings to the vagina and urethra. A rich supply of blood vessels gives the labia minora a pink color.

During sexual stimulation, these blood vessels become engorged with blood, causing the labia minora to swell and become more sensitive to stimulation.

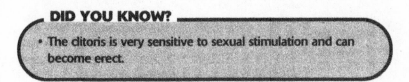

DID YOU KNOW?

• The clitoris is very sensitive to sexual stimulation and can become erect.

The area between the vaginal opening and the anus, at the back of the labia majora, is called the perineum. It varies in length from almost 1 to more than 2 inches (2 to 5 centimeters). A long perineum is less likely to tear during childbirth.

The labia majora and the perineum are covered with skin similar to that on the rest of the body. The skin is thick, dry, and sometimes scaly. In contrast, the labia minora are lined with a mucous membrane, whose surface is kept moist by fluid secreted by specialized cells.

The opening to the vagina is called the introitus. The vaginal opening is the entryway for the penis during sexual intercourse and the exit for menstrual blood and vaginal discharge as well as a baby. When stimulated, Bartholin's glands (located beside the vaginal opening) secrete a thick fluid that supplies lubrication for intercourse. The opening to the urethra, which carries urine from the bladder to the outside, is located above and in front of the vaginal opening.

The clitoris, located between the labia minora, is a small protrusion that corresponds to the penis in the male. The clitoris, like the penis, is very sensitive to sexual stimulation and can become erect. Stimulating the clitoris can result in an orgasm.

Internal Genital Organs

The internal genital organs form a pathway (the genital tract). This pathway consists of the following:

• The vagina (part of the birth canal), where sperm are deposited and from which a baby can emerge

- The uterus, where an embryo can develop into a fetus
- The fallopian tubes (oviducts), where a sperm can fertilize an egg
- The ovaries, which produce and release eggs.

Sperm travel up the tract, and eggs down the tract.

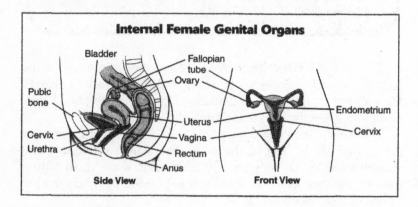

Internal Female Genital Organs

Side View — Bladder, Fallopian tube, Ovary, Pubic bone, Uterus, Cervix, Vagina, Urethra, Rectum, Anus

Front View — Endometrium, Cervix

At the beginning of the tract, just inside the vaginal opening is the hymen, a mucous membrane. In virgins, the hymen usually encircles the opening like a tight ring, but it may completely cover the opening. The hymen helps protect the genital tract but is not necessary for health. It may tear at the first attempt at sexual intercourse, or it may be so soft and pliable that no tearing occurs. The hymen may also be torn during exercise or insertion of a tampon or diaphragm. Tearing usually causes slight bleeding. In women who have had intercourse, the hymen may be unnoticeable or may form small tags of tissue around the vaginal opening.

The vagina is a narrow, muscular but elastic organ about 4 to 5 inches long in an adult woman. It connects the external genital organs with the uterus. The vagina is the main female organ of sexual intercourse, into which the penis is inserted. It is the passageway for sperm to the egg and for menstrual bleeding or a baby to the outside.

Usually, there is no space inside the vagina unless it is stretched open—for example, during an examination or sexual intercourse. The lower third of the vagina is surrounded by elastic muscles that control the diameter of its opening. These muscles contract rhythmically during sexual intercourse and can be toned by Kegel exercises.

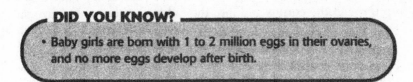

DID YOU KNOW?

• Baby girls are born with 1 to 2 million eggs in their ovaries, and no more eggs develop after birth.

The vagina is lined with a mucous membrane, kept moist by fluids oozing from cells on its surface and by secretions from glands in the cervix (the lower part of the uterus). These fluids may pass to the outside as a vaginal discharge, which is normal. During a woman's reproductive years, the lining of the vagina has folds and wrinkles. Before puberty and after menopause (if the woman is not taking estrogen), the lining is smooth.

The uterus is a thick-walled, muscular, pear-shaped organ located in the middle of the pelvis, behind the bladder, and in front of the rectum. The uterus is anchored in position by several ligaments. The main function of the uterus is to sustain a developing fetus. The uterus consists of the cervix and the main body (the corpus).

The cervix, the lower part of the uterus, protrudes into the upper end of the vagina and can be seen during a pelvic examination. Like the vagina, the cervix is lined with a mucous membrane, but the mucous membrane of the cervix is smooth.

Sperm can enter and menstrual blood can exit the uterus through a channel in the cervix. The channel is narrow. During labor, the channel widens to let the baby through. The cervix is usually a good barrier against bacteria, except during the menstrual period, around the time an egg is released by the ovaries (ovulation), or during labor. Bacteria can enter the uterus through the cervix during sexual intercourse. Unlike the bacteria that cause sexually transmitted diseases (see page 64), bacteria normally found in the vagina rarely cause problems.

The channel through the cervix is lined with glands that secrete mucus. This mucus is thick and impenetrable to sperm until just before ovulation. At ovulation, the consistency of the mucus changes so that sperm can swim through it and fertilization can occur. At this time, the mucus-secreting glands of the cervix can store live sperm for 2 or 3 days. These sperm can later move up through the corpus and into the fallopian tubes to fertilize an egg. Thus, intercourse 1 or 2 days before ovulation can lead to pregnancy. For some women, the time between a menstrual period and ovulation varies from month to month. Consequently, pregnancy can occur at different times during a menstrual cycle.

The corpus of the uterus, which is highly muscular, can stretch to accommodate a growing fetus. Its muscular walls contract during labor to push the baby out through the cervix and the vagina. During the reproductive years, the corpus is twice as long as the cervix. After menopause, the reverse is true.

As part of a woman's reproductive cycle (which usually lasts about a month), the lining of the corpus (endometrium) thickens. If the woman does not become pregnant during that cycle, most of the endometrium is shed and bleeding occurs, resulting in the menstrual period.

The two fallopian tubes, which are about 2 to 3 inches long, extend from the upper edges of the uterus toward the ovaries. The tubes do not connect with the ovaries. Instead, the end of each tube flares into a funnel shape with fingerlike extensions (fimbriae). When an egg is released from an ovary, the fimbriae guide the egg into the relatively large opening of a fallopian tube.

The fallopian tubes are lined with tiny hairlike projections (cilia). The cilia and the muscles in the tube's wall propel an egg downward through the tube to the uterus. The egg may be fertilized by a sperm in the fallopian tube (see page 270).

The ovaries are usually pearl-colored, oblong, and somewhat smaller than a chicken egg. They are attached to the uterus by ligaments. In addition to producing female sex hormones (estrogen and progesterone) and male sex hormones, the ovaries produce and release eggs. The developing egg cells (oocytes) are contained in fluid-filled cavities (follicles) in the wall of the ovaries. Each follicle contains one oocyte.

HOW MANY EGGS?

A baby girl is born with egg cells (oocytes) in her ovaries. Between 16 and 20 weeks of pregnancy, the ovaries of a female fetus contain 6 to 7 million oocytes. Most of the oocytes gradually waste away, leaving about 1 to 2 million present at birth. No new oocytes develop after birth. At puberty, only about 300,000—more than enough for a lifetime of fertility—remain. Only a small percentage of oocytes mature into eggs. The many thousands of oocytes that do not mature degenerate. Degeneration progresses more rapidly in the 10 to 15 years before menopause. All are gone by menopause.

Only about 400 eggs are released during a woman's reproductive life, usually one during each menstrual cycle. Until released, an egg remains dormant in its follicle—suspended in the middle of a cell division. Thus, the egg is one of the longest-lived cells in the body. Because a dormant egg cannot perform the usual cellular repair processes, the opportunity for damage increases as a woman ages. A chromosomal or genetic abnormality is thus more likely when a woman conceives a baby later in life.

Puberty

The physical changes that occur at puberty are regulated by changes in levels of hormones that are produced by the pituitary gland—luteinizing hormone and follicle-stimulating hormone. At birth, the levels of these hormones are high, but they decrease within a few months and remain low until puberty. Early in puberty, levels of luteinizing hormone and follicle-stimulating hormone increase, stimulating the production of sex hormones. The increased levels of sex hormones result in physical changes, including maturation of the breasts, ovaries, uterus, and vagina. Normally, these changes occur sequentially during puberty, resulting in sexual maturity.

The first change of puberty is usually the start of breast development (breast budding). In girls who live in the United States, this change usually occurs around age 9 to 11. Shortly afterward, pubic and underarm hair begin to grow. The interval from breast budding to the first menstrual period is usually about 2 ½ years. In the United

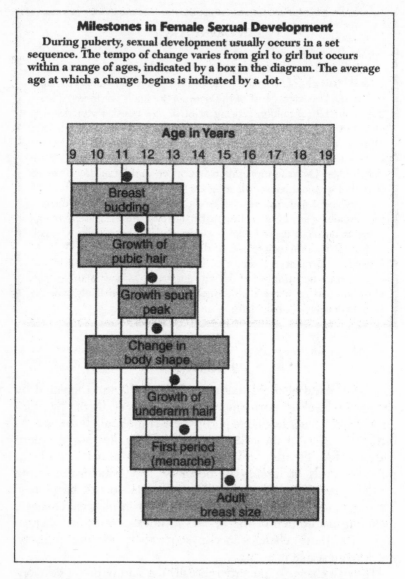

Milestones in Female Sexual Development

During puberty, sexual development usually occurs in a set sequence. The tempo of change varies from girl to girl but occurs within a range of ages, indicated by a box in the diagram. The average age at which a change begins is indicated by a dot.

Age in Years

9 10 11 12 13 14 15 16 17 18 19

Breast budding

Growth of pubic hair

Growth spurt peak

Change in body shape

Growth of underarm hair

First period (menarche)

Adult breast size

States, girls, on average, have their first period when they are almost 13. The girl's body shape changes, and the percentage of body fat increases. The growth spurt accompanying puberty typically begins even before the breasts start to develop. Growth is fastest relatively early in puberty (before menstrual periods begin) and peaks at about age 12. Then growth slows considerably, usually stopping between the ages of 14 and 16.

Menstrual Cycle

- When pregnancy does not occur, the uterine lining (endometrium) is shed, and bleeding from the uterus into the vagina occurs.
- A menstrual cycle (from the first day of bleeding to just before the next menstrual period) normally lasts 21 to 40 days.
- Hormones regulate the cycle.
- The ovary releases an egg during the middle of the cycle, around day 15.

Menstruation is the shedding of the lining of the uterus (endometrium) accompanied by bleeding. It occurs in approximately monthly cycles except during pregnancy and after menopause. Menstruation marks the reproductive years of a woman's life, from the start of menstruation (menarche) during puberty until its cessation (menopause—see page 133).

By definition, the first day of bleeding is counted as the beginning of each menstrual cycle (day 1). The cycle ends just before the next menstrual period. Menstrual cycles range from about 21 to 40 days. Only 10 to 15% of women have cycles that are exactly 28 days. The intervals between periods are usually longest in the years immediately after menarche and before menopause.

The menstrual cycle is regulated by hormones: luteinizing hormone and follicle-stimulating hormone, which are produced by the pituitary gland, and estrogen and progesterone, which are produced by the ovaries. The cycle has three phases: follicular, ovulatory, and luteal.

The **follicular phase** lasts from the first day of bleeding to immediately before a surge in the level of luteinizing hormone. The surge results in release of the egg (ovulation). During this phase, the follicles in the ovaries develop. The follicular phase varies in length, averaging about 13 days of the cycle. This phase tends to become shorter at the end of the reproductive years, near menopause.

Changes During the Menstrual Cycle

A menstrual cycle is regulated by the complex interaction of hormones: luteinizing hormone and follicle-stimulating hormone, which are produced by the pituitary gland, and the female sex hormones estrogen and progesterone, which are produced by the ovaries.

The menstrual cycle begins with menstrual bleeding (menstruation), which marks the first day of the follicular phase. Bleeding occurs when levels of estrogen and progesterone decrease, causing the thickened lining of the uterus (endometrium) to degenerate and be shed. During the first half of this phase, the follicle-stimulating hormone level increases slightly, stimulating the development of several follicles. Each follicle contains an egg. Later, as the follicle-stimulating hormone level decreases, only one follicle continues to develop. This follicle produces estrogen.

The ovulatory phase begins with a surge in luteinizing hormone and follicle-stimulating hormone levels. Luteinizing hormone stimulates egg release (ovulation), which usually occurs 16 to 32 hours after the surge begins. The estrogen level peaks during the surge, and the progesterone level starts to increase.

During the luteal phase, levels of luteinizing hormone and follicle-stimulating hormone decrease. The ruptured follicle closes after releasing the egg and forms a corpus luteum, which produces progesterone. Later in this phase, the level of estrogen increases. Progesterone and estrogen cause the lining of the uterus to thicken more. If the egg is not fertilized, the corpus luteum degenerates and no longer produces progesterone, the estrogen level decreases, the lining degenerates and is shed, and a new menstrual cycle begins.

Pituitary Hormone Cycle

Ovarian Cycle

Sex Hormone Cycle

Endometrial Cycle

At the beginning of the follicular phase, the lining of the uterus (endometrium) thickens with fluids and nutrients designed to nourish an embryo. If no egg has been fertilized, estrogen and progesterone levels decrease, the endometrium is shed, and menstrual bleeding occurs. Menstrual bleeding lasts 3 to 7 days, averaging 5 days. Blood loss during a cycle ranges from ½ to 10 ounces, averaging 4½ ounces. A sanitary pad or tampon, depending on the type, can hold up to an ounce of blood. Menstrual blood, unlike blood resulting from an injury, usually does not clot unless the bleeding is very heavy.

During the first part of the follicular phase, the pituitary gland increases slightly its production of follicle-stimulating hormone. This hormone then stimulates the growth of 3 to 30 follicles, each containing an egg. Later in the phase, as the level of this hormone decreases, only one of these follicles—the dominant follicle—continues to grow. It soon begins to produce estrogen, and the other stimulated follicles begin to degenerate.

The **ovulatory phase** starts with a surge in the levels of luteinizing hormone and, to a lesser degree, follicle-stimulating hormone. Luteinizing hormone stimulates the dominant follicle to bulge from the surface of the ovary and finally rupture, releasing the egg. (The function of the increase in follicle-stimulating hormone is not understood.)

The ovulatory phase ends with the release of the egg, usually 36 hours after the surge in luteinizing hormone begins. About 12 to 24 hours after the egg is released, this surge can be detected by measuring the luteinizing hormone level in the urine. The egg can be fertilized for only a short period (up to about 12 hours) after its release. Fertilization is more likely when sperm are present in the reproductive tract before the egg is released.

DID YOU KNOW?

- The first menstrual period usually occurs about 2½ years after breasts start to develop.
- Around the time of ovulation, normally some women feel a pain in one side of the lower abdomen.

Around the time of ovulation, some women feel a dull pain on one side of the lower abdomen. This pain is known as mittelschmerz (literally, middle pain). The pain may last for a few minutes to a few hours. The pain is felt on the same side as the ovary that released the egg, but the precise cause of the pain is unknown. The pain may precede or follow the rupture of the follicle and may not occur in all cycles. Egg release does not alternate between the two ovaries and appears to be random. If one ovary is removed, the remaining ovary releases an egg every month.

The **luteal phase** follows ovulation. It lasts about 14 days, unless fertilization occurs, and ends just before a menstrual period. In the luteal phase, the ruptured follicle closes after releasing the egg and forms a structure called a corpus luteum, which produces increasing quantities of progesterone. The function of the corpus luteum is to prepare the uterus in case fertilization occurs. The progesterone produced by the corpus luteum causes the endometrium to thicken, filling with fluids and nutrients in preparation for a potential fetus. Progesterone causes the mucus in the cervix to thicken, making the entry of sperm or bacteria into the uterus less likely. Progesterone also causes body temperature to increase slightly during the luteal phase and remain elevated until a menstrual period begins. This increase in temperature can be used to estimate whether ovulation has occurred (see page 55). In the second part of the luteal phase, the estrogen level increases, also stimulating the endometrium to thicken.

In response to the increase in estrogen and progesterone levels, the milk ducts in the breasts increase. As a result, the breasts may swell and become tender.

If the egg is not fertilized, the corpus luteum degenerates after 14 days, and a new menstrual cycle begins. If the egg is fertilized, the cells around the developing embryo begin to produce a hormone called human chorionic gonadotropin. This hormone maintains the corpus luteum, which continues to produce progesterone, until the growing fetus can produce its own hormones. Pregnancy tests are based on detecting an increase in the human chorionic gonadotropin level.

Effects of Aging

Around menopause (see page 133), changes in the genital organs occur rapidly. Menstrual cycles stop, and the ovaries stop producing estrogen. After menopause, the tissues of the labia minora, clitoris, vagina, and urethra thin (atrophy). This thinning can result in chronic irritation, dryness, and a discharge from the vagina. Vaginal infections are more likely to develop. Also after menopause, the uterus, fallopian tubes, and ovaries become smaller.

With aging, there is a decrease in the amount of muscle and connective tissue, including that in muscles, ligaments, and other tissues that support the bladder, uterus, vagina, and rectum. As a result, these organs may sag or drop down (prolapse), sometimes causing difficulty urinating, loss of control over urination or bowel movements (incontinence), or pain during sexual intercourse.

DID YOU KNOW?

- After menopause, the ovaries continue to produce male sex hormones, which help maintain sex drive, slow the loss of muscle tissue, and contribute to a sense of well-being.

Because there is less estrogen to stimulate milk ducts, the breasts decrease in size and may sag. The connective tissue that supports the breast also decreases, contributing to sagging. Fibrous tissue in the breasts is replaced with fat, making the breasts less firm.

Despite these changes, many women enjoy sexual activity more after menopause, possibly because they are no longer able to become pregnant. In addition, after menopause, the ovaries continue to produce male sex hormones. Male sex hormones help maintain the sex drive, slow the loss of muscle tissue, and contribute to an overall sense of well-being.

CHAPTER 8

Symptoms and Diagnosis of Gynecologic Disorders

Disorders that affect the female reproductive system, including the breasts, are called gynecologic disorders. Various diagnostic procedures are performed when a woman has specific symptoms (to determine the cause) or when a woman has a routine physical examination (to check for certain disorders). These procedures help prevent problems and maintain a woman's health.

Symptoms

- Common symptoms, such as vaginal itching, vaginal discharge, pelvic pain, and breast pain, have many causes, which are often not abnormal.
- Vaginal itching is considered a problem only when it persists, is severe, or recurs.
- A vaginal discharge is considered a problem only when it appears different from usual (is colored, bloody, or clumpy), has an odor, or is accompanied by itching or other symptoms.
- Vaginal bleeding is considered abnormal only when menstrual periods are too heavy or too light, last too long, occur

too frequently, or are irregular or when bleeding occurs before puberty, during pregnancy, or after menopause.

The most common symptoms due to gynecologic disorders include vaginal itching, a vaginal discharge, abnormal bleeding from the vagina, pain in the pelvic area, and breast pain. The significance of gynecologic symptoms often depends on the age of the woman, because hormonal changes that occur with age may be involved.

VAGINAL ITCHING

Vaginal itching may involve the area containing the external genital organs (vulva) as well as the vagina. Many women have occasional vaginal itching that resolves without treatment. Itching is considered a problem only when it is persistent, is severe, or recurs.

Vaginal itching may result from irritation by chemicals, such as those in laundry detergents, bleaches, fabric softeners, synthetic fibers, bubble baths, soaps, feminine hygiene sprays, perfumes, menstrual pads, fabric dyes, toilet tissue, vaginal creams, douches, and contraceptive foams. Vaginal itching may result from an infection (see page 176), such as bacterial vaginosis, candidiasis (a yeast infection), or trichomoniasis (a protozoan infection). Vaginal itching may also result from vaginal dryness due to hormonal changes at menopause. Other causes include skin disorders such as psoriasis or lichen sclerosus. Lichen sclerosus is characterized by thin white patches that develop around the opening of the vagina. If untreated, lichen sclerosus can cause scarring and may increase the risk of cancer. Treatment consists of a cream or an ointment containing a high dose of a corticosteroid (such as clobetasol).

Itching may be accompanied by a discharge. If itching persists or is accompanied by a vaginal discharge that looks or smells abnormal, a woman should see her doctor.

DID YOU KNOW?

- Normal newborn baby girls may have a normal vaginal discharge of mucus mixed with a little blood.

ABNORMAL VAGINAL DISCHARGE

A small amount of vaginal discharge is usually normal. The discharge consists of secretions (mucus) produced mainly by the cervix but also in the vagina. The discharge is usually thin and clear, milky white, or yellowish. Its amount and appearance vary with age. Typically, the discharge has no odor. It is not accompanied by itching or burning.

Newborn girls normally have a vaginal discharge of mucus, often mixed with a small amount of blood. This discharge is due to estrogen absorbed from the mother before birth. It usually stops within 2 weeks, as the level of estrogen in the blood decreases. Normally, older infants and girls, except those near puberty, do not have any significant vaginal discharge.

During a woman's reproductive years, the amount and appearance of the normal vaginal discharge vary with the menstrual cycle. For example, at the middle of the cycle (at ovulation), more mucus is usually produced and the mucus is thinner. Pregnancy, use of oral contraceptives, and sexual arousal also affect the amount and appearance of the discharge. After menopause, the estrogen level decreases, often reducing the amount of normal discharge.

A vaginal discharge is considered abnormal if it is:

- Heavier than usual
- Thicker than usual
- Puslike
- White and clumpy (like cottage cheese)
- Grayish, greenish, yellowish, or blood-tinged
- Foul-smelling (fishy)
- Accompanied by itching, burning, a rash, or soreness.

A discharge may indicate inflammation of the vagina (vaginitis), which may be due to a chemical irritant (as for vaginal itching) or to an infection (see page 176). In some women, spermicides, vaginal lubricants or creams, or diaphragms can irritate the vagina or vulva, causing inflammation. For women who are allergic to latex, contact with latex condoms can irritate the area. In young girls, a foreign object in the vagina can cause inflammation of the vagina, with a vaginal discharge that may contain blood. Most commonly, the foreign object is a piece of toilet paper that has worked its way into the vagina. Sometimes it is a toy.

A white, gray, or yellowish cloudy discharge with a foul or fishy odor is typically caused by bacterial vaginosis. A thick, white, and clumpy discharge (which looks like cottage cheese) is typically caused by candidiasis, a yeast infection. A heavy, greenish yellow, frothy discharge that may have a bad odor is typically caused by trichomoniasis, a protozoan infection.

A watery, blood-tinged discharge may be caused by cancer of the vagina, cervix, or lining of the uterus (endometrium). Radiation therapy to the pelvis may also cause an abnormal discharge.

Doctors may identify the cause of the abnormal discharge based on the appearance of the discharge, the woman's age, and other symptoms. A sample of the discharge is examined under a microscope to check for an infection and to identify it. Treatment depends on the cause. If a product (such as a cream, powder, soap, feminine hygiene spray, or brand of condom) causes persistent irritation, it should not be used.

ABNORMAL VAGINAL BLEEDING

Bleeding from the vagina may originate in the vagina or another reproductive organ, particularly the uterus. Abnormal vaginal bleeding includes menstrual bleeding that is excessively heavy or light, occurs too frequently, or is irregular. Any vaginal bleeding that is not associated with a menstrual period or that occurs before puberty, during pregnancy, or after menopause is also considered abnormal (see page 146).

Abnormal vaginal bleeding may result from a disorder (such as an injury, infection, or cancer) or from changes in the normal hormonal control of menstruation. Such hormonal changes are more likely to occur when menstrual periods are just starting (in teenagers) or nearing an end (in women in their 40s—see page 146).

DID YOU KNOW?

• In postmenopausal women, excess body hair may grow if levels of female hormones are too low or levels of male hormones are too high.

EXCESSIVE HAIRINESS

Excessive body hair, particularly on the face and trunk (in a male pattern) and on the limbs, is called hirsutism. Excessive hairiness may not seem like a gynecologic disorder, but it is considered one. It usually results from abnormal levels of female and male hormones.

Hirsutism is more common among postmenopausal women, because levels of female hormones have decreased. Hirsutism may be due to a disorder of the pituitary gland or adrenal glands that results in overproduction of male hormones (such as testosterone). Sometimes exaggerated masculine characteristics (virilization) result. Hirsutism may also be due to polycystic ovary syndrome (see page 161). Rare causes include tumors in the ovaries, porphyria cutanea tarda (a form of porphyria that affects the skin), and use of drugs such as anabolic steroids, corticosteroids, and minoxidil.

Blood tests may be performed to measure male and female hormone levels. Drugs that may be the cause are discontinued. Temporary solutions include shaving, plucking, waxing, and using depilatories. Eflornithine, a topical cream available by prescription, may be used. It can slow the growth of hair, causing a gradual reduction of unwanted facial hair. This drug may temporarily irritate the skin, causing redness, burning, stinging, or a rash. Bleaching may be effective if the hair is fine. Laser phototherapy is temporarily effective. The only safe permanent treatment is electrolysis, which destroys the hair follicles. The disorder causing hirsutism is treated when possible.

PELVIC PAIN

Many women experience pelvic pain—pain that occurs in the lowest part of the trunk, below the abdomen and between the hip bones. Pelvic pain may be caused by problems related to any of the organs in the pelvis: the reproductive organs (the uterus, fallopian tubes, ovaries, and vagina), bladder, rectum, or appendix. However, pelvic pain sometimes originates in organs outside the pelvis, such as the intestine, ureters, and gallbladder. Psychologic factors, especially stress and depression, may contribute to pelvic pain.

The pain may be sharp, intermittent, or crampy (like menstrual cramps). It may be sudden and excruciating, or it may be dull and constant. The pain may gradually increase in intensity. The area may feel tender to the touch. The pain may be accompanied by fever, nausea, and vomiting.

When a woman suddenly develops very severe pain in the lower abdomen or pelvis, doctors must quickly decide whether

---

WHAT CAUSES PELVIC PAIN?

Disorders related to the reproductive organs

- Ectopic pregnancy
- Endometriosis
- Fibroids
- Mittelschmerz (pain that occurs in the middle of the menstrual cycle and is caused by ovulation)
- Engorgement of blood vessels in the pelvis with blood about a week before the menstrual period (pelvic congestion syndrome)
- Ovarian cysts that are large, that rupture, or that twist
- Pelvic inflammatory disease

Disorders not related to the reproductive organs

- Appendicitis
- Urinary tract infections, such as cystitis
- Diverticulitis
- Gastroenteritis
- Ulcer disease
- Inflammatory bowel disease
- Inflammation of the lymph nodes in the abdomen (mesenteric lymphadenitis)
- Stones in the urinary tract, such as kidney stones

the cause requires emergency surgery. Examples of emergencies are appendicitis, a perforated ulcer, an aortic aneurysm, a twisted ovarian cyst, pelvic infections due to sexually transmitted diseases, and a pregnancy that develops outside of the uterus (ectopic pregnancy), usually in a fallopian tube.

To identify the cause, doctors may ask the woman to describe the pain, including its duration and location, and other symptoms. Doctors also ask about previous episodes of similar pain. Information about the timing of the pain in relation to eating, sleeping, sexual intercourse, activity, urination, and defecation may also be useful, as is information about any other factors that worsen or ease the pain.

Doctors gently feel the entire abdomen, checking for tenderness and abnormal growths. A pelvic examination helps doctors determine which organs are affected and whether an infection is present. Other procedures may include a complete blood cell count, urine tests, a pregnancy test, ultrasonography, computed tomography (CT), magnetic resonance imaging (MRI), and cultures to check for infections. Sometimes surgery or laparoscopy (use of a viewing tube to examine the abdominal and pelvic cavities) is needed to identify the cause of the pain.

Treating the disorder causing the pain, if identified, may relieve the pain. If a psychologic disorder is contributing to the pain, counseling or other therapy may help.

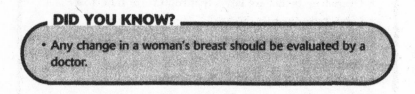

DID YOU KNOW?

- Any change in a woman's breast should be evaluated by a doctor.

BREAST SYMPTOMS

Symptoms related to the breast are common. They include breast pain, lumps (including solid masses and cysts), pitting or dimpling in the skin of the breast, and a discharge from the nipple (see page 206). Breast symptoms may or may not indicate a serious disorder. For example, diffuse breast pain that is related to hormonal changes before a menstrual period does not indicate a serious disorder. However, because breast cancer is a concern and because early detection is essential to the successful treatment of breast cancer, any change in the breast should be evaluated by a doctor. In addition, women should examine their breasts themselves once a month (see page 220).

Gynecologic Evaluation

- Regular gynecologic examinations and screening tests, particularly for cervical and breast cancer, can help keep women healthy.
- Women should report any symptoms to her doctor.
- A gynecologic examination includes examination of the breasts and pelvic organs.
- Occasionally, diagnostic procedures are done to view an abnormal area or to remove a sample of tissue from it.
- Many diagnostic procedures can be done in the doctor's office.

A healthy lifestyle includes having regular gynecologic examinations and screening tests for disorders that can be prevented or treated effectively if detected early. The main tests specific to women are the Papanicolaou (Pap) test or other similar tests to detect cancer of the cervix and mammography to detect breast cancer.

For gynecologic care, a woman should choose a health care practitioner with whom she can comfortably discuss sensitive topics, such as sex, birth control, pregnancy, and problems related to menopause. The practitioner may be a gynecologist, an internist, a nurse-midwife, or a general, family, or nurse practitioner. During the gynecologic visit, a woman can ask this practitioner any questions she has about reproductive and sexual function and anatomy, including safe sex practices.

GYNECOLOGIC HISTORY

A gynecologic evaluation starts with a series of questions related to reproductive function, which usually focus on the reason for the visit to the doctor's office. The answers form the gynecologic history. A complete gynecologic history includes information about the age at which menstrual bleeding began (menarche); the frequency, regularity, and duration of menstrual periods; the amount of flow; and the dates of the last two menstrual periods. Questions about abnormal bleeding—too much, too little, or between menstrual periods—are included.

A doctor may ask about sexual activity to assess the possibility of gynecologic infections, injuries, and pregnancy. A woman is asked whether she uses or wants to use birth control and whether she is interested in counseling or other information. The number of pregnancies, dates that they occurred, outcomes, and complications are recorded.

The doctor asks the woman whether she has pain during menstrual periods, during intercourse, or under other circumstances. If the woman has pain, she is asked how severe it is and what provides relief. Questions are also asked about breast problems, such as pain, lumps, areas of tenderness or redness, and discharge from the nipples. The woman is asked whether she is examining her breasts, how often, and whether she needs any instruction on technique.

The doctor reviews the woman's history of past gynecologic disorders and usually obtains a medical and surgical history that includes all previous health problems. The doctor reviews all the drugs a woman is taking, including prescription and nonprescription drugs, illicit drugs, tobacco, and alcohol, because many of them affect gynecologic function. The woman is asked about mental, physical, or sexual abuse in the present and the past. Some questions about urination are asked to find out whether the woman has a urinary tract infection or has problems with leakage of urine (incontinence).

GYNECOLOGIC EXAMINATION

If a woman has any questions or fears about the gynecologic examination, she should talk with the doctor beforehand about her concerns. If any part of the examination causes pain, the woman should let the doctor know. A woman is usually asked to empty her bladder before the physical examination and may be asked to collect a urine sample for analysis.

A breast examination may be performed before or after the pelvic examination. With the woman sitting, the doctor inspects the breasts for irregularities, dimpling, tightened skin, lumps, and a discharge. The woman then sits or lies down, with her arms above her head, while the doctor feels (palpates) each breast with a flat hand and examines each armpit for enlarged lymph nodes. The doctor also feels the neck and the thyroid gland for lumps and abnormalities. While performing the examination, the doctor can review the technique for breast self-examination with the woman (see page 220).

The doctor gently feels the entire abdomen, looking for abnormal growths or enlarged organs, especially the liver and spleen. Although the woman may experience some discomfort when the doctor presses deeply, the examination should not be painful. To estimate the size of the liver and spleen, the doctor may tap with the fingers (percuss) and listen for differences in sound between hollow-sounding and dull-sounding areas. A stethoscope may be used to listen for the activity of the intestines and for any abnormal noises made by blood flowing through narrowed blood vessels.

During the pelvic examination, the woman lies on her back with her hips and knees bent and her buttocks moved to the edge of the examining table. Most examining tables have heel stirrups that help a woman maintain this position. If a woman wants to observe the pelvic examination, she should let the doctor know ahead of time. The doctor can provide a mirror as well as explanations or a diagram. First, the doctor inspects the external genital area and notes the distribution of hair and any abnormalities, discoloration, discharge, or inflammation. This examination may indicate that all is well or give clues to hormonal problems, cancer, infections, injury, or physical abuse.

The doctor spreads the tissues around the opening of the vagina (labia) and examines the opening. Using a speculum (a metal or plastic instrument that spreads the walls of the vagina apart), the doctor examines the deeper areas of the vagina and the cervix. The cervix is examined closely for signs of irritation or cancer. The doctor checks for a protrusion of the bladder, rectum, or intestine into the vagina (see page 187).

For a Papanicolaou (Pap) test or another similar test, the doctor collects cells from the surface of the cervix with a plastic spatula similar to a tongue depressor. Then, a small bristle brush is used to obtain cells from the cervix. Usually, these tests feel

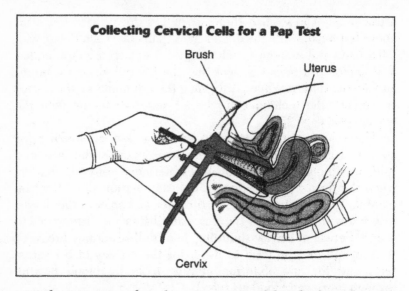

Collecting Cervical Cells for a Pap Test

Brush

Uterus

Cervix

scratchy or crampy, but they are not painful and take only a few seconds. The cells removed with the spatula or brush are placed on a glass slide and sprayed with a preservative or rinsed into a vial of liquid. The sample is sent to a laboratory, where it is examined under a microscope for abnormal cells, which may indicate cervical cancer. Such tests identify 80 to 85% of cervical cancers, even in their earliest stages. They can also detect changes in cells of the cervix that can lead to cancer. The changes can be treated, thus helping prevent cancer.

Pap and similar tests are most accurate if the woman is not having her period and does not douche or use vaginal creams for at least 24 hours before the examination. Most women should have such a test once a year. The first test is usually performed when a woman becomes sexually active or reaches age 18. If test results are normal for 3 consecutive years, the woman can discuss with her health care practitioner whether scheduling tests every 1, 2, or 3 years is appropriate.

If an infection is suspected, the doctor uses a swab to obtain a small amount of vaginal discharge from the vagina and cervix. The sample is sent to a laboratory for culture and evaluation. Tests for sexually transmitted diseases are not part of a routine examination. If a woman thinks she may have one of these diseases, she can request testing.

After removing the speculum, the doctor feels the vaginal wall to determine its strength and support. The doctor inserts the index and middle fingers of one gloved hand into the vagina and places the fingers of the other hand on the lower abdomen above the pubic bone. Between the two hands, the uterus can usually be felt as a pear-shaped, smooth, firm structure, and its position, size, consistency, and degree of tenderness (if any) can be determined. Then the doctor attempts to feel the ovaries by moving the hand on the abdomen more to the side and exerting slightly more pressure. More pressure is required because the ovaries are small and much more difficult to feel than the uterus. The woman may find this part of the examination to be slightly uncomfortable, but it should not be painful. The doctor determines how large the ovaries are and whether they are tender. The doctor also feels for growths or tender areas within the vagina.

Finally, the doctor performs a rectovaginal examination by inserting the index finger into the vagina and the middle finger into the rectum. In this way, the back wall of the vagina can be examined for abnormal growths or thickness. In addition, the doctor can examine the rectum for hemorrhoids, fissures, polyps, and lumps. A small sample of stool can be obtained with a gloved finger and tested for unseen (occult) blood. A woman may be given a take-home kit to test for occult blood in the stool.

DIAGNOSTIC PROCEDURES

Occasionally, more extensive diagnostic procedures are needed.

Colposcopy

For colposcopy, a binocular magnifying lens (similar to that of a microscope) can be used to inspect the cervix for signs of cancer. The procedure is often performed after an abnormal Pap test result. A speculum is used to spread the walls of the vagina so that the cervix can be seen. Colposcopy is painless and requires no anesthetic. It takes 15 to 30 minutes to perform.

Biopsy

A biopsy consists of removing a small sample of tissue for examination under a microscope. This procedure is performed when a precancerous condition (a condition that is likely to eventually lead to cancer) or cancer is suspected. A biopsy of the vulva can usually be performed in the doctor's office with use of a local anesthetic. A biopsy of the cervix and vagina is usually performed during colposcopy. Colposcopy enables doctors to take tissue samples from the area that looks most abnormal. Usually, biopsy of the cervix or vagina does not require an anesthetic. Typically, this procedure feels like a pinch or a cramp.

For biopsy of the lining of the uterus (endometrial biopsy), a small metal or plastic tube is inserted through the cervix into the uterus. The tube is moved back and forth and around to dislodge and suction out tissue from the uterine lining. This procedure is usually performed to determine the cause of abnormal vaginal bleeding. Also, infertility specialists use this procedure to determine whether ovulation is occurring normally or whether the uterus is ready for implantation of embryos. An endometrial biopsy can be performed in a doctor's office and usually does not require an anesthetic. Typically, it feels like strong menstrual cramps.

Endocervical Curettage

Endocervical curettage consists of inserting a small, sharp instrument (curet) inside the cervix to obtain tissue. This tissue is examined under a microscope by a pathologist. It is performed when endometrial or cervical cancer is suspected or needs to be ruled out. This procedure is usually performed during colposcopy and usually does not require an anesthetic.

Loop Electrical Excision Procedure

In a loop electrical excision procedure (LEEP), a thin wire loop through which an electrical current can pass is used to remove a piece of tissue. This procedure may be performed after an abnormal Pap test result to evaluate the abnormality more accurately and to remove the abnormal tissue. LEEP requires an anesthetic (often a local one), takes about 5 to 10 minutes, and can be performed in a doctor's office. Afterward, a woman may feel mild discomfort and have a small amount of bleeding.

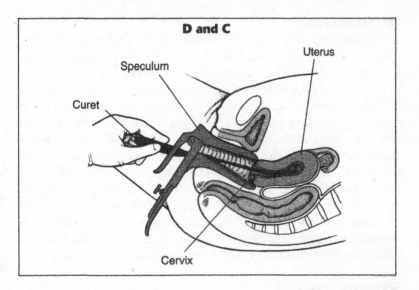

D and C

Uterus

Speculum

Curet

Cervix

Dilation and Curettage

For dilation and curettage (D and C), the cervix is stretched open (dilated) with metal rods so that a small, sharp instrument (curet) can be inserted to remove tissue lining the uterus. This procedure may be used to identify abnormalities of the uterine lining if biopsy results are inconclusive or to treat women who have had an incomplete miscarriage. D and C is often performed in a hospital, and a general anesthetic may be used. However, most women do not have to stay overnight in the hospital.

Hysteroscopy

To view the interior of the uterus, doctors can insert a thin viewing tube (hysteroscope) through the vagina and cervix into the uterus. The tube is about 1/4 inch in diameter and contains cables that transmit light. A biopsy, an electrocautery (heat), or a surgical instrument may be threaded through the tube. The site of abnormal bleeding or other abnormalities can usually be seen and can be sampled for a biopsy, sealed off using heat, or removed. This procedure may be performed in a doctor's office or in a hospital at the same time as a dilation and curettage.

Ultrasonography

Ultrasonography uses ultrasound waves, produced at a frequency too high to be heard. The ultrasound waves are emitted by a handheld device that is placed on the abdomen or inside the vagina. The waves reflect off internal structures, and the pattern of this reflection can be displayed on a monitor. In pregnant women, ultrasonography can help determine the condition and size of a fetus and can detect the presence of more than one fetus. It can often identify the sex of the fetus. Ultrasonography can also be used to monitor the fetus and to detect fetal abnormalities. It can be used to guide the placement of instruments during amniocentesis and chorionic villus sampling, which are used to detect genetic disorders in the fetus. Ultrasonography can detect an ectopic pregnancy, tumors, cysts, and other abnormalities in the pelvic organs. Ultrasonography is painless and has no known risks.

Sonohysterography

For sonohysterography, fluid is placed in the uterus through a thin tube (catheter) inserted through the vagina. Then ultrasonography is performed. The fluid fills and stretches (distends) the uterus so that abnormalities inside the uterus, such as polyps or fibroids, can be more easily detected. The procedure is performed in a doctor's office and may require a local anesthetic. A nonsteroidal anti-inflammatory drug (NSAID), such as ibuprofen, may be taken 20 minutes before the procedure to help relieve the cramping that may occur.

Laparoscopy

To directly examine the uterus, fallopian tubes, or ovaries, doctors use a viewing tube called a laparoscope. The laparoscope is attached to a thin cable containing flexible plastic or glass rods that transmit light. The laparoscope is inserted into the abdominal cavity through a small incision just below the navel. A probe is inserted through the vagina and into the uterus. The probe enables doctors to manipulate the organs for better viewing. Carbon dioxide is pumped through the laparoscope to inflate the abdomen, so that organs in the abdomen and pelvis can be seen clearly. Laparoscopy is performed in a hospital and requires an anesthetic, usually a general anesthetic. An overnight stay in the hospital is usually not required. Laparoscopy may cause mild abdominal discomfort, but normal activities can usually be resumed in 1 or 2 days.

Often, laparoscopy is used to determine the cause of pelvic pain, infertility, and other gynecologic disorders. Instruments can be threaded through the laparoscope to perform some surgical procedures, such as biopsies, sterilization procedures, and removal of an ectopic pregnancy in a fallopian tube or an ovary.

Hysterosalpingography

For hysterosalpingography, x-rays are taken after a radiopaque dye, which can be seen on x-rays, is injected through the cervix to outline the interior of the uterus and fallopian tubes. The procedure is often used to help determine the cause of infertility. The procedure is performed in a place where x-rays can be taken, such as a hospital or the radiology suite of a doctor's office. Hysterosalpingography usually causes discomfort, such as cramps.

Mammography

For mammography, x-rays of the breasts are taken to detect abnormal areas (see page 222). A technician positions the woman's breast on top of an x-ray plate. An adjustable plastic cover is lowered on top of the breast, firmly compressing the breast. Thus, the breast is flattened so that the maximum amount of tissue can be imaged and examined. X-rays are aimed downward through the breast, producing an image on the x-ray plate. Two x-rays are taken of each breast in this position. Then plates may be placed vertically on either side of the breast, and x-rays are aimed from the side. This position produces a side view of the breast.

Mammography is one of the best ways to detect breast cancer early. It is designed to detect the possibility of cancer at an early stage, years before it can be felt. All women aged 50 and older should have mammograms once a year to check for breast cancer. Many authorities recommend that women aged 40 to 49 have mammograms every 1 to 2 years.

The dose of radiation used is very low and is considered safe. This procedure may cause some discomfort, but the discomfort

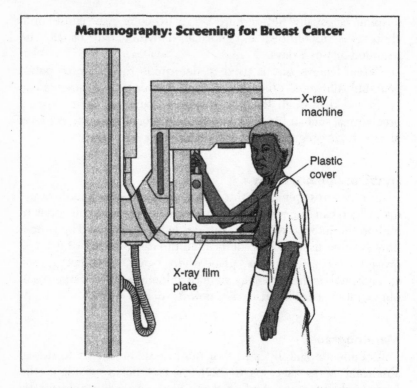

Mammography: Screening for Breast Cancer

X-ray machine

Plastic cover

X-ray film plate

lasts only a few seconds. Mammography should be scheduled at a time during the menstrual period when the breasts are less likely to be tender. Deodorants should not be used on the day of the procedure, because they can affect it. The entire procedure takes about 15 minutes.

CHAPTER 9

Menopause

Menopause is the permanent end of cyclic functioning of the ovaries and thus of menstrual periods.

- At menopause, menstrual periods and fertility end permanently, on average, around age 51 to 52.
- For up to several years before and just after menopause, estrogen levels fluctuate widely and symptoms may occur.
- Periods become irregular, and women may have hot flashes and mood changes, often lose their concentration, and feel depressed or unusually tired.
- After menopause, bone density decreases.
- Menopause is usually obvious, but blood tests may be done to confirm it.
- Hormones may be taken for a short time to relieve hot flashes and other symptoms, but long-term use has risks.

Menopause occurs because as women age, the ovaries produce smaller and smaller amounts of estrogen and progesterone. Estrogen and progesterone are the hormones that control the monthly cycle of egg release (ovulation—see page 111). Thus, as women approach menopause, an egg is released in fewer and fewer cycles, and eventually, egg release stops. As a result, menstrual periods end and pregnancy is no longer possible. A woman's last period can be identified only later, after she has had no periods for at least 6 months. (Women who do not wish to become pregnant should use birth control until 1 year has passed since their last menstrual period.)

A distinctive transitional period called perimenopause occurs before and just after menopause. During perimenopause, estrogen and progesterone levels fluctuate widely. Estrogen levels may be high at the beginning of this transitional period, but for short intervals, no estrogen may be produced. These fluctuations explain why many women in their 40s report bouts of menopausal symptoms, which may subside without treatment.

In the United States, the average age at which menopause occurs is about 51 to 52. However, menopause may occur normally in women as young as 40. Premature menopause is menopause occurring before age 40 (see page 144).

Artificial menopause results from a medical treatment that reduces or stops hormone production by the ovaries. Examples are surgery to remove the ovaries, surgery that unintentionally reduces the blood supply to the ovaries, and chemotherapy or radiation therapy to the pelvis, including the ovaries, to treat cancer. Surgery to remove the uterus (hysterectomy) ends menstrual periods but does not cause menopause as long as the ovaries are functioning.

Symptoms

During perimenopause, symptoms may be nonexistent, mild, moderate, or severe. Perimenopausal symptoms are thought to be caused by the fluctuations in hormone levels that occur as women approach menopause.

Irregular menstrual periods, which occur more or less often, may be the first symptom of perimenopause. Periods may be shorter or longer, lighter or heavier. They may not occur for months, then become regular again. However, periods may occur regularly until menopause.

Hot flashes affect three of four women. Most women have hot flashes for more than 1 year, and up to one half of women have them for more than 5 years. What causes hot flashes is unknown, but they may be related to fluctuations in hormone levels. Hot flashes seem to result in the widening (dilating) of blood vessels near the skin's surface. As a result, blood flow increases, causing the skin, especially on the head and neck, to become red and warm (flushed). Perspiration may be profuse. Hot flashes are sometimes called hot flushes because of this warming effect. A hot flash lasts from 30 seconds to 5 minutes and may be followed by chills.

> **DID YOU KNOW?**
>
> * Symptoms of menopause can start years before menstrual periods end.
> * Avoiding spicy foods, hot beverages, caffeine, and alcohol may help prevent or minimize hot flashes.

Other symptoms that may occur around the time of menopause include mood changes, depression, irritability, anxiety, nervousness, insomnia, loss of concentration, headache, and fatigue. These symptoms may be related to the decreases in estrogen levels occurring at the same time. But the precise relationship between estrogen levels and symptoms is unclear. Night sweats, which are related to hot flashes, may disturb sleep, contributing to fatigue and irritability. However, sleep disorders are common even among women who do not seem to have hot flashes.

Women may feel dizzy occasionally or have tingling (pins-and-needles) sensations. They may feel the heart beating very forcefully or rapidly (have palpitations). Weight gain may occur during perimenopause and continue after menopause. But this weight gain is unrelated to the changes in hormone levels and is most likely part of normal aging.

Many of the symptoms of perimenopause, although disturbing, become less frequent and less intense after menopause. In contrast, the complications of menopause, which result from the decrease in estrogen, are progressive, unless measures to prevent them are taken.

After menopause, the decrease in estrogen causes changes in the reproductive tract over a period of months or years. The lining of the vagina becomes thinner, drier, and less elastic (a condition called vaginal atrophy). These changes may make sexual intercourse painful and may increase the risk of inflammation (vaginitis). Other genital organs—the labia minora, clitoris, uterus, and ovaries—decrease in size. Sex drive (libido) commonly decreases. The effect of menopause on the ability to have an orgasm varies from woman to woman. In many women, the ability is unaffected. It improves in some women but is lost in others.

The lining of the urethra becomes thinner, and the muscles that control the outflow of urine (around the bladder outlet) become weaker. As a result, a burning sensation may occur when urinating, and urinary tract infections may develop more easily. Many postmenopausal women have stress incontinence, in which small amounts of urine escape from the bladder during laughing, coughing, or other activities that put pressure on the bladder. Some women develop urge incontinence, which is an abrupt, intense urge to urinate that cannot be suppressed.

The amount of collagen, a protein that makes skin strong, and elastin, a protein that makes skin elastic, also decrease. Thus, the skin may become thinner, drier, less elastic, and more vulnerable to injury. However, this may be more related to aging than menopause.

The decrease in estrogen often leads to a decrease in bone density and sometimes to osteoporosis, because estrogen helps maintain bone. Bone becomes less dense and weaker, making fractures more likely. During the first 2 years after menopause, bone density decreases by about 3 to 5% each year. After that, it decreases by about 1 to 2% each year.

After menopause, levels of lipids, particularly LDL cholesterol, increase in women; this probably results more from aging itself than from menopause. The increase in lipid levels may partly explain why coronary artery disease becomes more common among women after menopause. Also, until menopause, the high estrogen levels seem to protect against the disease.

Diagnosis

In about three fourths of women, menopause is obvious. If menopause needs to be confirmed (particularly in younger women), blood tests are performed to measure levels of estrogen and follicle-stimulating hormone (which stimulates the ovaries to produce estrogen and progesterone).

Before any treatment is started, doctors ask women about their medical and family history and perform a physical examination, including breast and pelvic examinations and measurement of blood pressure. Mammography is also performed. Blood tests may be performed, and bone density may be measured. The information thus obtained helps doctors determine the woman's risk of developing disorders after menopause. For women with a history of abnormal bleeding from the vagina, an endometrial biopsy (see page 128) may be performed to check for signs of cancer. A small sample of tissue is removed from the lining of the uterus (endometrium) and is examined under a microscope.

Treatment

Not consuming spicy foods, hot beverages, caffeine, and alcohol may help prevent hot flashes, because these substances can trigger hot flashes. Eating foods rich in B vitamins or vitamin E or foods rich in plant estrogens (phytoestrogens), such as tofu, soy milk, tempeh, and miso, may also help. Not smoking, avoiding stress, and exercising regularly may help improve sleep as well as relieve hot flashes. Wearing layers of clothing, which can be taken off when a woman feels hot and put on when she feels cold, can help her cope with hot flashes. Wearing clothing that breathes, such as cotton underwear and sleepwear, may enhance comfort.

Aerobic exercise, relaxation techniques, meditation, massage, and yoga may help relieve depression, irritability, and fatigue. Reducing the number of calories consumed and exercising more can help prevent weight gain. Weight-bearing exercise (such as walking, jogging, and weight lifting) and taking calcium and vitamin D supplements slow the loss of bone density.

Many of these measures—losing weight if needed, stopping smoking, and exercising regularly—plus decreasing the total amount of fat and cholesterol in the diet may be recommended to help lower cholesterol levels and thus reduce the risk of atherosclerosis.

If vaginal dryness makes sexual intercourse painful, an over-the-counter vaginal lubricant may help. Staying sexually active also helps by stimulating blood flow to the vagina and surrounding tissues and by keeping tissues flexible. Kegel exercises may help with bladder control (see page 198). For these exercises, a woman tightens the pelvic muscles as if stopping urine flow.

Hormone Therapy

For women who have a uterus, hormone therapy usually includes a progestin, such as medroxyprogesterone, as well as estrogen. Estrogen plus a progestin is called combination hormone therapy. A progestin is a drug similar to the hormone progesterone.

Doctors first decide whether hormonal therapy should include an estrogen, a progestin, or both. Estrogen used alone increases the risk of cancer of the uterine lining (endometrial cancer). The risk is higher with higher doses and longer use of estrogen. In contrast, taking a progestin with estrogen does not increase the risk of endometrial cancer. Women whose uterus has been removed have no risk of developing this cancer and thus do not need to take a progestin.

Whether to take hormone therapy is a difficult decision that must be made by a woman and her doctor based on the woman's individual situation. For many women, risks outweigh benefits, so this therapy is not a good choice. However, depending on what medical problems and risk factors a woman has, benefits sometimes outweigh risks. Symptoms may be intolerable, and the benefit of hot flash reduction may outweigh the risks.

Estrogen is the most effective treatment for hot flashes. It can prevent the drying and thinning of vaginal and urinary tract tissues, thus improving sexual function and helping prevent infections. Progestins may relieve hot flashes but not vaginal dryness.

Estrogen and progestins, taken individually or as combination therapy, help prevent or slow the progression of bone loss. However, women have the option of using other therapies such as raloxifene or bisphosphonates instead. Taking hormone therapy with the sole purpose of preventing osteoporosis is an option in women who have significant bone loss, cannot tolerate other medications, and understand the risk.

Combination therapy increases the risk of breast cancer, coronary heart disease, stroke, blood clots in the legs and lungs, dementia, and urinary incontinence. Combination therapy lowers the risk of hip fracture and colorectal cancer. Taking estrogen alone does not change the risk of coronary artery disease but increases the risk of stroke and urinary incontinence and decreases the risk of hip fracture. Estrogen alone does not increase the risk of breast cancer and does not decrease the risk of colorectal cancer. The effects of estrogen alone on the risk of blood clots and dementia are less clear.

Risk of all of these disorders with a progestin alone is unknown. Synthetic progestins increase the LDL (the bad) cholesterol level and decrease the HDL (the good) cholesterol level and may increase the risk of atherosclerosis. However, a type of progestin called micronized progesterone appears to have fewer side effects and may not adversely affect cholesterol levels.

Estrogen and progestins, especially at high doses, may cause certain symptoms, including nausea, breast tenderness, headache, fluid retention, and mood changes.

Estrogen and a progestin can be taken in several ways. They may be taken as two tablets or a combination tablet daily. This schedule typically causes irregular vaginal bleeding for the first year or more of therapy. Alternatively, a cyclic monthly schedule may be followed causing monthly vaginal bleeding: Estrogen is taken daily, and a progestin is taken for 12 to 14 days each month.

Other forms include an estrogen or estrogen-progestin skin patch (transdermal estrogen), and estrogen gel or cream. Treatment for only vaginal atrophy comes in multiple forms: An estrogen cream or tablet may be applied to or an estrogen tablet may be inserted into the vagina, or a ring may be inserted into the vagina (similar to a diaphragm). Applied in these ways, estrogen may help prevent thinning and drying of the vaginal lining. Such treatment helps prevent intercourse from being painful. Some of the estrogen cream is absorbed into the bloodstream, particularly as the vaginal lining becomes healthier. Theoretically, the cream form of estrogen, because it enters the bloodstream in much higher amounts than the tablet or ring, can increase the risk of endometrial cancer. Therefore, if women use this form, they should also take a progestin. The vaginal tablet and ring forms (which do not enter the bloodstream in substantial amounts) may be suggested for women who have had breast cancer or a high risk of developing it.

Selective Estrogen Receptor Modulators (SERMs): These drugs function like estrogen in some parts of the body and like an anti-estrogen in other areas. The only SERM currently used to prevent problems related to menopause is raloxifene. Like estrogen, raloxifene helps prevent bone density from decreasing in postmenopausal women and increases the chance of developing blood clots (from 1 to 2 or 3 in 10,000 women). Raloxifene also prevents fractures of the bones in the spine (vertebrae). However, hot flashes worsen in about 1 in 10 women. It also does not appear to increase the risk of endometrial cancer, and it inhibits the growth of breast tissue.

Tamoxifen, another SERM, is used to treat breast cancer and prevent its recurrence and to prevent breast cancer in women who have a high risk of developing it. Raloxifene has recently been shown to be effective for the prevention of breast cancer in high risk postmenopausal women.

Other Drugs: Several other types of drugs can help reduce the severity of some of the symptoms associated with menopause. Clonidine, which is used to treat high blood pressure, can reduce the intensity of hot flashes. An antidepressant, such as fluoxetine, paroxetine, sertraline, or venlafaxine, may relieve hot flashes. Antidepressants may also help relieve depression, anxiety, and irritability. Sleep aids may help relieve insomnia.

Lipid-lowering drugs may be taken to lower cholesterol levels, reducing the risk of atherosclerosis. Bisphosphonates can be taken to reduce the risk of osteoporosis. They increase bone density and are the only drugs proved to reduce the risk of spine and hip fractures.

Testosterone, the main male sex hormone, taken with estrogen is an option for relief of some symptoms of menopause. Taking testosterone may help increase sex drive, increase bone density, improve mood, and increase energy. Testosterone is available as a tablet (combined with estrogen). Testosterone is also available as an injection or a cream, but it's not approved for use in women. Side effects include decreasing the HDL (the good) cholesterol level. When taken in usual doses, testosterone may have some masculinizing effects such as deepening of the voice, hair growth, and liver problems, including cancer.

Some Drugs Used to Treat Symptoms and Complications of Menopause

DRUG	ADVANTAGES	DISADVANTAGES
Female hormones		
Estrogen	Relieves hot flashes, night sweats, and vaginal dryness Helps prevent osteoporosis	Increases the risk of endometrial cancer if not taken with a progestin in women with a uterus Increases the risk of stroke Increases the risk of developing gallstones Increases the risk of urinary incontinence
A progestin, such as medroxy-progesterone	Reduces the risk of endometrial cancer associated with taking estrogen alone May help relieve hot flashes May help prevent osteoporosis	Does not relieve vaginal dryness May increase the risk of atherosclerosis Unknown effects on the risks on coronary artery disease, stroke, blood clots, and breast cancer May have negative effects on cholesterol levels
Combination therapy (estrogen plus a progestin)	Helps relieve hot flashes Decreases risk of osteoporosis and colorectal cancer	Increases risk of coronary artery disease, stroke, breast cancer, blood clots, dementia, and most types of urinary incontinence
Selective estrogen receptor modulators (SERMs)		
Raloxifene	Prevents and treats osteoporosis Does not appear to increase the risk of endometrial cancer Decreases the risk of breast cancer in high risk postmenopausal women	Increases the risk of blood clots May mildly worsen hot flashes Leg cramps

(Continued)

Some Drugs Used to Treat Symptoms and Complications of Menopause (Continued)

DRUG	ADVANTAGES	DISADVANTAGES
Bisphosphonates		
Alendronate Risedronate	Prevents and treats osteoporosis	Must be taken with a glass of water after awakening, followed by 30 minutes without consuming any food, liquid, or drug and without lying down Can irritate the lining of the esophagus if taken improperly
Ibandronate	Prevents osteoporosis	Must be taken with a glass of water after awakening, followed by 30 minutes without consuming any food, liquid, or drug and without lying down Can irritate the lining of the esophagus if taken improperly
Antidepressants		
Selective serotonin reuptake inhibitors (for example, fluoxetine, sertraline, sustained-release paroxetine) and serotonin-norepinephrine reuptake inhibitors (for example, venlafaxine)	Relieve depression, anxiety, irritability, and insomnia May relieve hot flashes	Depending on the drug, can cause side effects, such as sexual dysfunction, nausea, diarrhea, weight loss (short-term), weight gain (long-term), sedation, dry mouth, confusion, increased or decreased blood pressure

Some Drugs Used to Treat Symptoms and Complications of Menopause (Continued)

DRUG	ADVANTAGES	DISADVANTAGES
Lipid-lowering drugs		
Statins (for example, atorvastatin, lovastatin, pravastatin, simvastatin), bile acid binders (for example, cholestyramine, colestipol), fibric acid derivatives (for example, fenofibrate, gemfibrozil), niacin	Prevent atherosclerosis (including coronary artery disease)	Depending on the drug, can cause side effects, such as constipation, loose stools, abdominal pain, nausea, bloating, rash, muscle inflammation, increased levels of liver enzymes, fatigue
One type of antihypertensive drug		
Clonidine	Lessens hot flashes	Can cause side effects, such as drowsiness, dry mouth, fatigue, an abnormally slow heart rate, rebound high blood pressure when the drug is withdrawn, and sexual dysfunction
Male hormone		
Testosterone (used in combination with estrogen)	May increase sex drive and energy. Prevents osteoporosis. Improves mood	Decreases the HDL (good) cholesterol level. May have some masculinizing effects, such as facial hair growth. Has not been studied extensively, so risks are unknown

Alternative Medicine: Some women take medicinal herbs and other supplements to relieve hot flashes, irritability, mood changes, and memory loss. Examples are black cohash, DHEA (dehydro-epiandrosterone), dong quai, evening primrose, ginseng, and St. John's wort. However, such remedies are not regulated. That is, they have not been shown to be safe or effective for this use, and what their ingredients are and how much of each ingredient a product contains are not standardized. Furthermore, some supplements can interact with other drugs and can worsen some disorders. Women who are considering taking such supplements are advised to discuss them with a doctor.

Premature Menopause

Premature menopause (premature ovarian failure) is the permanent end of the cyclic functioning of the ovaries and thus of menstrual periods before age 40.

- Premature menopause is the permanent end of menstrual periods and of fertility before age 40.
- Causes include genetic abnormalities, autoimmune and metabolic disorders, and cancer chemotherapy.
- Symptoms are the same as those of natural menopause, including hot flashes and mood swings.
- Tests are done to identify the cause.
- Various measures, including estrogen (used only for a few years) and other drugs, can relieve or reduce symptoms.
- If pregnancy is desired, having eggs from another woman implanted in the uterus provides the best chance of success.

Hormonally, premature menopause resembles natural menopause. Estrogen levels are low.

Premature menopause may result from genetic abnormalities, including chromosomal abnormalities, or from an autoimmune disorder, in which the body produces abnormal antibodies that attack the body's tissues (including the ovaries). Other possible causes of premature menopause include metabolic disorders and chemotherapy for cancer. Premature menopause has the same symptoms as natural menopause, such as hot flashes and mood swings.

Diagnosis and Treatment

Identifying the cause of premature menopause can help doctors evaluate a woman's health risks and recommend treatment.

For women younger than 30, a chromosome analysis may be performed. If a chromosomal abnormality is detected, additional procedures and treatment may be required.

Estrogen or other therapies used during natural menopause can usually prevent or reverse symptoms. However, a woman with premature menopause has less than a 10% chance of becoming pregnant. She has up to a 50% chance of becoming pregnant by having another woman's eggs (donor eggs) implanted in her uterus after they have been fertilized in the laboratory (see page 62).

CHAPTER 10

Menstrual Disorders and Abnormal Vaginal Bleeding

Complex interactions among hormones control the start of menstruation during puberty, the rhythms and duration of menstrual cycles during the reproductive years, and the end of menstruation at menopause. Hormonal control of menstruation begins in the hypothalamus (the part of the brain that coordinates and controls hormonal activity). The hypothalamus releases gonadotropin-releasing hormone in pulses. This hormone stimulates the pituitary gland to produce two hormones called gonadotropins: luteinizing hormone and follicle-stimulating hormone. These hormones stimulate the ovaries. The ovaries produce the female hormones estrogen and progesterone (see page 111), which ultimately control menstruation. Hormones produced by other glands, such as the adrenal glands and the thyroid gland, can also affect the functioning of the ovaries and menstruation.

Menstrual disorders include premenstrual syndrome, dysmenorrhea, and amenorrhea. Vaginal bleeding may be abnormal during the reproductive years when menstrual periods are too heavy or too light, last too long, occur too often, or are irregular. Any vaginal bleeding that occurs before puberty or after menopause is abnormal until proven otherwise.

Deciphering Medical Terms for Menstrual Disorders

TERM	DESCRIPTION
Amenorrhea	Absence of periods
Dysmenorrhea	Painful periods
Hypomenorrhea	Unusually light periods
Menometrorrhagia	Prolonged bleeding that occurs at irregular intervals
Menorrhagia	Unusually long and heavy periods
Metrorrhagia	Bleeding that occurs at frequent, irregular intervals
Oligomenorrhea	Unusually infrequent periods
Polymenorrhea	Unusually frequent periods
Postmenopausal bleeding	Bleeding that occurs after menopause
Premenstrual syndrome (PMS)	Physical and psychologic symptoms that occur before the start of a period
Primary amenorrhea	No periods ever starting at puberty
Secondary amenorrhea	Periods that have stopped

Premenstrual Syndrome

Premenstrual syndrome (PMS) is a group of physical and psychologic symptoms that occur before a menstrual period begins.

- Many women have physical and psychologic symptoms just before a menstrual period begins.
- Symptoms include aches, bloating, breast fullness and pain, fatigue, skin problems, swelling, weight gain, agitation, depression, and mood swings.
- Reducing salt and caffeine in the diet, exercising, using stress reduction techniques, or taking nonsteroidal anti-inflammatory drugs (NSAIDs) or an oral contraceptive may help relieve symptoms.

Because so many monthly symptoms, such as bad mood, irritability, bloating, and breast tenderness, have been ascribed to PMS, defining and identifying PMS can be difficult. PMS affects 20 to 50% of women. About 5% of women of reproductive age have a severe form of PMS called premenstrual dysphoric disorder.

PMS may occur partly because estrogen and progesterone levels fluctuate during the menstrual cycle. Also, in some women with PMS, progesterone may be broken down differently. Progesterone is usually broken down into two components that have opposite effects on mood. Women with PMS may produce less of the component that tends to reduce anxiety and more of the component that tends to increase anxiety.

DID YOU KNOW?

- Many women, particularly teenagers, who have premenstrual syndrome (PMS) also have painful periods.
- Other disorders that a woman has may worsen when PMS symptoms occur.
- Calcium and magnesium have each been shown to be effective in the treatment of PMS.
- Taking vitamin B_6 in high doses for PMS can cause nerve damage.

Symptoms and Diagnosis

The type and intensity of symptoms vary from woman to woman and from month to month in the same woman. The various physical and psychologic symptoms of PMS can temporarily upset a woman's life.

Symptoms may begin a few hours up to about 14 days before a menstrual period, and they usually disappear completely after the period begins. Women who are approaching menopause may have symptoms that persist through and after the menstrual period. The symptoms of PMS are often followed each month by a painful period (dysmenorrhea), particularly in teenagers.

Other disorders may worsen while PMS symptoms are occurring. Women who have a seizure disorder may have more seizures than usual. Women who have a connective tissue disease, such as lupus or rheumatoid arthritis, may have flare-ups. Respiratory disorders (such as allergies and congestion of the nose and airways) and eye disorders (such as conjunctivitis) may worsen.

In premenstrual dysphoric disorder, premenstrual symptoms are so severe that they interfere with work, social activities, and relationships.

The diagnosis is based on symptoms. To identify it, doctors ask a woman to keep a daily record of her symptoms. This record helps the woman be aware of changes in her body and moods and helps doctors determine what treatment is best. Premenstrual dysphoric disorder cannot be diagnosed until a woman has recorded her symptoms for at least two menstrual cycles. Doctors can distinguish premenstrual syndrome and premenstrual dysphoric disorder from mood disorders, such as depression, because the symptoms disappear soon after the menstrual period begins.

SYMPTOMS OF PREMENSTRUAL SYNDROME

Physical

- Awareness of heartbeats (palpitations)
- Backache
- Bloating
- Breast fullness and pain
- Changes in appetite and cravings for certain foods
- Constipation
- Cramps, heaviness, or pressure in the lower abdomen
- Dizziness
- Easy bruising
- Fainting
- Fatigue
- Headaches
- Hot flashes
- Insomnia, including difficulty falling or staying asleep at night
- Joint and muscle pain
- Lack of energy
- Nausea and vomiting

(Continued)

SYMPTOMS OF PREMENSTRUAL SYNDROME (Continued)

- Pins-and-needles sensations in the hands and feet
- Skin problems, such as acne and localized scratch dermatitis
- Swelling of hands and feet
- Weight gain

Psychologic

- Agitation
- Confusion
- Crying spells
- Depression
- Difficulty concentrating
- Emotional hypersensitivity
- Forgetfulness or memory loss
- Irritability
- Mood swings
- Nervousness
- Short temper
- Social withdrawal

Treatment

Treatment involves relieving symptoms. Reducing the intake of salt often reduces fluid retention and relieves bloating. Diuretics (which help the kidneys eliminate salt and water from the body) may be prescribed to help reduce the buildup of fluid. For most women who have mild to moderate symptoms, exercise and stress reduction techniques (meditation or relaxation exercises) help relieve nervousness and agitation. Reducing the consumption of beverages and foods containing caffeine (including chocolate) may also help. Taking calcium supplements (1,000 milligrams a day) lessens the physical and emotional symptoms of PMS. There are claims that other supplements such as magnesium and the B vitamins, especially B_6 (pyridoxine), taken daily, lessen symptoms. However, the usefulness of these supplements has not been confirmed. Taking vitamin B_6 in high doses may be harmful. Nerve damage has been reported with as little as 100 milligrams a day.

Taking nonsteroidal anti-inflammatory drugs (NSAIDs) may help relieve headaches, pain due to abdominal cramps, and joint pain. Taking combination oral contraceptives (birth control pills that contain estrogen and a progestin) reduces pain, breast tenderness, and changes in appetite in some women but worsens these symptoms in a few. Taking oral contraceptives that contain only a progestin does not help.

Women who have more severe symptoms may benefit from taking fluoxetine, paroxetine, or sertraline, which are antidepressants. They are most effective for reducing irritability, depression, and some of the other psychologic and physical symptoms of PMS. Buspirone or alprazolam (both antianxiety drugs) may reduce irritability and nervousness and help reduce stress. However, taking alprazolam can result in drug dependency. Doctors may ask a woman to continue keeping a record of her symptoms so that they can judge the effectiveness of treatment.

Women who have premenstrual dysphoric disorder may benefit from taking antidepressants. Taking a gonadotropin-releasing hormone (GnRH) agonist (such as leuprolide or goserelin—see page 170), given by injection, plus estrogen, given in a low dose by mouth or patch, may control symptoms. GnRH agonists cause the body to produce less estrogen and progesterone.

Dysmenorrhea

Dysmenorrhea is pelvic pain during a menstrual period.

- The cause is often unknown.
- The pain is often accompanied by bloating, headache, nausea, constipation, and diarrhea.
- Doctors may do tests to look for endometriosis, fibroids, or other possible causes.
- Nonsteroidal anti-inflammatory drugs (NSAIDs) or sometimes low-dose oral contraceptives can relieve pain.

About three fourths of women with dysmenorrhea have primary dysmenorrhea, for which no cause can be identified. The rest have secondary dysmenorrhea, for which a cause is identified.

Primary dysmenorrhea may affect more than 50% of women, usually starting during adolescence. In about 5 to 15%, primary dysmenorrhea is sometimes severe, interfering with daily activities and resulting in absence from school or work. Primary dysmenorrhea may become less severe with age and after pregnancy.

In primary dysmenorrhea, the pain occurs only during menstrual cycles in which an egg is released. The pain is thought to result from prostaglandins released during menstruation. Prostaglandins are hormonelike substances that cause the uterus to contract, reduce the blood supply to the uterus, and increase the sensitivity of nerve endings in the uterus to pain. Women who have primary dysmenorrhea have higher levels of prostaglandins.

DID YOU KNOW?

- More than half of women sometimes have painful periods.
- Taking nonsteroidal anti-inflammatory drugs (NSAIDs) 1 or 2 days before a period begins may relieve pain better than taking them after a period begins.

Common causes of secondary dysmenorrhea include endometriosis, fibroids, adenomyosis, pelvic congestion syndrome, and pelvic infection. In a few women, the pain results from passage of menstrual blood through a narrow cervix (cervical stenosis). A narrow cervix may be present at birth or result from removal of polyps or treatment of a precancerous condition (dysplasia) or cancer of the cervix. Abdominal pain due to other disorders, such as inflammation of the fallopian tubes or abnormal bands of fibrous tissue (adhesions) between structures in the abdomen, may be worse during a menstrual period.

Symptoms and Diagnosis

Pain occurs in the lower abdomen and may extend to the lower back or legs. The pain is usually crampy and comes and goes, but it may be a dull, constant ache. Usually, the pain starts shortly before or during the menstrual period, peaks after 24 hours, and subsides after 2 days. Other common symptoms include headache, nausea, constipation, diarrhea, and an urge to urinate frequently. Occasionally, vomiting occurs. Premenstrual irritability,

ADENOMYOSIS: NONCANCEROUS GROWTH OF THE UTERUS

In adenomyosis, glandular tissue from the lining of the uterus (endometrium) grows into the muscular wall of the uterus. The uterus becomes enlarged, sometimes doubling or tripling in size. This common disorder causes symptoms in only a small percentage of women, usually between the ages of 35 and 50. It is-more common among women who have had children. The cause is unknown.

Symptoms include heavy and painful periods, bleeding between periods, vague pain in the pelvic area, and a feeling of pressure on the bladder and rectum. Sometimes sexual intercourse is painful.

Doctors suspect adenomyosis when they perform a pelvic examination and discover that the uterus is enlarged, round, and softer than normal. Pelvic ultrasound or magnetic resonance imaging (MRI) helps confirm the diagnosis. Sometimes when adenomyosis causes abnormal bleeding, a biopsy is performed. Usually, no treatment is effective, although oral contraceptives and gonadotropin-releasing hormone agonists (such as leuprolide or goserelin) may be tried. Analgesics may be taken for pain. In some cases, a hysterectomy may be performed.

nervousness, depression, and abdominal bloating may persist during part or all of the menstrual period.

Diagnosis is based on symptoms and the results of a physical examination. To identify possible causes (such as fibroids), doctors may examine the abdominal cavity using a viewing tube (laparoscope) inserted through a small incision just below the navel. They may examine the interior of the uterus using a similar tube (hysteroscope) inserted through the vagina and cervix. Other procedures may include dilation and curettage (D and C) and hysterosalpingography (see page 129 and page 131).

Treatment

Nonsteroidal anti-inflammatory drugs (NSAIDs) usually relieve pain effectively. NSAIDs may be more effective if started 1 or 2 days before a menstrual period begins and continued for 1 or 2 days after it begins. An antiemetic drug may relieve nausea and vomiting, but these symptoms usually disappear without treatment as the pain subsides. Getting enough rest and sleep and exercising regularly may also help relieve symptoms.

If the pain continues to interfere with daily activities, oral contraceptives that contain estrogen in a low dose plus a progestin may be prescribed to suppress the release of eggs from the ovaries (ovulation). If these treatments are ineffective, procedures to identify the cause of the pain may be performed.

When dysmenorrhea results from another disorder, that disorder is treated if possible. A narrow cervical canal can be widened surgically. However, this operation usually relieves the pain only temporarily. If needed, fibroids or misplaced endometrial tissue (due to endometriosis) is surgically removed.

When other treatments are ineffective and the pain is severe, the nerves to the uterus may be cut surgically. However, this operation occasionally injures other pelvic organs, such as the ureters. Alternatively, hypnosis or acupuncture may be tried.

WHAT IS PELVIC CONGESTION SYNDROME?

Sometimes pain that occurs before or during menstrual periods results from a problem with veins in the pelvis. The veins may widen and become convoluted and blood accumulates in them. The result is varicose veins in the pelvis—a disorder called pelvic congestion syndrome. Pain, sometimes debilitating, can result. Estrogen may contribute because it causes some veins supplying the ovaries and uterus to widen. Up to 15% of women of reproductive age have varicose veins in their pelvis, but not all of them have symptoms.

Typically, the pain is dull and aching, but it may be sharp or throbbing. It is worse at the end of the day (after a woman has been sitting or standing a long time) and is relieved when she lies down. The pain is also worse during or after sexual intercourse. It is often accompanied by low back pain, aches in the legs, abnormal menstrual bleeding, and a vaginal discharge. Occasionally, fatigue, mood swings, headache, and abdominal bloating occur.

Doctors may suspect pelvic congestion syndrome when a woman has pelvic pain but a pelvic examination does not detect inflammation or another abnormality. Ultrasonography can help doctors confirm the diagnosis. Alternatively, the veins can be viewed with a viewing tube inserted through a small incision just below the navel in a procedure called laparoscopy. Nonsteroidal anti-inflammatory drugs (NSAIDs) usually relieve the pain.

Amenorrhea

Amenorrhea is the absence of menstrual periods.

- Menstrual periods may never start or may start, then stop.
- Amenorrhea may be caused by birth defects, chromosomal disorders, malfunction of the brain or glands, tumors, autoimmune or hormonal disorders, drugs, or stress.
- A physical examination and various tests are done to try to determine the cause.
- The underlying disorder is treated if possible.

Some women never go through puberty, so periods never start. This disorder is called primary amenorrhea. In other women, periods start at puberty, then stop. This disorder is called secondary amenorrhea. Amenorrhea is normal only before puberty, during pregnancy, while breastfeeding, and after menopause.

Causes

Primary amenorrhea may be caused by a birth defect in which the uterus or fallopian tubes do not develop normally or by a chromosomal disorder, such as Turner syndrome (in which the cells contain one X chromosome instead of the usual two). Primary amenorrhea can also result from malfunction of the hypothalamus (a part of the brain), pituitary gland, or ovaries. Sometimes it results from malfunction of the thyroid gland (hyperthyroidism or hypothyroidism). Young women who are very thin, particularly those who have anorexia nervosa, may never menstruate.

Secondary amenorrhea can result from malfunction of the hypothalamus, pituitary gland, ovaries, thyroid gland, adrenal glands, or almost any part of the reproductive tract. Malfunction of these organs may result from a tumor, an autoimmune disorder, or use of certain drugs (including hallucinogenic drugs, chemotherapy drugs, antipsychotic drugs, and antidepressants). Cushing's syndrome and polycystic ovary syndrome (both of which involve hormonal abnormalities) may cause periods to stop or to be irregular. Other causes of secondary amenorrhea include a hydatidiform mole (a tumor that develops from an abnormal fertilized egg or the placenta) and Asherman's syndrome (scarring of the lining of the uterus resulting from an infection or surgery).

DID YOU KNOW?

• Experiencing excessive stress, exercising too much, or eating too little may cause periods to stop.

Stress due to internal or situational concerns can cause secondary amenorrhea, because stress interferes with the brain's control (through hormones) of the ovaries. Exercising too much or eating too little (as in anorexia nervosa) also affects the brain's control of the ovaries. Either behavior can cause the brain to signal the pituitary gland to decrease its production of the hormones that stimulate the ovaries. As a result, the ovaries produce less estrogen and periods stop.

Symptoms and Diagnosis

Amenorrhea may or may not be accompanied by other symptoms, depending on the cause.

Primary amenorrhea is diagnosed when periods have not started by age 16. Girls who have no signs of puberty by age 13 or who have not started having periods within 5 years of starting puberty are evaluated for possible problems.

Secondary amenorrhea is diagnosed when a woman of reproductive age (who is not pregnant or breastfeeding) has had no menstrual periods for at least 3 months. A physical examination can help doctors determine whether puberty occurred normally and may provide evidence of the cause of amenorrhea. But other procedures may be needed to confirm or identify the cause. Hormone levels in the blood may be measured. X-rays of the skull may be taken to look for a pituitary tumor. Computed tomography (CT), magnetic resonance imaging (MRI), or ultrasonography may be used to look for a tumor in the ovaries or adrenal glands.

Treatment

The underlying disorder is treated if possible. For example, a tumor is removed. Some disorders, such as Turner syndrome and other genetic disorders, cannot be cured.

If a girl's periods have never started and all test results are normal, she is examined every 3 to 6 months to monitor the progression of puberty. A progestin and sometimes estrogen may be given to start her periods and to stimulate the development of secondary sexual characteristics, such as breasts.

Abnormal Vaginal Bleeding

- Vaginal bleeding is abnormal when menstrual periods are too heavy or too light, last too long, occur too frequently, or are irregular or when bleeding occurs before puberty, during pregnancy, or after menopause.
- Causes vary and include hormonal imbalances, use of oral contraceptives, tumors, and injuries.
- Symptoms and results of a physical examination may suggest the cause, but tests may be needed to confirm it.
- Treatment depends on the cause.

During the reproductive years, bleeding from the vagina may be abnormal when menstrual periods are too heavy or too light, last too long, occur too frequently, or are irregular. Any vaginal bleeding that occurs before puberty or after menopause is abnormal. Bleeding from the vagina may originate in the vagina or other reproductive organs, particularly the uterus.

Many disorders, including inflammation, infection, and cancer, can cause bleeding from the vagina. Injuries, including that due to sexual abuse, can also cause bleeding. The cause may be hormonal changes, resulting in a type of bleeding called dysfunctional uterine bleeding. Some causes are more common among certain age groups.

In children, vaginal bleeding is rare and should be evaluated by a doctor. The most common cause is injury to the vulva or vagina (sometimes due to insertion of an object, such as a toy). Vaginal bleeding may also result from prolapse of the urethra (in which the urethra bulges outside of the body) or tumors of the reproductive tract. Tumors of the ovaries usually cause bleeding only if they produce hormones. Bleeding may also be caused by vaginal adenosis (overgrowth of glandular tissue in the vagina). Having vaginal adenosis increases the risk of developing clear cell adenocarcinoma (a cancer of the cervix and vagina) later in life.

Bleeding in children may also result from puberty that starts very early (precocious puberty. This cause can be easily recognized because pubic hair and breasts also develop.

In women of reproductive age, abnormal bleeding may be caused by birth control methods, such as oral contraceptives (a combination of a progestin and estrogen or a progestin alone) or an intrauterine device (IUD). Abnormal bleeding may also be caused by complications of pregnancy, such as an ectopic pregnancy, or by infections of the uterus, usually after delivery of a baby or an abortion.

DID YOU KNOW?

- Any bleeding that occurs before puberty or after menopause should be evaluated.
- An imbalance in female hormones is a common cause of abnormal bleeding from the vagina.

Other causes of bleeding include blood disorders involving abnormal clotting (such as leukemia or a low platelet count), a hydatidiform mole, endometriosis, and noncancerous growths (such as adenomyosis, fibroids, cysts, and polyps). Cancer may cause bleeding in women of reproductive age, but not commonly. Bleeding from the vulva is usually due to injury. Thyroid disorders can cause menstrual periods to be irregular, to be heavy and occur more frequently, or to occur less frequently (as well as to stop).

In postmenopausal women, bleeding from the vagina may be due to thinning of the lining of the vagina (atrophic vaginitis), thinning or thickening (hyperplasia) of the lining of the uterus, or polyps in the uterus. Cancer, such as cancer of the cervix, vagina, or lining of the uterus (endometrial cancer) can also cause bleeding.

Diagnosis and Treatment

The cause of abnormal bleeding may be suggested by symptoms and the results of a physical examination (including a pelvic examination). But additional procedures may be needed. If doctors suspect vaginal adenosis, a biopsy of the vagina is performed. Usually, women who have abnormal bleeding from the vagina, particularly after menopause, are evaluated to determine whether they have cancer of the vagina, cervix, or lining of the uterus (see page 236). Procedures may include a Papanicolaou (Pap) test, a biopsy of the cervix, and dilation and curettage (D and C). Ultrasonography using an ultrasound device inserted through the vagina into the uterus (transvaginal ultrasonography) can determine whether the uterine lining is thickened. A biopsy of cells obtained during dilation and curettage can determine if the thickening is due to cancer.

Treatment varies, depending on the cause. Usually, a girl who has vaginal adenosis does not need to be treated unless cancer is detected. However, she is reexamined at regular intervals for signs of cancer. Uterine polyps, fibroids, and cancers may be surgically removed.

Dysfunctional Uterine Bleeding

Dysfunctional uterine bleeding is abnormal bleeding resulting from changes in the normal hormonal control of menstruation.

- Dysfunctional uterine bleeding is irregular, prolonged, and sometimes heavy bleeding.
- It is due to changes in the normal hormonal control of menstruation.
- This type of bleeding usually occurs in adolescent girls, women older than 45, or women with polycystic ovary syndrome.
- Doctors identify it by doing tests to exclude other possible causes.
- Oral contraceptives, estrogen (sometimes with a progestin), or clomiphene (if pregnancy is desired) may correct the abnormal bleeding.

Dysfunctional uterine bleeding occurs most commonly at the beginning and end of the reproductive years: 20% of cases occur in adolescent girls, and more than 50% occur in women older than 45.

Dysfunctional uterine bleeding commonly results when the level of estrogen remains high. The high level of estrogen is not balanced by an appropriate level of progesterone, and release of an egg (ovulation) does not occur. As a result, the lining of the

uterus (endometrium) thickens. This condition is called endometrial hyperplasia. The lining is then shed incompletely and irregularly, causing bleeding. Bleeding is irregular, prolonged, and
sometimes heavy. This type of bleeding is common among women
who have polycystic ovary syndrome.

Diagnosis and Treatment

Dysfunctional uterine bleeding is diagnosed when all other
possible causes of vaginal bleeding have been excluded. The
results of a blood test can help doctors estimate the extent of the
blood loss. Transvaginal ultrasonography may be used to determine whether the uterine lining is thickened. If the risk of cancer
of the uterine lining (endometrial cancer) is high, an endometrial
biopsy is performed before drug treatment is started. Women at
risk include those who are 35 or older, those who are substantially
overweight, and those who have polycystic ovary syndrome, high
blood pressure, or diabetes.

Treatment depends on how old the woman is, how heavy the
bleeding is, whether the uterine lining is thickened, and whether
the woman wishes to become pregnant.

When the uterine lining is thickened but its cells are normal,
hormones may be used. Women who have heavy bleeding may be
treated with an oral contraceptive containing estrogen and a
progestin. When bleeding is very heavy, estrogen may be given
intravenously until the bleeding stops. Sometimes a progestin is
given by mouth at the same time or started 2 or 3 days later.
Bleeding usually stops in 12 to 24 hours. Low doses of the oral
contraceptive may then be prescribed for at least 3 months.

Treatment with an oral contraceptive or estrogen given intravenously is inappropriate for some women (such as postmenopausal women and women with significant risk factors for heart or
blood vessel disease). These women may be given a progestin
alone by mouth for 10 to 14 days each month. For women who
wish to become pregnant, clomiphene may be given by mouth
instead. It stimulates ovulation.

If the uterine lining remains thickened or the bleeding persists
despite treatment with hormones, dilation and curettage (D and C)
is usually needed. In this procedure, tissue from the uterine lining
is removed by scraping. When the uterine lining is thickened and

contains abnormal cells (particularly in women who are older than 35 and do not want to become pregnant), treatment begins with a high dose of a progestin. If the cells continue to be abnormal after treatment, a hysterectomy is performed, because the abnormal cells may become cancerous.

Polycystic Ovary Syndrome

Polycystic ovary syndrome (Stein-Leventhal syndrome) involves enlarged ovaries, which contain many fluid-filled sacs (cysts), and a tendency to have high levels of male hormones (androgens).

- Levels of male hormones (androgens) are abnormally high, sometimes causing deepening of a woman's voice, decreased breast size, increased muscle size, increased body hair, weight gain, and irregular periods.
- The risk of cancer of the uterine lining (endometrial cancer) may be increased.
- Blood tests and sometimes ultrasonography of the ovaries can confirm the diagnosis.
- Losing weight and taking a progestin or oral contraceptive may help reduce body hair, normalize periods, and decrease the risk of endometrial cancer.

Polycystic ovary syndrome affects about 7 to 10% of women. A common cause is excess production of luteinizing hormone by the pituitary gland. The excess luteinizing hormone increases the production of male hormones (androgens). If the disorder is not treated, some of the male hormones may be converted to estrogen. Not enough progesterone is produced to balance the estrogen's effects. If this situation continues a long time, the lining of the uterus (endometrium) may become extremely thickened (a condition called endometrial hyperplasia). Also, the risk of cancer of the lining of the uterus (endometrial cancer) may be increased.

Symptoms and Diagnosis

Symptoms typically develop during puberty. In some women, menstrual periods do not start at puberty. Thus, these women do not release an egg from the ovaries (ovulate). These women also develop symptoms related to the high levels of male hormones—a process called masculinization or virilization. Symptoms include acne, a deepened voice, a decrease in breast size, and an increase in muscle size and in body hair (hirsutism) growing in a male pattern, such as on the chest and face. Many women with polycystic ovary syndrome produce too much insulin, or the insulin they produce does not function normally. Consequently, these women tend to gain weight or have a hard time losing weight. Most women are obese. Other women have irregular vaginal bleeding, with no increase in weight or body hair. Women with polycystic ovary syndrome also have an increased risk of heart disease, diabetes, and high blood pressure.

Often, the diagnosis is based on symptoms. Blood tests to measure levels of luteinizing hormone and male hormones are performed, and ultrasonography of the ovaries may be performed. Ultrasonography or computed tomography (CT) may be used to determine whether the male hormones are being produced by a tumor in an ovary or adrenal gland.

DID YOU KNOW?

* As many as 10% of women have polycystic ovary syndrome, which can cause women to develop masculine traits (such as a deepened voice and increased muscle tissue) and gain weight.

Treatment

No ideal treatment is available. The choice of treatment depends on the type and severity of symptoms, the woman's age, and her plans regarding pregnancy. Often, a biopsy of the uterine lining is performed to make sure no cancer is present.

If insulin levels are high, lowering them may help. Exercising (at least 30 minutes a day) and reducing consumption of carbohydrates (found in breads, pasta, potatoes, and sweets) can help lower insulin levels. In some women, weight loss lowers insulin levels enough that ovulation can begin. Weight loss may help reduce hair growth and the risk of thickening of the uterine lining.

Women who do not wish to become pregnant may take a progestin by mouth or a combination oral contraceptive (which contains estrogen and a progestin). Either treatment may reduce the risk of cancer of the uterine lining due to the high estrogen level and help lower the levels of male hormones. However, oral contraceptives are not given to women who have reached menopause or who have other significant risk factors for heart or blood vessel disorders.

Women who wish to become pregnant may take clomiphene. This drug stimulates ovulation. If clomiphene is not effective, other hormones may be tried. They include follicle-stimulating hormone (to stimulate the ovaries), a gonadotropin-releasing hormone agonist (to stimulate the release of follicle-stimulating hormone), and human chorionic gonadotropin (to trigger ovulation).

Increased body hair can be bleached or removed by electrolysis, plucking, waxing, hair-removing liquids or creams (depilatories), or laser. No drug treatment for removing excess hair is ideal or completely effective. Oral contraceptives may help, but they must be taken for several months before any effect, which is often slight, can be seen. Spironolactone, a drug that blocks the production and action of male hormones, can reduce unwanted body hair. Side effects include increased urine production and low blood pressure (sometimes causing fainting). Spironolactone may not be safe for a developing fetus, so sexually active women taking the drug are advised to use effective birth control methods. Cyproterone, a strong progestin that blocks the action of male hormones, reduces unwanted body hair in 50 to 75% of affected women. It is used in many countries but is not approved in the United States. Gonadotropin-releasing hormone agonists and antagonists are being studied as treatment for unwanted body hair. Both types of drugs inhibit the production of sex hormones by the ovaries. But both can cause bone loss and lead to osteoporosis.

CHAPTER 11

Endometriosis

Endometriosis is a noncancerous disorder in which pieces of endometrial tissue—normally occurring only in the lining of the uterus (endometrium)—grow outside the uterus.

- Pain occurs in the lower abdomen and pelvis, sometimes with spotting or heavy menstrual bleeding.
- The only way to confirm the diagnosis is by viewing the tissue through a laparoscope.
- Oral contraceptives, progestins, danazol, or gonadotropin-releasing hormone agonists may relieve symptoms, but surgery to remove the endometriosis tissue may also be needed.
- Endometriosis tends to recur.

Endometriosis is a chronic disorder that may be painful. Exactly how many women have endometriosis is unknown because it can usually be diagnosed only by directly viewing the endometrial tissue (which requires a surgical procedure). Endometriosis probably affects about 10 to 15% of menstruating women aged 25 to 44. It can also affect teenagers.

Endometriosis sometimes runs in families. It is more likely to occur in women who have their first baby after age 30, who have never had a baby, who are of Asian descent, or who have structural abnormalities of the uterus.

The cause of endometriosis is unclear, but there are several theories: Small pieces of the uterine lining that are shed during

Endometriosis: Misplaced Tissue

In endometriosis, small or large patches of tissue that usually occurs only in the lining of the uterus (endometrium) appear in other parts of the body. How and why the tissue appears in other locations is unclear. The misplaced endometrial tissue may adhere to the ovaries, the ligaments supporting the uterus, the small and large intestines, the ureters, the bladder, the vagina, surgical scars, or the lining of the chest cavity. The misplaced endometrial tissue can irritate nearby tissues, causing large bands of scar tissue (adhesions) to form between structures in the abdomen.

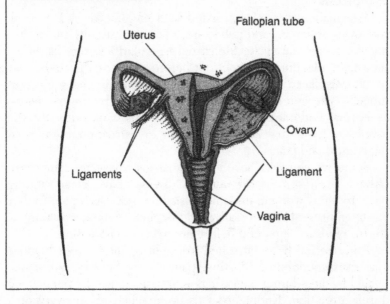

menstruation may flow backward through the fallopian tubes toward the ovaries into the abdominal cavity, rather than flow through the vagina and out of the body with the menstrual period. Cells from the uterine lining (endometrial cells) may be transported through the blood or lymphatic vessels to another location. Or cells located outside the uterus may change into endometrial cells.

Common locations of misplaced endometrial tissue are the ovaries and the ligaments that support the uterus. Less common locations are the outer surface of the small and large intestines, the ureters (tubes leading from the kidneys to the bladder), the bladder, the vagina, and surgical scars in the abdomen. Rarely, endometrial tissue grows on the membranes covering the lungs (pleura), the sac that envelops the heart (pericardium), the vulva, or the cervix.

As the disorder progresses, the misplaced endometrial tissue tends to gradually increase in size. It may also spread to new locations.

Symptoms

The main symptom associated with endometriosis is pain in the lower abdomen and pelvic area. The pain usually varies during the menstrual cycle. Menstrual irregularities, such as heavy menstrual bleeding and spotting before menstrual periods, may occur. Misplaced endometrial tissue responds to the same hormones—estrogen and progesterone (produced by the ovaries)—as normal endometrial tissue in the uterus. Consequently, the misplaced tissue may also bleed during menstruation, often causing cramps and pain.

Some women with severe endometriosis have no symptoms. Others, even some with minimal disease, have incapacitating pain. In many women, endometriosis does not cause pain until it has been present for several years. For such women, sexual intercourse tends to be painful before or during menstruation.

Endometrial tissue attached to the large intestine or bladder may cause abdominal bloating, pain during bowel movements, rectal bleeding during menstruation, or pain above the pubic bone during urination. Endometrial tissue attached to an ovary or a nearby structure can form a blood-filled mass (endometrioma). Occasionally, an endometrioma ruptures or leaks, causing sudden, sharp abdominal pain.

The misplaced endometrial tissue may irritate nearby tissues. As a result, scar tissue may form, sometimes as bands of fibrous tissue (adhesions) between structures in the abdomen. The misplaced endometrial tissue and adhesions can interfere with the functioning of organs. Rarely, adhesions block the intestine.

Severe endometriosis may block the egg's passage from the ovary into the uterus, causing infertility. Mild endometriosis may also cause infertility, but how it does so is less clear. Endometriosis affects as many as 25 to 50% of infertile women.

DID YOU KNOW?

- About 7 to 10% of women and as many as 25 to 50% of infertile women have endometriosis.
- A third of women with chronic pelvic pain have endometriosis.
- Severe endometriosis may cause no symptoms, and mild endometriosis may cause incapacitating symptoms.

Diagnosis

A doctor may suspect endometriosis in a woman who has certain symptoms or unexplained infertility. Occasionally, during a pelvic examination, a woman may feel pain or tenderness or a doctor may feel a mass of tissue behind the uterus or near the ovaries.

However, the diagnosis can usually be confirmed only if a doctor examines the abdominal cavity and sees pieces of endometrial tissue. For this examination, a viewing tube (laparoscope) is usually used. It is inserted into the abdominal cavity through a small incision just below the navel. Carbon dioxide gas is injected into the abdominal cavity to distend it so that organs can be viewed more easily. Laparoscopy usually requires a general anesthetic, so that the entire abdominal cavity can be examined. An overnight stay in the hospital is not required. Laparoscopy may cause mild abdominal discomfort, but normal activities can usually be resumed in 1 or 2 days.

Sometimes a biopsy is necessary. A small sample of tissue is removed, usually through the laparoscope, and examined under a microscope.

Other procedures, such as ultrasonography, barium enemas with x-ray, computed tomography (CT), and magnetic resonance imaging (MRI), may be used to determine the extent of endometriosis and follow its course, but their usefulness for diagnosis is limited. Blood tests may be performed to measure levels of substances (called markers) that increase when endometriosis is present. Markers include cancer antigen 125 and antibodies to endometrial tissue. Such measurements may help a doctor follow the course of endometriosis. However, because these markers may be increased in several other disorders, they are not useful in establishing the diagnosis. Tests may also be performed to determine whether the endometriosis is affecting the woman's fertility (see page 60).

Treatment

Treatment depends on a woman's symptoms, pregnancy plans, and age, as well as the extent of endometriosis.

Drugs can be given to suppress the activity of the ovaries and thus slow the growth of the misplaced endometrial tissue and reduce bleeding and pain. However, these drugs do not eliminate endometriosis. They include combination oral contraceptives (estrogen plus a progestin), progestins (such as medroxyprogesterone), danazol (a synthetic hormone related to testosterone), and gonadotropin-releasing hormone agonists (GnRH agonists—such as buserelin, goserelin, leuprolide, and nafarelin). GnRH agonists turn off the brain's signal to the ovaries to produce estrogen and progesterone. As a result, production of these hormones decreases. Continued use of GnRH agonists causes a decrease in bone density and may lead to osteoporosis unless small doses of estrogen plus a progestin or of a progestin alone are also taken. Even when taken this way, GnRH agonists are not usually given for longer than 1 year. New types of drugs, such as GnRH antagonists, antiprogestins, and aromatase inhibitors, are being studied for the treatment of endometriosis.

Nonsteroidal anti-inflammatory drugs (NSAIDs) may be given to relieve pain. For persistent pain, options include surgery to remove the misplaced endometrial tissue, surgery to interrupt the nerve pathways that conduct pain sensation from the pelvic area to the brain, and surgery to do both.

Often, misplaced endometrial tissue can be removed during laparoscopy when the diagnosis is made. However, if endometriosis is moderate to severe, more extensive surgery requiring an incision into the abdomen (abdominal surgery) may be necessary. This type of surgery is usually necessary when pieces of endometrial tissue are larger than 1½ to 2 inches in diameter, when adhesions in the lower abdomen or pelvis cause significant symptoms, when endometrial tissue blocks one or both fallopian tubes, or when drugs cannot relieve severe lower abdominal or pelvic pain.

Sometimes electrocautery (a device that uses an electrical current to produce heat), an ultrasound device, or a laser (which concentrates light into an intense beam to produce heat) is used to destroy or remove endometrial tissue during laparoscopic or abdominal surgery. Doctors remove as much misplaced endometrial tissue as possible without damaging the ovaries. Thus, the woman's ability to have children may be preserved. Depending on the extent of the endometriosis, 40 to 70% of women who have surgery may become pregnant.

Surgical removal of misplaced endometrial tissue is only a temporary measure. After treatment, endometriosis recurs in most women, although the use of oral contraceptives or other drugs may slow its progression. The drugs used to suppress endometriosis may be started immediately after surgery.

Some women who have endometriosis can become pregnant through the use of assisted reproductive techniques, such as in vitro fertilization (see page 62).

Both ovaries and the uterus are removed only when drugs do not relieve abdominal or pelvic pain and the woman does not plan to become pregnant. Because removal of the ovaries and uterus has the same effects as menopause (effects that result from the decrease in estrogen levels—see page 133), estrogen therapy may

Drugs Commonly Used to Treat Endometriosis

DRUG	SOME SIDE EFFECTS AND COMPLICATIONS	COMMENTS
Combination estrogen-progestin oral contraceptives	Abdominal bloating, breast tenderness, increased appetite, ankle swelling, nausea, bleeding between periods, and deep vein thrombosis	Oral contraceptives may be useful for women who wish to delay childbearing. They may be taken cyclically or continuously.
Progestins	Bleeding between periods, mood swings, depression, and atrophic vaginitis	Progestins are drugs similar to the hormone progesterone. They can be given by mouth or by injection into a muscle.

(Continued)

Drugs Commonly Used to Treat Endometriosis (Continued)

DRUG	SOME SIDE EFFECTS AND COMPLICATIONS	COMMENTS
Danazol	Weight gain, acne, a lowered voice, an increase in body hair, hot flashes, vaginal dryness, ankle swelling, muscle cramps, bleeding between periods, decreased breast size, mood swings, liver malfunction, carpal tunnel syndrome, and adverse effects on cholesterol levels in the blood	Danazol, a synthetic hormone related to testosterone, inhibits the activity of estrogen and progesterone. It is given by mouth. The usefulness of danazol may be limited by its side effects.
GnRH agonists	Hot flashes, vaginal dryness, a decrease in bone density, and mood swings	GnRH agonists may be injected into a muscle once a month, used as a nasal spray, or implanted as a pellet under the skin. These drugs are often given with estrogen, a progestin, or both to reduce the side effects of a decrease in estrogen levels, including decreased bone density. (This use of estrogen and a progestin or of a progestin alone is called add-back therapy.)

GnRH = gonadotropin-releasing hormone.

be started. Some experts recommend the use of estrogen plus a progestin (because a progestin can suppress the growth of endometriosis). When estrogen is given alone, it may be started after a delay of 4 to 6 months after surgery, because estrogen may stimulate any remaining pieces of endometrial tissue. The delay gives the endometrial tissue time to disappear.

CHAPTER 12

Fibroids

A fibroid is a noncancerous tumor composed of muscle and fibrous tissue.

- Fibroids may cause no symptoms or cause pain, pressure, or a feeling of heaviness in the pelvic area or heavy menstrual bleeding.
- Fibroids may be diagnosed during a pelvic examination.
- Oral contraceptives or gonadotropin-releasing hormone agonists may temporarily relieve symptoms, but surgical procedures to remove or destroy the fibroids or remove the uterus may also be needed.

Fibroids are also known as fibromyomas, fibromas, myofibromas, leiomyomas, and myomas. Fibroids in the uterus are the most common noncancerous tumor of the female reproductive tract. They occur in one fourth of white women and one half of black women.

What causes fibroids to grow in the uterus is unknown. High estrogen levels seem to stimulate their growth. Thus, fibroids often grow larger during pregnancy and shrink after menopause. If fibroids grow too large, they may not be able to get enough blood. As a result, they begin to degenerate.

Fibroids may be microscopic or as large as a basketball. They may grow in the wall of the uterus, from the wall into the interior of the uterus (sometimes from a stalk), under the lining of the uterus, or on the outside of the uterus. Usually, more than one fibroid is present. Large fibroids that grow in the wall or under the lining of the uterus can distort the shape or interior of the uterus.

Symptoms

Symptoms depend on the number of fibroids present, their size, and their location in the uterus. Many fibroids, even large ones, do not cause symptoms. However, large fibroids, particularly those that grow in the wall of the uterus, may cause pain, pressure, or a feeling of heaviness in the pelvic area during or between menstrual periods. Fibroids may press on the bladder, making a woman need to urinate more frequently or more urgently. They may press on the rectum, causing discomfort and constipation. Large fibroids may cause the abdomen to enlarge. A fibroid growing from a stalk inside the uterus may twist and cause severe pain. Fibroids that are growing or degenerating usually cause pressure or pain. Pain due to degenerating fibroids can last as long as they continue to degenerate.

Fibroids, particularly those just under the lining of the uterus, commonly cause menstrual bleeding to be heavier or to last longer than usual. Anemia may result from the loss of blood. Less often, fibroids cause bleeding between menstrual periods, after sexual intercourse, or after menopause. Rarely, fibroids cause infertility by blocking the fallopian tubes or distorting the shape of the uterus, making implantation of a fertilized egg difficult or impossible.

Fibroids that cause no symptoms before pregnancy may cause problems during pregnancy. Problems include miscarriage, early (preterm) labor, abnormal positioning (presentation) of the baby before delivery, and excessive blood loss after delivery (postpartum hemorrhage).

Rarely, cancerous tumors that resemble fibroids (sarcomas) develop in the uterus (see page 239).

DID YOU KNOW?

- Fibroids occur in one fourth of white women and one half of black women.
- Fibroids may be microscopic or as large as a basketball.
- Infertility may result from fibroids.
- Fibroids that cause no symptoms before pregnancy may cause serious complications during pregnancy.

Diagnosis

Doctors can often detect fibroids during a pelvic examination. Several procedures that enable doctors to examine the uterus can confirm the diagnosis. For transvaginal ultrasonography, an ultrasound device is inserted into the vagina. For saline infusion sonohysterography, ultrasonography is performed after a small amount of fluid is infused into the uterus to outline its interior. For hysteroscopy, a flexible viewing tube is inserted through the vagina and cervix into the uterus. A local, regional, or general anesthetic is used. Sometimes magnetic resonance imaging (MRI) or computed tomography (CT) is also performed. Additional tests are usually unnecessary.

If bleeding (other than menstrual) has occurred, doctors may want to exclude cancer of the uterus. So they may perform a Papanicolaou (Pap) test, biopsy of the uterine lining (endometrial biopsy), ultrasonography, sonohysterography, or hysteroscopy.

Treatment

For most women who have fibroids but no symptoms, treatment is not required. They are reexamined every 6 to 12 months to determine whether the fibroid is growing.

Several treatment options, including drugs and surgery, are available if bleeding or other symptoms worsen or if fibroids enlarge substantially.

Drugs: Drugs may be used to relieve symptoms or to shrink fibroids, but only temporarily. No drug can permanently shrink a fibroid. Nonsteroidal anti-inflammatory drugs (NSAIDs), alone or given with a progestin (a drug similar to the hormone progesterone), can reduce bleeding caused by fibroids. Both are usually taken by mouth, but the progestin may be injected into muscle. Danazol (a synthetic hormone related to testosterone) can suppress the growth of a fibroid, but it is rarely used because of its side effects (see page 170). Hormonal contraceptives (see page 31) can control bleeding in some women. However, when women discontinue contraceptives, abnormal bleeding and pain tend to recur. Also, when some women are treated with contraceptives, the fibroids grow.

Synthetic forms of gonadotropin-releasing hormone (GnRH agonists) can shrink fibroids and reduce bleeding by causing the body to produce less estrogen (and progesterone). GnRH agonists may be given before surgery to make removal of fibroids easier. They are injected once a month, used as a nasal spray, or implanted as a pellet under the skin. They can be given only for a few months, because if taken for a long time, they may cause a decrease in bone density and increase the risk of osteoporosis (see page 170). Estrogen may be given in low doses with GnRH agonists to help prevent side effects. Fibroids often regrow within 6 months after the GnRH agonist is discontinued.

Surgery: Surgery may involve removal of the fibroids (myomectomy) or removal of the entire uterus (hysterectomy). In contrast with hysterectomy, myomectomy usually preserves the ability to have children and avoids the psychologic effects of removing the uterus. However, fibroids regrow in up to 50% of women.

For myomectomy, an incision may be made in the abdomen. Or a viewing tube with surgical attachments may be inserted through a small incision just below the navel (laparoscopy) or through the vagina into the uterus (hysteroscopy). Which method is used depends on the size, number, and location of fibroids. Laparoscopy and hysteroscopy are outpatient procedures, and recovery is faster than recovery after an abdominal incision. However, laparoscopy often cannot be used to remove large fibroids, and the risk of complications after laparoscopy can be higher.

Hysterectomy is usually considered when symptoms, such as pain and bleeding, are severe enough to interfere with daily activities and other treatments have been ineffective. If a woman is bothered by large fibroids that she can feel, she may choose to have a hysterectomy. Hysterectomy is performed only in women who do not wish to become pregnant. It is the only permanent solution to fibroids. For treatment of fibroids, only the uterus is removed, not the ovaries.

Other Treatments: New procedures that destroy rather than remove fibroids appear to shrink fibroids. In myolysis, a needle that transmits an electrical current is inserted into the fibroid during laparoscopy. The current is used to destroy the core of the fibroid, causing the fibroid to shrink. In cryomyolysis, a similar procedure, a cold probe (containing liquid nitrogen) is used to destroy the core of the fibroid. Whether these procedures affect the ability to become pregnant is unknown. Also, fibroids tend to grow back after these procedures.

In uterine artery embolization, a thin tubular, flexible instrument (catheter) is inserted into the main artery of the thigh (femoral artery) through a puncture made with a needle or through a tiny incision. Before the procedure, a local anesthetic is given to numb the insertion site. The catheter is threaded to the artery that supplies the fibroid. Small synthetic particles are injected. They travel to the small arteries supplying the fibroid. There, they block blood flow, causing the fibroid to shrink. Whether the fibroid will regrow (because blocked arteries reopen or new arteries form) and whether the woman can become pregnant are unknown. The most common problems after this procedure are pain and infection.

After these procedures, fibroids may grow back, or if they could not be completely removed, they may continue to grow. In such cases, a woman may need to have a hysterectomy.

CHAPTER 13

Vaginal Infections

- Vaginal infections are more likely to occur just before and during menstrual periods and during pregnancy.
- Typically, women have a discharge from the vagina and sometimes itching, soreness, sores, odor, and pain during urination.
- Doctors take a sample of the discharge to examine under a microscope or to culture.
- Antibiotics or antifungal drugs, applied topically or taken by mouth, can cure the infection.

In the United States, vaginal infections are one of the most common reasons women see their doctor, accounting for more than 10 million visits each year. Usually, vaginal infections cause only discomfort, although the discomfort may be substantial. However, these infections occasionally are or become serious.

Vaginal infections are a type of vaginitis, or inflammation of the lining (mucosa) of the vagina. Inflammation may result from chemical or mechanical irritants, such as hygiene products, bubble bath, laundry detergents, contraceptive foams and jellies, and synthetic underwear, as well as from bacterial, yeast, and viral infections.

In women, anything that reduces the acidity (increases the pH) of the vagina increases the likelihood of infection. Acidity may be reduced by hormonal changes shortly before and during menstrual periods or during pregnancy. Frequent douching, use of spermicides, and semen can also reduce acidity.

Many bacteria normally reside in the vagina. One type, called lactobacilli, normally maintains the acidity of the vagina. By doing so, lactobacilli help keep the lining of the vagina healthy and prevent the growth of bacteria or yeasts that cause infections. Bacterial vaginosis, the most common vaginal infection, results when the number of protective lactobacilli decreases and the number of other normally occurring bacteria (such as *Gardnerella* and *Peptostreptococcus*) increases. The reason for these changes is unknown. Bacterial vaginosis is more common among women who have a sexually transmitted disease, who have several sex partners, or who use an intrauterine device (IUD). But it is not a sexually transmitted disease. It can also occur in sexually inexperienced, lesbian, or monogamous women.

In women, yeast infections due to the fungus *Candida albicans* (candidiasis) are particularly common. Candida albicans normally resides on the skin or in the intestines. From these areas, the organism can spread to the vagina. Yeast infections are not transmitted sexually. They are common among pregnant women, obese women, and women who have diabetes. Yeast infections are more likely to occur during menstrual periods. Yeast infections are also more likely to develop if the immune system is suppressed by drugs (such as corticosteroids or chemotherapy drugs) or impaired by a disorder (such as AIDS). Antibiotics taken by mouth tend to kill the bacteria in the vagina that normally suppress the growth of yeast. Thus, the use of antibiotics increases the risk of developing vaginal infections. After menopause, women who take hormone replacement therapy are more likely to develop yeast infections.

DID YOU KNOW?

- Vaginal infections, including bacterial vaginosis (which is not sexually transmitted), are more common among sexually active women, and having several sex partners increases the risk even more.
- If a vaginal discharge looks like cottage cheese, it is probably caused by a yeast infection.
- Common sense measures, including keeping the genital area clean and dry and wearing loose, absorbent clothing, help prevent vaginal infections.

Some vaginal infections are sexually transmitted (see page 64). Sexually transmitted diseases that can affect the vagina include chlamydial infections, genital herpes, gonorrhea, syphilis, and trichomoniasis (a protozoan infection). Genital warts usually develop on the vulva but can develop in the vagina or on the cervix.

Tight, nonabsorbent underclothing may irritate the genital area and trap moisture, making infection by bacteria or yeast more likely. Not keeping the genital area clean (for example, inadequately or improperly cleaning it after urinating or defecating) and fingering the genital area may make infection more likely.

Some Vaginal Infections

INFECTION	SYMPTOMS	COMPLICATIONS	TREATMENT
Bacterial vaginosis	A thin, white, gray or yellowish cloudy discharge with a foul or fishy odor that may become stronger after sexual intercourse Itching and irritation	Pelvic inflammatory disease Infections of the membranes around the fetus Infections of the uterus after delivery of a baby or after surgery	Metronidazole (used first; taken as a vaginal gel or by mouth) Clindamycin
Chlamydial infection	Usually, no symptoms A yellow, puslike discharge A frequent need to urinate Pain during urination Abnormal vaginal bleeding	Pelvic inflammatory disease Infection and scarring of the fallopian tubes	Azithromycin Doxycycline Ofloxacin Tetracycline
Genital herpes	Painful blisters that form sores in the genital area, in the vagina, and on the cervix Itching Sometimes a fever and flu-like symptoms	If present during delivery, possibly serious infection in the newborn	Acyclovir Famciclovir Valacyclovir

Some Vaginal Infections (Continued)

INFECTION	SYMPTOMS	COMPLICATIONS	TREATMENT
Gonorrhea	A puslike discharge A frequent need to urinate Pain during urination Fever Pelvic pain	Pelvic inflammatory disease Infection of the fallopian tubes Arthritis	Ceftriaxone with azithromycin or doxycycline
Syphilis	Painless sore on the vagina or vulva Later, a fever and flu-like symptoms	Rarely, serious heart or brain disorders	Penicillin
Trichomoniasis	A usually profuse, greenish yellow, frothy, fishy-smelling discharge Itching and irritation	No known serious complications	Metronidazole (given by mouth only)
Yeast infection (candidiasis)	Thick, white, clumpy discharge (like cottage cheese) Moderate to severe itching and burning (but not always) Redness and swelling of the genital area	No serious complications	Butoconazole Clotrimazole Econazole Fluconazole Ketoconazole Miconazole Terconazole Tioconazole

Symptoms and Diagnosis

Typically, vaginal infections produce a vaginal discharge and irritation in the genital area. The appearance and amount of the discharge vary depending on the cause. Soreness and swelling are less common. Some infections can make sexual intercourse painful and make urination painful and more frequent. Rarely, the folds of skin around the vaginal and urethral openings become stuck together. However, vaginal infections sometimes produce minimal or no symptoms. Some vaginal infections, if untreated, may lead to complications that are sometimes serious.

NEARBY INFECTIONS: VULVITIS AND BARTHOLINITIS

The vulva is the area surrounding the opening of the vagina and containing the external female genital organs. Vulvitis is inflammation of the vulva. When both the vulva and vagina are inflamed, the disorder is called vulvovaginitis. Vulvitis may result from allergic reactions to substances that come in contact with the vulva (such as soaps, bubble bath, fabrics, and perfumes), from skin disorders (such as dermatitis), or from infections, including candidiasis and sexually transmitted diseases (such as herpes). The vulva may be infested by pubic lice (a disorder called pediculosis pubis).

Vulvitis causes itching, soreness, and redness. Rarely, the folds of skin around the vaginal and urethral openings (labia) become stuck together. Long-standing (chronic) vulvitis may result in sore, scaly, thickened, or whitish patches on the vulva. If chronic vulvitis does not respond to treatment, doctors usually perform a biopsy to look for the cause, such as cancer.

Bartholin's glands are located beside the opening of the vagina. Bartholinitis—infection of one or both glands or their ducts—may develop when bacteria from the vagina enter the glands. Rarely, bartholinitis is due to a sexually transmitted disease. The surrounding tissues (vulva) may swell. Pus accumulates in the gland, causing a painful abscess. Taking an antibiotic usually clears the infection in a few days, but the infection may recur. Analgesics may relieve the pain. An abscess or cyst needs to be drained.

If the ducts become blocked, the gland may swell but cause no pain—a disorder called Bartholin's cyst. In women younger than 50, a cyst that causes no symptoms does not require treatment. In women 50 and older, a biopsy of the cyst is recommended.

Because a vaginal discharge, itching, and odor may have different causes, women who have such symptoms should see a doctor. Information about a vaginal discharge, if present, can help the doctor determine the cause. The doctor may ask about possible causes of the discharge, such as lotions or creams used to try to relieve the symptoms (including home remedies), as well as hygiene. Other questions include when the discharge began, whether it is accompanied by itching, burning, pain, or a sore in the genital area, when it occurs in relation to the menstrual period, whether the discharge comes and goes or is always present, and, if the woman has had an abnormal discharge before, how it responded to treatment. The woman may be asked about her past and current use of birth control, pain after sexual intercourse, previous vaginal infections, and the possibility of sexually transmitted diseases. The doctor also asks whether the sex partner has symptoms and whether anyone else in the household has itching in the genital area. This information helps the doctor identify the cause of the woman's symptoms and determine whether other people require treatment.

A pelvic examination is performed. While examining the vagina, the doctor takes a sample of the discharge, if present, with a cotton-tipped swab. The sample is examined under a microscope or cultured to identify bacteria or other organisms. To determine whether the infection has spread outside the vagina, the doctor checks the uterus and ovaries by inserting the index and middle fingers of one gloved hand into the vagina and pressing on the outside of the lower abdomen with the other hand. If this maneuver causes substantial pain or if a fever is present, the infection may have spread.

Prevention

Keeping the genital area clean and dry can help prevent infections. Washing every day with a mild soap (such as glycerin soap) and rinsing and drying thoroughly are recommended. Wiping front to back after urinating or defecating prevents bacteria from the anus from being moved to the vagina.

Wearing loose, absorbent clothing, such as cotton or cotton-lined underpants, allows air to circulate and helps keep the genital area dry. Douching frequently and using medicated douches are discouraged. These measures can reduce the acidity of the vagina, making infections, including pelvic inflammatory disease, more likely. Practicing safe sex and limiting the number of sex partners are important preventive measures.

Treatment

Treatment varies according to the cause.

Bacterial vaginosis is treated with an antibiotic taken by mouth or applied as a vaginal gel or cream. Bacterial vaginosis usually resolves in a few days but commonly recurs. If it recurs often, antibiotics may have to be taken for a long time. Propionic acid jelly may be used to make the vaginal secretions more acidic and thus discourage the growth of bacteria. For sexually transmitted diseases, both sex partners are treated at the same time to prevent reinfection.

Yeast infections are treated with antifungal drugs applied as a cream to the affected area, inserted into the vagina as a suppository, or taken by mouth. Several antifungal creams and suppositories are available without a prescription. A single dose of an antifungal drug taken by mouth is usually as effective as vaginal creams and suppositories. However, if infections recur often, several doses may be needed.

For trichomoniasis, a single dose of metronidazole cures up to 95% of women. However, a single dose is more likely to cause nausea and vomiting than treatment with several smaller doses. During sexual intercourse, condoms should be used until the infection resolves.

To relieve symptoms, a woman can use a premeasured vinegar-and-water douche, but only for a brief time. Occasionally, placing ice packs against the genital area, applying cool compresses, or sitting in a cool sitz bath may reduce soreness and itching. A sitz bath is taken in the sitting position with the water covering only the genital and rectal area. Flushing the genital area with luke-warm water squeezed from a water bottle may also provide relief.

Women who are at high risk of a yeast infection, such as those who have an impaired immune system, who have diabetes, or who are taking antibiotics for a long time (as for a urinary tract infection), may need to take an antifungal drug to prevent other infections from developing.

CHAPTER 14

Pelvic Inflammatory Disease

Pelvic inflammatory disease is an infection of the upper female reproductive organs.

- Pelvic inflammatory disease is infection of the cervix, uterus, fallopian tubes, or ovaries.
- Usually, the disease is caused by the same bacteria that cause the sexually transmitted diseases gonorrhea or chlamydial infection.
- The disease can cause abdominal pain, irregular vaginal bleeding, fever, and a vaginal discharge with a bad odor.
- Doctors take a sample of the discharge for culture so that the bacteria can be identified.
- Antibiotics are given as soon as possible.

Pelvic inflammatory disease can affect the cervix (causing mucopurulent cervicitis), the uterus (causing endometritis), the fallopian tubes (causing salpingitis), and sometimes the ovaries (causing oophoritis). Pelvic inflammatory disease is the most common preventable cause of infertility in the United States. Infertility occurs in about one of five women with pelvic inflammatory disease. About one third of women who have had pelvic inflammatory disease develop the infection again.

Pelvic inflammatory disease usually occurs in sexually active women. It rarely affects girls before their first menstrual period (menarche) or women during pregnancy or after menopause. Risk is increased for women who are younger than 24 and who do not use a barrier contraceptive (such as a condom or diaphragm), who have many sex partners, who have a sexually transmitted disease or bacterial vaginosis, or who use an intrauterine device (IUD).

Infection is usually caused by bacteria that enter the vagina, most commonly, during sexual intercourse. Usually, pelvic inflammatory disease is caused by the bacteria that cause gonorrhea (*Neisseria gonorrhoeae*) or chlamydial infection (*Chlamydia trachomatis*), which are sexually transmitted diseases (see page 71 and page 74). Bacteria may also enter the vagina during douching. Less commonly, bacteria enter the vagina during a vaginal delivery, an abortion, or a medical procedure, such as dilation and curettage (D and C).

Pelvic inflammatory disease typically starts in the cervix and uterus. Usually, both fallopian tubes are infected, although symptoms may be worse on one side. The ovaries are not usually infected, unless the infection is severe.

Symptoms

Pelvic inflammatory disease tends to cause symptoms cyclically, toward the end of the menstrual period or for a few days afterward. For many women, the first symptoms are a low fever, mild to moderate abdominal pain (often aching), irregular vaginal bleeding, and a vaginal discharge with a bad odor. As the infection spreads, pain in the lower abdomen becomes increasingly severe and may be accompanied by nausea or vomiting. Later, the fever becomes higher, and the discharge often becomes puslike and yellow-green. However, a chlamydial infection may not produce a discharge or any other noticeable symptoms.

Sometimes infected fallopian tubes become blocked. Blocked tubes may swell because fluid is trapped. If the infection is not treated, pain in the lower abdomen may persist and irregular bleeding may occur. The infection can spread to surrounding structures, including the membrane that lines the abdominal cavity and covers the abdominal organs (causing peritonitis). Peritonitis can cause sudden, severe pain in the entire abdomen.

If infection of the fallopian tubes is due to gonorrhea or a chlamydial infection, it may spread to the tissues around the liver. Such an infection may cause pain in the upper right side of the abdomen that resembles a gallbladder disorder or stones. This complication is called the Fitz-Hugh-Curtis syndrome.

A collection of pus (abscess) forms in the fallopian tubes or ovaries of about 15% of women who have infected fallopian tubes. An abscess sometimes ruptures, and pus spills into the pelvic cavity (causing peritonitis). A rupture causes severe pain in the lower abdomen, quickly followed by nausea, vomiting, and very low blood pressure (shock). The infection may spread to the bloodstream (a condition called sepsis) and can be fatal.

Pelvic inflammatory disease often produces a puslike fluid, which can result in scarring and the formation of abnormal bands of scar tissue (adhesions) in the reproductive organs or between organs in the abdomen. Infertility may result. The longer and more severe the inflammation and the more often it recurs, the higher the risk of infertility and other complications. The risk increases each time a woman develops the infection.

Women who have had pelvic inflammatory disease are 6 to 10 times more likely to have a tubal pregnancy, in which the fetus grows in a fallopian tube rather than in the uterus. This type of pregnancy threatens the life of the woman, and the fetus cannot survive.

DID YOU KNOW?

- Pelvic inflammatory disease is the most common preventable cause of infertility in the United States.
- Women who have had this disease are more likely to have a tubal pregnancy than are other women.
- The risk of getting pelvic inflammatory disease can be decreased by abstaining from sex, by limiting the number of sex partners, and by using a condom or diaphragm plus contraceptive vaginal foam or jelly during sexual intercourse.
- Pelvic inflammatory disease may cause serious damage, including infertility, even when symptoms are mild or absent.
- Pelvic inflammatory disease sometimes causes pain in the upper abdomen around the liver.

Prevention

Prevention of pelvic inflammatory disease is essential to the health and fertility of a woman. The best way to prevent the infection is abstaining from sex. However, if a woman has sexual intercourse with only one partner, the risk of pelvic inflammatory disease is very low, as long as neither person has a sexually transmitted disease. Refraining from douching is also helpful.

Barrier methods of birth control (such as condoms) and spermicides (such as vaginal foams) used with a barrier method can help prevent pelvic inflammatory disease.

Diagnosis and Treatment

A doctor suspects the diagnosis based mainly on the severity and location of the pain. A physical examination, including a pelvic examination, is performed. A sample is usually taken from the cervix and tested to determine whether the woman has gonorrhea or a chlamydial infection. Other symptoms and laboratory test results help confirm the diagnosis. The white blood cell count is usually high. Ultrasonography of the pelvis may be performed. If the diagnosis is still uncertain or if the woman does not respond to treatment, the doctor may insert a viewing tube (laparoscope) through a small incision near the navel to view the inside of the abdominal cavity.

As soon as possible, antibiotics are usually given. Typically, two different antibiotics that are effective against a variety of organisms are used. Most women are treated at home. However, hospitalization is usually necessary if the infection does not improve within 48 hours, if symptoms are severe, if the woman may be pregnant, or if an abscess is detected.

If abscesses persist despite treatment with antibiotics, surgery may be necessary. A ruptured abscess requires emergency surgery.

Women should refrain from sexual intercourse until antibiotic therapy is completed and a doctor confirms that the infection is completely eliminated, even if symptoms disappear. All recent sex partners should be tested for infection and treated. If pelvic inflammatory disease is diagnosed and treated promptly, a full recovery is more likely.

CHAPTER 15

Pelvic Floor Disorders

Pelvic floor (pelvic support) disorders involve a dropping down (prolapse) of the bladder, rectum, or uterus caused by weakness of or injury to the ligaments, connective tissue, and muscles of the pelvis.

- Pregnancy, vaginal delivery, excessive straining, certain disorders, or aging may weaken or damage the pelvic muscles, ligaments, and connective tissues that hold the bladder, rectum, or uterus in place.
- Women experience heaviness, pressure, or pain in the pelvic area and sometimes urinary or fecal incontinence or constipation.
- Doctors can diagnose these disorders during a pelvic examination.
- Kegel exercises and use of a pessary (inserted into the vagina) can relieve symptoms, but sometimes surgery is needed.

Pelvic floor disorders occur only in women and become more common with age. About 1 of 11 women needs surgery for a pelvic floor disorder during her lifetime.

The pelvic floor is a network of muscles, ligaments, and tissues that act like a hammock to support the organs of the pelvis: the uterus, bladder, and rectum. If the muscles become weak or the ligaments or tissues are stretched or damaged, the pelvic organs may drop down and protrude into the wall of the vagina. If the disorder is severe, tissues may protrude all the way through the vagina and outside the body.

Pelvic floor disorders usually result from a combination of factors. Being pregnant and having a vaginal delivery may weaken or stretch some of the supporting structures in the pelvis. Pelvic floor disorders are more common among women who have had several vaginal deliveries, and the risk may increase with each delivery. The delivery itself may damage nerves, leading to muscle weakness. Delivery by cesarean section may reduce the risk of developing a pelvic floor disorder.

DID YOU KNOW?

- Having a baby can weaken or damage the muscles and other tissues that hold the bladder, rectum, and uterus in place.
- About 1 of 11 women needs surgery for a pelvic floor disorder during her lifetime.

Obesity, chronic coughing (for example, due to a lung disorder or smoking), frequent straining during bowel movements, and heavy lifting can also contribute to pelvic floor disorders. Other causes include a hysterectomy, nerve disorders, injuries, and tumors. Some women are born with weak pelvic tissues. As women age, the supporting structures in the pelvis may weaken, making pelvic floor disorders more likely to develop.

Types and Symptoms

All pelvic floor disorders are essentially hernias, in which tissue protrudes abnormally because another tissue is weakened. The different types of pelvic floor disorders are named according to the organ affected. Often, a woman has more than one type. In all types, the most common symptom is a feeling of heaviness or pressure in the area of the vagina—a feeling that the uterus, bladder, or rectum is dropping out.

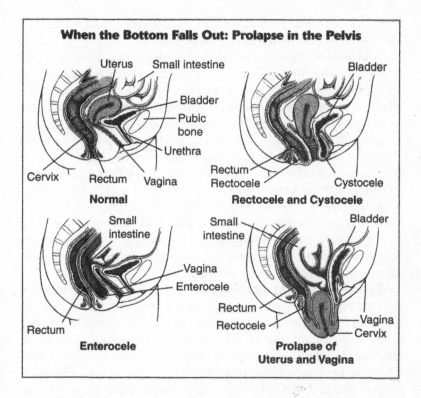

When the Bottom Falls Out: Prolapse in the Pelvis

Symptoms tend to occur when the woman is upright and to disappear when she is lying down. For some women, sexual intercourse is painful. Mild cases may not cause symptoms until a woman is older.

A **rectocele** develops when the rectum drops down and protrudes into the back wall of the vagina. It results from weakening of the muscular wall of the rectum and the connective tissue around the rectum. A rectocele can make having a bowel movement difficult and may cause a sensation of constipation. Some women need to place a finger in the vagina to have a bowel movement.

An **enterocele** develops when the small intestine and the lining of the abdominal cavity (peritoneum) bulge downward between the uterus and the rectum or, if the uterus has been removed, between the bladder and the rectum. It results from weakening of the connective tissue and ligaments supporting the uterus. An enterocele often causes no symptoms. But some women have a sense of fullness or feel pressure or pain in the pelvis. Pain may also be felt in the lower back.

A **cystocele** develops when the bladder drops down and protrudes into the front wall of the vagina. It results from weakening of the connective tissue and supporting structures around the bladder. A **cystourethrocele** is similar but develops when the upper part of the urethra (bladder neck) also drops down. Either of these disorders may cause stress incontinence (passage of urine during coughing, laughing, or any other maneuver that suddenly increases pressure within the abdomen) or overflow incontinence (passage of urine when the bladder becomes too full). After urination, the bladder may not feel completely empty. Sometimes a urinary tract infection develops. Because the nerves to the bladder or urethra can be damaged, women who have these disorders may develop urge incontinence (an intense, irrepressible urge to urinate, resulting in passage of urine).

In **prolapse of the uterus** (procidentia), the uterus drops down into the vagina. It usually results from weakening of the connective tissue and ligaments supporting the uterus. The uterus may bulge only into the upper part of the vagina, into the middle part, or all the way through the opening of the vagina, causing total uterine prolapse. Prolapse of the uterus may cause pain in the lower back or over the tailbone, although many women have no symptoms. Total uterine prolapse, which is obvious, can cause pain during walking. Sores may develop on the protruding cervix and cause bleeding, a discharge, and infection. Prolapse of the uterus may cause a kink in the urethra. A kink may hide urinary incontinence if present or make urinating difficult. Women with total uterine prolapse may also have difficulty having a bowel movement.

In **prolapse of the vagina**, the upper part of the vagina drops down into the lower part, so that the vagina turns inside out. The upper part may drop partway through the vagina or all the way through, protruding outside the body and causing total vaginal prolapse. Prolapse of the vagina occurs only in women who have had a hysterectomy. Total vaginal prolapse may cause pain while sitting or walking. Sores may develop on the protruding vagina and cause bleeding and a discharge. Prolapse of the vagina may cause a compelling or frequent need to urinate. Or it may cause a kink in the urethra. A kink may hide urinary incontinence if present or make urinating difficult. Having a bowel movement may also be difficult.

Diagnosis

Doctors can usually diagnose pelvic floor disorders by performing a pelvic examination, using a speculum (an instrument that spreads the walls of the vagina apart). A doctor may insert one finger in the vagina and one finger in the rectum to determine how severe a rectocele is.

A woman may be asked to bear down (as when having a bowel movement) or to cough while standing. She may be examined while standing. The resulting pressure in the pelvis may make a pelvic floor disorder more obvious.

Procedures to determine how well the bladder and rectum are functioning, such as urine tests, may be performed. These procedures help doctors determine whether drugs or surgery is the best treatment. If a woman has a problem with the passage of urine or urinary incontinence, doctors may use a flexible viewing tube to view the inside of the bladder (a procedure called cystoscopy) or the urethra (a procedure called urethroscopy). Also, the amount of urine that the bladder can hold without leakage and the rate of urine flow may be measured. Doctors may determine whether prolapse of the uterus may be preventing urinary incontinence.

Treatment

If prolapse is mild, performing Kegel exercises can help by strengthening the pelvic floor muscles. Kegel exercises target the muscles around the vagina, urethra, and rectum—the muscles used to stop a stream of urine. These muscles are tightly squeezed, held tight for about 10 seconds, then relaxed for about 10 seconds. The exercise is repeated 10 to 20 times in a row. Performing the exercises several times a day is recommended. Women can do Kegel exercises when sitting, standing, or lying down.

If prolapse is severe, a pessary may be used to support the pelvic organs. A pessary may be shaped like a diaphragm, cube, or doughnut. Pessaries are especially useful for women who are waiting for surgery or who cannot have surgery. A doctor fits the pessary to the woman by inserting and removing different sizes until the right one is found. A pessary can be worn for many weeks before it needs to be removed and cleaned with soap and water. Women are taught how to insert and remove the pessary for monthly cleaning. If they prefer, they may go to the doctor's office periodically to have the pessary cleaned. Pessaries can irritate the vaginal tissues and cause a foul-smelling discharge. Women who have this problem can use a vaginal deodorizer to mask the odor. As long as no other problems occur, these women may continue to use the pessary, removing it for cleaning each month. These women should also see their doctor every 6 to 12 months.

Estrogen vaginal suppositories or cream may be used. These preparations can help keep vaginal tissues healthy and can prevent sores from forming.

Surgery is often needed but is usually performed only after a woman has decided not to have any more children. Surgery usually involves inserting instruments into the vagina. The weakened area is located, and the tissues around it are built up to prevent the organ from dropping through the weakened area.

For severe prolapse of the uterus or vagina, the surgery may require an incision in the abdomen. The upper part of the vagina is attached with stitches to a nearby bone in the pelvis. Often, a catheter is inserted to drain the urine for 1 to 2 days. If urinary incontinence is a problem or would occur after prolapse of the uterus is repaired, surgery to correct incontinence can usually be performed at the same time. In such cases, the catheter may be left in place longer. Heavy lifting, straining, and standing for a long time should be avoided for at least 3 months after surgery.

If prolapse of the rectum makes having a bowel movement difficult, surgery may be necessary.

CHAPTER 16

Sexual Dysfunction in Women

Normal sexual function involves mind (thoughts and emotions) and body (including the nervous, circulatory, and endocrine systems), leading to a sexual response. Sexual response consists of desire, arousal, orgasm, and resolution.

Desire is the wish to engage in sexual activity. Desire may be triggered by thoughts, words, sights, smells, or touch.

Arousal is sexual excitement. It involves an increase in blood flow to the genital area. In women, arousal leads to enlargement of the clitoris, engorgement of the vaginal walls, and an increase in vaginal secretions.

Orgasm is the peak or climax of sexual excitement. In women, orgasm involves rhythmic contraction of the muscles surrounding the vagina. At orgasm, muscle tension throughout the body increases, and the pelvic muscles contract.

Resolution is a sense of well-being and widespread muscular relaxation that follow orgasm. Many women can respond to additional stimulation almost immediately after resolution.

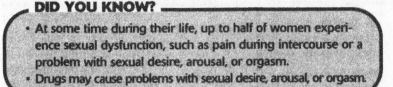

DID YOU KNOW?

- At some time during their life, up to half of women experience sexual dysfunction, such as pain during intercourse or a problem with sexual desire, arousal, or orgasm.
- Drugs may cause problems with sexual desire, arousal, or orgasm.

Sexual function is affected by physical and psychologic factors. It may be affected by culture, emotions, age, previous sexual experiences, use of drugs, and the presence of disorders. Sexual dysfunction may involve pain during intercourse or a disturbance in sexual response, affecting desire, arousal, or orgasm. About 30 to 50% of women experience sexual dysfunction at some time during their life.

Dyspareunia

Dyspareunia is pain during sexual intercourse.

- Pain may be caused by vaginal dryness, use of some contraceptives, inflammation, infections, injuries, tumors, or psychologic factors.
- Treatment depends on the cause.
- Women should abstain from painful sexual intercourse until the pain resolves.

The pain of dyspareunia may be superficial, occurring in the genital area (in the vulva, including the opening of the vagina), or deep, occurring within the pelvis due to pressure on internal organs. The pain may be burning, sharp, or cramping.

Superficial pain during sexual intercourse has many causes. When women have sexual intercourse the first time, the membrane that covers the opening of the vagina (hymen), if still intact, may tear as the penis enters the vagina, causing pain and sometimes bleeding. When the vagina is inadequately lubricated, intercourse may be painful. (Inadequate lubrication usually results from insufficient foreplay or from the decrease in estrogen levels after menopause.) Inflammation or infection in the genital area (for example, affecting the vulva, vagina, or Bartholin's glands) or in the urinary tract can make intercourse painful. Herpes can cause severe genital pain. Other causes include injuries in the genital area, a diaphragm or cervical cap that does not fit properly, an allergic reaction to contraceptive foams or jellies or to latex condoms, a congenital abnormality (such as a rigid hymen or an abnormal wall within the vagina), and involuntary contraction of the vaginal muscles (vaginismus). Sexual intercourse may be painful for women who have had surgery that narrows the vagina (for example, to repair tissues torn during childbirth or to correct a pelvic floor disorder (see page 187). Taking antihistamines can cause slight, temporary dryness of the vagina. During breastfeeding, the vagina may become dry because estrogen levels are low.

As women age, the lining of the vagina thins and becomes dry because estrogen levels decrease. This condition is called atrophic vaginitis. As a result, intercourse may be painful.

DID YOU KNOW?

- A poorly fitting diaphragm can make sexual intercourse painful.
- Changes in vaginal tissues after menopause can make sexual intercourse painful.

Deep pain after sexual intercourse may result from an infection of the cervix, uterus, or fallopian tubes. Other causes include endometriosis, pelvic inflammatory disease (including pelvic abscess), pelvic tumors (including ovarian cysts), and bands of scar tissue (adhesions) that have formed between organs in the pelvis after an infection or surgery. Sometimes one of these disorders results in the uterus bending backward (retroversion). The ligaments, muscles, and other tissues that hold the uterus in place may weaken, resulting in the uterus dropping down toward the vagina (prolapse—see pages 189 and 190). Such changes in position can result in pain during intercourse. Radiation therapy for cancer may cause changes in the tissues that make intercourse painful.

Psychologic factors can cause superficial or deep pain. Examples are anger or repulsion toward a sex partner, fear of intimacy or pregnancy, a negative self-image, and a traumatic sexual experience (including rape). However, psychologic factors may be difficult to identify.

Diagnosis and Treatment

The diagnosis is based on symptoms: when and where the pain occurs and when intercourse began to be painful. To try to identify the cause, a doctor asks the woman about her medical and sexual history and performs a pelvic examination.

Women should abstain from intercourse until the problem resolves. However, sexual activity that does not involve vaginal penetration can continue.

Superficial pain can be reduced by applying an anesthetic ointment and by taking sitz baths. Liberally applying a lubricant before intercourse may help. Water-based lubricants rather than petroleum jelly or other oil-based lubricants are preferable. Oil-based products tend to dry the vagina and can damage latex contraceptive devices such as condoms and diaphragms. Spending more time in foreplay may increase vaginal lubrication. Deep pain may be reduced by using a different position for intercourse. For example, a position that gives the woman more control of penetration (such as being on top) or that involves less deep thrusting may help.

More specific treatment depends on the cause. If the cause is thinning and drying of the vagina after menopause, using a topical estrogen cream or suppository or taking estrogen by mouth (as part of hormone therapy—see page 138) can help.

Inflammation and infection are treated with antibiotics, antifungal drugs, and other drugs as appropriate (see page 178). If the cause is inflammation of the vulva (vulvitis), applying wet dressings of aluminum acetate solution may help. Surgery may be needed to remove cysts or abscesses, open a rigid hymen, or repair an anatomic abnormality. A poorly fitting diaphragm should be replaced with one that fits and is comfortable, or a different method of birth control should be tried.

If the cause of pain is the position of the uterus, a pessary, which resembles a diaphragm and is inserted into the vagina, can support and reposition the uterus. Using a pessary reduces the pain in some women.

Vaginismus

Vaginismus is an involuntary contraction of muscles around the opening of the vagina that makes sexual intercourse painful or impossible.

- The vagina may contract involuntarily and painfully because a woman has an unconscious desire to prevent sexual intercourse or because she has a physical disorder.

- Doing Kegel exercises and using techniques to relax the vaginal muscles can help women control the involuntary contractions of the vagina.

Vaginismus may result from a woman's unconscious desire to prevent sexual intercourse. Pain experienced in the past during sexual intercourse can lead to vaginismus. Other reasons women do not want to engage in intercourse include fear of becoming pregnant, of being controlled by their partner, or of losing control. Sometimes vaginismus is caused by a physical disorder, such as a pelvic infection or scarring of the vaginal opening (due to injury, childbirth, or surgery). Irritation (due to douches, spermicides, or latex in condoms) may also cause vaginismus.

Because of the pain, some women who have vaginismus cannot tolerate sexual intercourse (that is, penetration of the vagina by the penis). However, sexual activity that does not involve penetration may be pleasurable. Some women cannot tolerate the insertion of a tampon and may need an anesthetic when a doctor performs a pelvic examination.

Diagnosis and Treatment

The diagnosis is based on the woman's description of the problem, her medical history, and the physical examination, including her reaction to a pelvic examination.

Physical disorders that may be causing or contributing to vaginismus are treated. If the cause is psychologic, counseling for the woman and her partner is usually helpful.

If vaginismus persists, the woman is taught a technique to relax the muscle spasms. The technique involves gradually widening (dilating) the vagina. The woman begins by inserting very small, lubricated plastic rods (dilators) into her vagina. The woman inserts slightly but progressively larger dilators as her level of comfort increases. Once the woman can tolerate having large dilators inserted without discomfort, she and her partner may try to have sexual intercourse again.

Kegel exercises, which strengthen the pelvic muscles, can be helpful if performed while the dilators are in place. For these exercises, the muscles around the vagina, urethra, and rectum—the muscles used to stop the flow of urine—are repeatedly squeezed hard and then relaxed 10 to 20 times. Performing the exercises several times a day is recommended. These exercises enable the woman to develop a sense of control over the muscles that were contracting involuntarily.

KEGEL EXERCISES: SQUEEZE AND RELAX

Kegel exercises help strengthen the pelvic muscles, primarily those around the vagina, urethra, and rectum. Performing them regularly can help improve sexual function and prevent or reduce the involuntary loss of urine (urinary incontinence) or stool (fecal incontinence).

To perform these exercises, a woman squeezes the muscles used to stop the flow of urine for about 10 seconds, then relaxes them for about 10 seconds. The exercise is repeated 10 to 20 times in a row at least 3 times a day. Muscle tone usually improves in 2 to 3 months. Kegel exercises can be performed anywhere, whether a woman is sitting, standing, or lying down.

Finding the right muscles to squeeze can be difficult. The muscles can be identified by inserting a finger into the vagina and squeezing or by trying to stop the flow of urine. If pressure is felt around the finger or urine flow stops, the right muscles are being squeezed.

Vulvodynia

Vulvodynia is chronic discomfort in the vulva—the area containing the external genital organs.

- Injuries, various disorders, and irritants (such as soaps or synthetic underclothing) may trigger vulvodynia.
- Avoiding potential irritants, doing pelvic muscle and relaxation exercises, and applying topical anesthetics or corticosteroids may relieve symptoms.

Vulvodynia typically begins suddenly, then becomes a chronic problem, lasting months to years. The cause is unknown. It may be triggered by irritation of or injury to the nerves supplying the vulva (as may occur during cryotherapy or laser therapy). Vulvodynia tends to be more common among women who have infections (especially yeast infections and sexually transmitted diseases), skin disorders, diabetes, precancerous conditions, cancer, or spasms of the muscles that support the pelvic organs. Certain substances (such as soaps, feminine hygiene sprays, menstrual pads, laundry detergents, and synthetic fibers) may cause an allergic reaction or irritate the area, increasing the likelihood of developing vulvodynia. Women who are undergoing hormonal changes or who have a history of sexual abuse are also more likely to develop vulvodynia. Eating certain foods, such as greens, chocolate, berries, beans, and nuts, produces urine that can be irritating.

DID YOU KNOW?

- Eating greens, chocolate, berries, beans, or nuts can result in urine that irritates the vulva.

The vulva may burn or sting. It may feel raw, irritated, or painful. The pain ranges from mild to debilitating and may be constant or intermittent. It can interfere with daily activities, limiting physical and sexual activity. It may make walking and sitting uncomfortable. The vulva may appear swollen and red, or it may appear normal.

Doctors diagnose vulvodynia by ruling out other disorders that can cause similar symptoms. The goal of treatment is to relieve symptoms. Potential irritants should be avoided. Wearing cotton underwear may help reduce irritation in the area. Tight-fitting, restrictive clothing, such as pantyhose, should not be worn. Foods that may produce irritating urine should not be eaten. Physical therapy, including exercises to improve tone in the pelvic muscles, biofeedback, and relaxation exercises, often help, as do support groups.

Topical anesthetics such as viscous lidocaine may reduce the pain. Topical corticosteroids may be rubbed into the skin 2 or 3 times a day to control symptoms.

Disorders that may be contributing to vulvodynia, such as infections, are treated. Some women benefit from tricyclic antidepressants or anticonvulsants.

Decreased Libido

Decreased libido is a reduction in the sex drive.

A temporary reduction in sex drive is common, often caused by temporary conditions, such as fatigue. Sex drive that continues to be reduced can distress a woman or her partner.

Sex drive is controlled in part by sex hormones, such as estrogen and testosterone. Fluctuations in the levels of these hormones, which occur monthly and during pregnancy, can affect sex drive. In postmenopausal women, sex drive may be reduced because estrogen levels decrease. Sex drive may also be reduced in women who have had both ovaries removed.

A reduction in sex drive may result from depression, anxiety, stress, or problems in a relationship. Use of certain drugs, including anticonvulsants, chemotherapy drugs (such as tamoxifen), beta-blockers, and oral contraceptives, can also reduce the sex drive, as can drinking excessive amounts of alcohol.

The diagnosis is based on the woman's description of the problem. A doctor asks the woman about stress and other lifestyle problems and her sexual and medical history, including use of drugs. Levels of sex hormones may be measured in a blood sample.

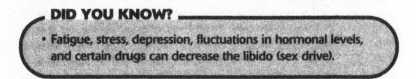

DID YOU KNOW?

• Fatigue, stress, depression, fluctuations in hormonal levels, and certain drugs can decrease the libido (sex drive).

Treatment depends on the cause. Drugs that may be contributing are discontinued if possible. If psychologic factors are involved, counseling may be recommended. If the cause is low levels of sex hormones, a low dose of testosterone combined with estrogen may be given by mouth. In addition to increasing sex drive, testosterone may also increase muscle strength, prevent loss of bone density, and improve energy.

Sexual Arousal Disorder

Sexual arousal disorder is the persistent or recurring inability to attain or to maintain adequate vaginal lubrication and other physical responses of sexual excitement before or during sexual intercourse.

- Psychologic factors, physical disorders, vaginal dryness, or certain drugs may interfere with arousal.
- Doctors base the diagnosis on the woman's description of the problem.
- Counseling, use of topical estrogen, sensate focus therapy, and Kegel exercises may help.

Usually, when a woman is sexually stimulated, the vagina releases lubricating secretions, the labia and clitoris of the vulva swell, and the breasts enlarge slightly. In sexual arousal disorder, these responses do not occur despite sufficiently long and intense sexual stimulation.

If the disorder has been present since puberty, the woman may not know how the genital organs (particularly the clitoris) function or what arousal techniques are effective. The lack of knowledge leads to anxiety, which worsens the problem. Many women who have sexual arousal disorder associate sex with sinfulness and sexual pleasure with guilt. Fear of intimacy and a negative self-image may also contribute.

If the disorder develops after a period of adequate sexual functioning, it may be due to a problem in the current sexual relationship, such as constant fighting or arguing. Depression is a common cause, and stress may contribute.

Physical causes include inflammation of the vagina (vaginitis), inflammation of the bladder (cystitis), endometriosis, an underactive thyroid gland (hypothyroidism), diabetes mellitus, multiple sclerosis, and muscular dystrophy.

Sexual arousal disorder may develop as women age. As menopause approaches, the lining of the vagina thins and becomes dry because the estrogen level decreases. As a result, the ability to become aroused declines, partly because sexual intercourse may be painful.

DID YOU KNOW?

- Taking oral contraceptives or drinking large amounts of alcohol can decrease the sex drive.
- Women who cannot be sexually aroused may also lack sexual desire.
- Couples can be taught techniques to help them be more comfortable with each other sexually.

Taking drugs such as oral contraceptives, antihypertensives, antidepressants, or sedatives can cause sexual arousal disorder. Surgical removal of the uterus (hysterectomy) or breast (mastectomy) may damage a woman's sexual self-image, contributing to sexual arousal disorder.

Many women with sexual arousal disorder also lack sexual desire. Because the vagina does not become lubricated, sexual intercourse is usually painful or uncomfortable.

Diagnosis and Treatment

The diagnosis is based on the woman's description of the problem. To determine the severity of the disorder and identify the cause, a doctor asks the woman about her sexual and medical history (including use of drugs) and performs a physical examination. Tests to detect physical disorders, if thought to be the cause, may be performed.

If the cause is psychologic, counseling for the woman, usually with her partner, often helps. Individual psychotherapy or group therapy is sometimes useful. Physical disorders, if present, are treated. Postmenopausal women may benefit from treatment with estrogen or male hormones such as testosterone. Estrogen creams and suppositories reduce the thinning and drying of the lining of the vagina and thus may help with lubrication during intercourse. The use of testosterone in treating women with sexual arousal disorder is controversial.

Sensate focus exercises for couples can help relieve a couple's anxiety about intimacy and sexual intercourse. Learning about how the genital organs function can help. A woman can learn which arousal techniques are effective for her and her partner. Performing Kegel exercises can help because they strengthen the muscles involved in sexual intercourse.

SEX THERAPY: SENSATE FOCUS TECHNIQUE

The sensate focus technique may help couples that are having sexual difficulties because of psychologic rather than physical factors. The technique aims to make both partners aware of what each finds pleasurable and to reduce anxiety about performance. It is often used in the treatment of decreased libido, sexual arousal disorder, orgasmic disorder, and erectile dysfunction (impotence).

The technique has three steps. Both partners must become comfortable at each level of intimacy before proceeding to the next step.

- The first step focuses on the sensation of touching, rather than the likelihood of sexual arousal or intercourse. Each partner takes turns touching any part of the other's body, except the genitals and breasts.

- The second step allows partners to touch any part of the other's body, including the genitals and breasts. However, the focus remains the same—on the sensation of touching, not on sexual response. Intercourse is not allowed.

- The third step involves mutual touching, eventually leading to sexual intercourse as the couple becomes more comfortable with touching and being touched. The focus is on enjoyment rather than on orgasm.

Orgasmic Disorder

Orgasmic disorder is the delay in or absence of sexual climax (orgasm) despite sufficiently long and intense sexual stimulation.

- Psychologic factors (commonly, depression), physical disorders, and some drugs may interfere with orgasm.
- Counseling, psychotherapy, sensate focus therapy, and Kegel exercises may help.

The amount and type of stimulation required for orgasm varies greatly from woman to woman. Most women can reach orgasm when the clitoris is stimulated, but only about half of women regularly reach orgasm during sexual intercourse. About 1 of 10 women never reach orgasm. Orgasmic disorder occurs when problems with orgasm are persistent and frequent, interfering with sexual function and causing distress.

Usually, women who have learned how to reach orgasm do not lose that ability unless poor sexual communication, conflict in a relationship, a traumatic experience, or a physical or psychologic disorder intervenes. Physical and psychologic causes are similar to those of sexual arousal disorder. Depression is a common cause.

Orgasmic disorder may result from lovemaking that consistently ends before the woman reaches orgasm. The woman may not reach orgasm because foreplay is inadequate, because one or both partners do not understand how the genital organs function, or because ejaculation is premature. Such lovemaking produces frustration and may result in resentment and occasionally in distaste for anything sexual. Some women who become aroused may not reach orgasm because they fear "letting go," especially during intercourse. This fear may be due to guilt after a pleasurable experience, fear of abandoning oneself to pleasure that depends on the partner, or fear of losing control.

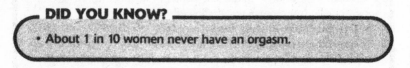

DID YOU KNOW?

- About 1 in 10 women never have an orgasm.

Certain drugs, particularly selective serotonin reuptake inhibitors such as fluoxetine, may inhibit orgasm.

Orgasmic disorder may be temporary, may occur after years of normal sexual function, or may be lifelong. It may occur all the time or only in certain situations. Most women who have a problem reaching orgasm also have a problem being aroused.

Diagnosis and Treatment

The diagnosis is based on the woman's description of the problem. To identify the cause, a doctor asks the woman about her sexual and medical history, including use of drugs, and performs a physical examination.

If the cause is psychologic, counseling for the woman, usually with her partner, often helps. Psychotherapy for the woman or the couple may be recommended. Physical disorders, if present, are treated.

Other useful measures include sensate focus exercises for couples, information about how the genital organs function, and Kegel exercises.

CHAPTER 17

Breast Disorders

Breast disorders may be noncancerous (benign) or cancerous (malignant). Most are noncancerous and not life threatening. Often, they do not require treatment. In contrast, breast cancer can mean loss of a breast or of life. Thus, for many women, breast cancer is their worst fear. However, potential problems can be detected early when women regularly examine their breasts themselves and have mammograms.

DID YOU KNOW?

- Breast symptoms require evaluation, but most breast disorders are not cancer.
- Breast pain without a lump is usually not cancer.
- Most women have some lumpiness in the breasts.
- Most breast lumps are not cancerous.
- A bloody discharge from the nipples may occur during pregnancy or breastfeeding or be caused by a tumor, usually a noncancerous tumor.

Symptoms

Common symptoms include breast pain, lumps, and a discharge from the nipple. Breast symptoms do not necessarily mean that a woman has breast cancer or another serious disorder.

However, if a woman has any of the following symptoms, she should see her doctor:

- A lump that feels distinctly different from other breast tissue or that does not go away
- Swelling that does not go away
- Puckering or dimpling in the skin of the breast
- Scaly skin around the nipple
- Changes in the shape of the breast
- Changes in the nipple, such as turning inward
- Discharge from the nipple, especially if it is bloody

Inside the Breast

The female breast is composed of milk-producing glands (lobules) surrounded by fatty tissue and some connective tissue. Milk secreted by the glands flows through ducts to the nipple. Around the nipple is an area of pigmented skin called the areola.

Collarbone

Rib

Muscle

Connective tissue

Fatty tissue

Areola

Nipple

Milk duct

Milk gland

Skin

Breast Pain: Many women experience breast pain (mastalgia). Breast pain may be related to hormonal changes. For example, it may occur during or just before a menstrual period (as part of the premenstrual syndrome) or early in pregnancy. Women who take oral contraceptives or who take hormone therapy after menopause commonly have this kind of pain. The pain is due to growth of breast tissue. Such pain is usually diffuse, making the breasts tender to touch. Pain related to the menstrual period may come and go for months or years.

Other causes of breast pain include breast cysts, infections, and abscesses. In these cases, breast pain is usually felt in a particular place. Fibrocystic breast disease can also cause breast pain. Breast pain is occasionally due to breast cancer, but breast cancer does not usually cause pain. Breast pain that persists for more than 1 month should be evaluated.

Mild breast pain usually disappears eventually, even without treatment. Pain that occurs during menstrual periods can usually be relieved by taking acetaminophen or a nonsteroidal anti-inflammatory drug (NSAID).

For certain types of severe pain, danazol (a synthetic hormone related to testosterone) or tamoxifen (a drug used to treat breast cancer) may be used. These drugs inhibit the activity of estrogen and progesterone, which affect the breast. Because long-term use of these drugs causes side effects, the drugs are usually given for only a short time. Tamoxifen has fewer side effects than danazol. Tamoxifen is used mainly for postmenopausal women but may benefit younger women.

If a specific disorder is identified as the cause, the disorder is treated. For example, if a cyst is the cause, draining the fluid from the cyst usually relieves the pain.

Breast Lumps: Lumps in the breasts are relatively common and are usually not cancerous. But because they may be cancerous, they should be evaluated by a doctor without delay. Lumps may be fluid-filled sacs (cysts) or solid masses, which are usually fibroadenomas (see page 210).

Other solid breast lumps include hardened glandular tissue (sclerosing adenosis) and scar tissue that has replaced injured fatty tissue (fat necrosis). Neither is cancerous. However, these lumps can be diagnosed only by biopsy. They require no treatment.

Nipple Discharge: One or both nipples sometimes discharge a fluid. A nipple discharge occurs normally during milk production (lactation) after childbirth or as a result of mechanical stimulation of the nipple by fondling, suckling, or irritation from clothing. During the last weeks of pregnancy, the breasts may produce a milky discharge (colostrum). A normal nipple discharge is a thin, cloudy, whitish or almost clear fluid that is not sticky. However, during pregnancy or breastfeeding, a slightly bloody discharge sometimes occurs normally.

Several disorders can cause an abnormal discharge. Abnormal discharges vary in appearance depending on the cause. A bloody discharge may be caused by a noncancerous breast tumor (such as a tumor in a milk duct, called an intraductal papilloma) or, less commonly, by breast cancer. Among women who have an abnormal discharge, breast cancer is the cause in fewer than 10%. A greenish discharge is usually due to a fibroadenoma, a noncancerous solid lump. A discharge that contains pus and smells foul may result from a breast infection. A large amount of milky discharge in women who are not breastfeeding (galactorrhea) may result from a pituitary gland disorder. Tumors of the pituitary gland or brain, encephalitis (a brain infection), and head injuries can also cause a nipple discharge. Taking certain drugs, such as antidepressants and certain antihypertensives, can cause a nipple discharge. Taking oral contraceptives may cause a watery discharge.

A discharge from one breast is likely to be caused by a problem with that breast, such as a noncancerous or cancerous breast tumor. A discharge from both breasts is more likely to be caused by a problem outside the breast, such as a pituitary tumor, or by drugs.

If a nipple discharge persists for more than one menstrual cycle or seems unusual to the woman, she should see a doctor. Postmenopausal women who have a nipple discharge should see a doctor promptly. Doctors examine the breast, looking for abnormalities. Mammography and blood tests to measure hormone levels may be performed. Computed tomography (CT) or magnetic resonance imaging (MRI) of the head may be performed. The woman is asked for a complete list of drugs she is taking. Sometimes a specific cause cannot be identified.

If a disorder is the cause, the disorder is treated. If a noncancerous tumor is causing a discharge from one breast, the duct that the discharge is coming from may be removed.

Breast Cysts

Breast cysts are fluid-filled sacs that develop in the breast.

Breast cysts are common. In some women, many cysts develop frequently, sometimes as part of fibrocystic breast disease. However, in other women, cysts never develop. The cause of breast cysts is unknown, although injury may be involved. Breast cysts can be tiny or several inches in diameter.

Cysts sometimes cause breast pain. To relieve the pain, a doctor may drain fluid from the cyst with a thin needle. The fluid is examined under a microscope to check for cancer. The color and amount are noted. If the fluid is bloody, brown, or cloudy or if the cyst does not disappear or reappears within 12 weeks after it is drained, the entire cyst is removed surgically, because cancer in the cyst wall, although rare, is possible.

Fibroadenomas

Fibroadenomas are small, solid, rubbery noncancerous lumps composed of fibrous and glandular tissue.

Fibroadenomas usually appear in young women, including teenagers. The cause is unknown.

The lumps are easy to move and have clearly defined edges that can be felt during self-examination. They may feel like small, slippery marbles. These characteristics indicate to a doctor that the lumps are less likely to be cancerous. Nonetheless, to be sure that they are not cancerous, the doctor usually removes the lumps. A local anesthetic is used. Fibroadenomas often recur. If several lumps have been removed and found to be noncancerous, a woman and her doctor may decide against removing new lumps that develop.

Fibrocystic Breast Disease

Fibrocystic breast disease is characterized by breast pain, cysts, and noncancerous lumpiness.

Most women have some general lumpiness in the breasts, usually in the upper outer part, near the armpit. In the United States, about 30% of women have this kind of lumpiness with breast pain and breast cysts—a condition called fibrocystic breast disease.

Normally, the levels of the female hormones estrogen and progesterone fluctuate during the menstrual cycle. Milk glands and ducts enlarge and breasts retain fluid when levels increase, and the breasts return to normal when levels decrease. (These fluctuations partly explain why breasts are swollen and more sensitive during a particular time of each menstrual cycle.) Fibrocystic changes may result from repeated stimulation by these hormones.

In women with fibrocystic breast disease, the lumpy areas may enlarge, causing a feeling of heaviness, discomfort, tenderness to the touch, or a burning pain. The symptoms tend to subside after menopause. Fibrocystic breast disease may increase the risk of breast cancer very slightly. Also, this condition may make breast cancer more difficult to detect.

Lumps may be removed and a biopsy may be performed. Sometimes cysts are drained, but they tend to recur. No specific treatment is available or required.

Breast Infection and Abscess

A breast infection (mastitis) is rare, except around the time of childbirth (see page 376) or after an injury or surgery. The most common symptom is a swollen, red area that feels warm and tender. An uncommon type of breast cancer called inflammatory breast cancer (see page 217) can produce similar symptoms. A breast infection is treated with antibiotics.

A breast abscess, which is even rarer, is a collection of pus in the breast. An abscess may develop if a breast infection is not treated. An abscess is treated with antibiotics and is usually drained surgically.

Breast Cancer

- Among women, breast cancer is the second most common cancer and the second most common cause of cancer deaths.
- Monthly self-examination, yearly breast examination by a doctor, and a yearly mammogram for women who are 50 or older or who are at increased risk are the most effective ways to prevent deaths due to breast cancer.
- Typically, the first symptom is a painless lump, usually noticed by the woman.
- If indicated, a biopsy is done using a needle to remove a few cells or surgery to remove the whole lump.
- Surgery is almost always required, sometimes with radiation therapy, chemotherapy, other drugs, or a combination.
- Women are monitored regularly for the return of the cancer.
- Outcome is hard to predict and depends partly on the characteristics and spread of the cancer.

Breast cancer is the second most common cancer among women after skin cancer and, of cancers, is the second most common cause of death among women after lung cancer. In 2001, breast cancer was diagnosed in about 200,000 women in the United States. About one fifth of them will die of it.

Many women fear breast cancer, because it is common. However, some of the fear about breast cancer is based on misunderstanding. For example, the statement, "One of every eight women will get breast cancer," is misleading. That figure is an estimate based on women from birth to age 95. It means that theoretically, one of eight women who live to age 95 or older will develop breast cancer. However, a 40-year-old woman has only a 1 in 1,200 chance of developing breast cancer during the next year and about a 1 in 120 chance of developing it during the next decade. But as she ages, her risk increases.

Other factors also affect the risk of developing breast cancer. Thus, for some women, the risk is much higher or lower than average. Most factors that increase risk, such as age, cannot be modified. However, regular exercise, particularly during adolescence and young adulthood, and possibly weight control may slightly reduce the risk of developing breast cancer. Regularly drinking alcoholic beverages may increase the risk.

Far more important than trying to modify risk factors is being vigilant about detecting breast cancer so that it can be diagnosed and treated early, when it is more likely to be cured. Early detection is more likely when women have mammograms and perform breast self-examinations regularly (see pages 220 and 222).

What Are the Risks of Developing or Dying of Breast Cancer?

| AGE (YEARS) | RISK (%) | | | | | |
| | IN 10 YEARS | | IN 20 YEARS | | IN 30 YEARS | |
	DEVELOP	DIE	DEVELOP	DIE	DEVELOP	DIE
30	0.4	0.1	2.0	0.6	4.3	1.2
40	1.6	0.5	3.9	1.1	7.1	2.0
50	2.4	0.7	5.7	1.6	9.0	2.6
60	3.6	1.0	7.1	2.0	9.1	2.6
70	4.1	1.2	6.5	1.9	7.1	2.0

Based on information from Feuer EJ et al.: "The lifetime risk of developing breast cancer." *Journal of the National Cancer Institute* 85(11):892-897, 1993.

Staging

Staging involves assigning a stage to a cancer when it is diagnosed. The stage is based on how advanced the cancer is. The stage helps doctors determine the most appropriate treatment and the prognosis. Stages of breast cancer may be generally described as in situ (not invasive), localized invasive, regional invasive, or distant (metastatic) invasive. Or, stages may be described in detail and designated by a number (0 through IV).

Carcinoma in situ means cancer in place. It is the earliest stage of breast cancer. Carcinoma in situ may be large and may even affect a substantial area of the breast, but it has not invaded the surrounding tissues or spread to other parts of the body. More than 15% of all breast cancers diagnosed in the United States are carcinoma in situ. It is usually detected during mammography.

RISK FACTORS FOR BREAST CANCER

Age

Increasing age is an important risk factor. About 60% of breast cancers occur in women older than 60. Risk is greatest after age 75.

Previous Breast Cancer

At highest risk are women who have had in situ or invasive breast cancer. After the diseased breast is removed, the risk of developing cancer in the remaining breast is about 0.5 to 1.0% each year.

Family History of Breast Cancer

Breast cancer in a first-degree relative (mother, sister, or daughter) increases a woman's risk by 2 to 3 times, but breast cancer in more distant relatives (grandmother, aunt, or cousin) increases the risk only slightly. Breast cancer in two or more first-degree relatives increases a woman's risk by 5 to 6 times.

Breast Cancer Gene

Recently, two separate genes for breast cancer (BRCA1 and BRCA2) have been identified in two separate small groups of women. These genes are present in fewer than 1% of women. If a woman has one of these genes, her chances of developing breast cancer are very high, possibly as high as 50 to 85% by age 80. However, if such a woman develops breast cancer, her chances of dying of breast cancer are not necessarily greater than those of any other woman with breast cancer. Women likely to have one of these genes are those who have a strong family history of breast cancer. Usually, several women in each of three generations have had breast cancer. For this reason, routine screening for these genes does not appear necessary, except in women who have such a family history. The incidence of ovarian cancer is increased in families with both breast cancer genes. The incidence of breast cancer in men is increased in families with the BRCA2 gene.

Fibrocystic Breast Disease

Having fibrocystic breast disease seems to increase risk only in women who have an increased number of cells in the milk ducts. For these women, the risk is moderate unless abnormal tissue structure (atypical hyperplasia) is detected during a biopsy or the woman has a family history of breast cancer.

Age at Puberty, First Pregnancy, and Menopause

The earlier menstruation begins, the greater the risk of developing breast cancer. The risk is 1.2 to 1.4 times greater for women who first menstruated before age 12 than for those who first menstruated after age 14. The later menopause occurs and the later the first pregnancy, the greater the risk. Never having had a baby also doubles the risk of developing breast cancer during a woman's lifetime. These factors probably increase risk because they involve longer exposure to estrogen, which stimulates the growth of certain cancers. (Pregnancy, although it results in high estrogen levels, may reduce the risk of breast cancer.)

Prolonged Use of Oral Contraceptives or Estrogen Therapy

Most studies do not show any relationship between the use of oral contraceptives and the later development of breast cancer, except possibly for women who took them for many years. After menopause, taking estrogen therapy for 5 to 10 years may slightly increase risk. Taking hormone therapy that combines estrogen with a progestin increases the risk (although it reduces the risk of cancer of the uterus).

Obesity After Menopause

Risk is somewhat higher for obese postmenopausal women. However, there is no proof that a high-fat diet contributes to the development of breast cancer. Some studies suggest that obese women who are still menstruating are less likely to develop breast cancer.

Radiation Exposure

Radiation exposure (such as radiation therapy for cancer or significant exposure to x-rays) before age 30 increases risk.

Localized invasive cancer has invaded surrounding tissues but is confined to the breast.

Regional invasive cancer has invaded tissues near the breasts, including the chest wall and lymph nodes.

Distant (metastatic) invasive cancer has spread from the breast to other parts of the body. Cancer tends to move into the lymphatic vessels in the breast. Most lymphatic vessels in the breast drain into lymph nodes in the armpit (axillary lymph nodes). One function of lymph nodes is to filter out and destroy abnormal or foreign cells, such as cancer cells. If cancer cells get past these lymph nodes, the cancer can spread any-where in the body. Breast cancer can also spread through the bloodstream to other parts of the body. Breast cancer tends to spread to bones and the brain but can spread to any area, includ-ing the lungs, liver, and skin. Breast cancer can appear in these areas years or even decades after it is first diagnosed and treated. If the cancer has spread to one area, it probably has spread to other areas, even if it is not detected right away.

DID YOU KNOW?

- Breast cancer rarely causes pain at first.
- Many experts recommend that women over age 40 have mammograms every 1 to 2 years.
- Mammography may miss up to 10% of breast cancers.
- If mammography shows an abnormality, the chance of cancer is about 1 in 10.
- Breast lumps that contain fluid are rarely cancerous.
- One or more lymph nodes under the arm are removed if doctors suspect the cancer has spread.
- Breast cancer that has spread beyond the lymph nodes is rarely cured, but treatment may improve quality of life and prolong life.

Types

Breast cancer is usually classified by the kind of tissue in which the cancer starts and by the extent of its spread. Breast cancer that starts in the milk ducts is called ductal carcinoma. About 90% of all breast cancers are this type. Breast cancer that starts in the milk-producing glands (lobules) is called lobular carcinoma. Breast cancer that starts in fatty or connective tissue, a rare type, is called sarcoma.

Ductal carcinoma in situ is confined to the milk ducts of the breast. It does not invade surrounding breast tissue, but it can spread along the ducts and gradually affect a substantial area of the breast. This type accounts for 20 to 30% of breast cancers.

Lobular carcinoma in situ grows within the milk-producing glands of the breast. It often occurs in several areas of both breasts.

Women with lobular carcinoma in situ have a 30% chance of developing invasive breast cancer in the same or other breast during the next 24 years. This type accounts for 1 to 2% of breast cancers.

Invasive ductal carcinoma begins in the milk ducts but breaks through the wall of the ducts, invading the surrounding breast tissue. It can also spread to other parts of the body. It accounts for 65 to 80% of breast cancers.

Invasive lobular carcinoma begins in the milk-producing glands of the breast but invades surrounding breast tissue and spreads to other parts of the body. It is more likely than other types of breast cancer to occur in both breasts. It accounts for 10 to 15% of breast cancers.

Inflammatory breast cancer is fast growing and often fatal. Cancer cells block the lymphatic vessels in the skin of the breast, causing the breast to appear inflamed: swollen, red, and warm. Usually, inflammatory breast cancer spreads to the lymph nodes in the armpit. The lymph nodes can be felt as hard lumps. However, often no lump may be felt in the breast itself because this cancer is dispersed throughout the breast. Inflammatory breast cancer accounts for about 1% of breast cancers.

Paget's disease of the nipple is a type of ductal breast cancer. The first symptom is a crusty or scaly nipple sore or a discharge from the nipple. Slightly more than half of the women who have this cancer also have a lump in the breast that can be felt. Paget's disease may be in situ or invasive. Because this disease usually causes little discomfort, a woman may ignore it for a year or more before seeing a doctor. The prognosis depends on how invasive and how large the cancer is as well as whether it has spread to the lymph nodes.

Less common types of invasive ductal breast cancers include medullary carcinoma, tubular carcinoma, and mucinous (colloid) carcinoma. Mucinous carcinoma tends to develop in older women and to be slow growing. Women with these types of breast cancer have a much better prognosis than women with other types of invasive breast cancer.

Cystosarcoma phyllodes is a relatively rare type of breast cancer. It originates in breast tissue around milk ducts and milk-producing glands. It spreads to other parts of the body in fewer than 5% of women who have it.

Stages of Breast Cancer

STAGE	DESCRIPTION
0	The tumor is confined to a milk duct or milk-producing gland and has not invaded surrounding breast tissue (in situ carcinoma).
I	The tumor is less than $3/4$ inch (2 cm) in diameter and has not spread beyond the breast.
II	The tumor is larger than $3/4$ inch but smaller than 2 inches (5 cm) in diameter and/or has spread to at least one lymph node in the armpit on the same side as the tumor.
III	The tumor is larger than 2 inches in diameter and/or has spread to lymph nodes that are stuck to one another or to surrounding tissues, or the tumor, regardless of size, has spread to the skin, the chest wall, or the lymph nodes that are beneath the breast inside the chest.
IV	The tumor, regardless of size, has spread to distant organs or tissues, such as the lungs or bones, or to lymph nodes distant from the breast.

Characteristics

All cells, including breast cancer cells, have molecules on their surfaces called receptors. A receptor has a specific structure that allows only particular substances to fit into it and thus affect the cell's activity. Whether breast cancer cells have certain receptors affects how quickly the cancer spreads and how it should be treated.

Some breast cancer cells have receptors for estrogen. The resulting cancer, described as estrogen receptor-positive, is stimulated by estrogen. This type of cancer is more common among postmenopausal women than among younger women. Some breast cancer cells have receptors for progesterone. The resulting cancer, described as progesterone receptor-positive, is stimulated by progesterone. Estrogen receptor-positive breast cancers grow more slowly than estrogen receptor-negative breast cancers, and the prognosis is better. The same is true for progesterone receptor-positive and progesterone receptor-negative breast cancers. The prognosis is better with cancer that is both estrogen and progesterone receptor-positive than with cancer that is one or the other.

Cells have receptors called HER-2/*neu* receptors that help them grow. Breast cancer cells with too many HER-2/*neu* receptors tend to be very fast growing. In about 20 to 30% of breast cancers, the cancer cells have too many HER-2/*neu* receptors.

Symptoms

At first, a woman who has breast cancer has no symptoms. Most commonly, the first symptom is a lump, which usually feels distinctly different from the surrounding breast tissue. In more than 80% of breast cancer cases, the woman discovers the lump herself. Usually, scattered lumpy changes in the breast, especially the upper outer region, are not cancerous and indicate fibrocystic breast disease. A firm, distinctive thickening that appears in one breast but not the other may indicate cancer.

In the early stages, the lump may move freely beneath the skin when it is pushed with the fingers. In more advanced stages, the lump usually adheres to the chest wall or the skin over it. In these cases, the lump cannot be moved at all or it cannot be moved separately from the skin over it. One way to detect even slight adherence of a cancer to the chest wall or skin is to lift the arms over the head while standing in front of a mirror. A breast containing cancer may show skin puckering or another shape abnormality compared with the other breast. In advanced cancer, swollen bumps or festering sores may develop on the skin. Sometimes the skin over the lump is dimpled and leathery and looks like the skin of an orange (peau d'orange) except in color.

The lump may be painful, but pain is an unreliable sign. Pain without a lump is rarely due to breast cancer.

Lymph nodes, particularly those in the armpit on the affected side, may feel like hard small lumps. The lymph nodes may be stuck together or adhere to the skin or chest wall. They are usually painless but may be slightly tender.

In inflammatory breast cancer, the breast is warm, red, and swollen, as if infected (but it is not). The skin of the breast may become dimpled and leathery, like the skin of an orange, or may have ridges. The nipple may turn inward (invert). A discharge from the nipple is common. Often, no lump can be felt in the breast.

Screening

Because breast cancer rarely produces symptoms in its early stages and because early treatment is more likely to be successful, screening is important. Screening is the hunt for a disorder before any symptoms occur.

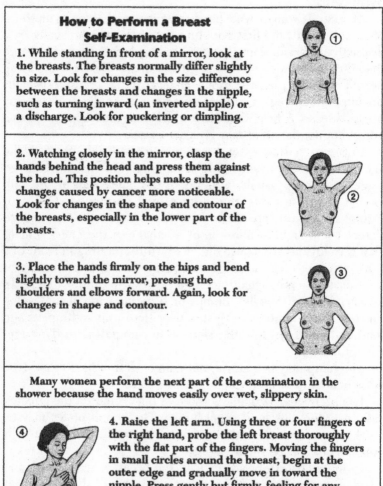

How to Perform a Breast Self-Examination

1. While standing in front of a mirror, look at the breasts. The breasts normally differ slightly in size. Look for changes in the size difference between the breasts and changes in the nipple, such as turning inward (an inverted nipple) or a discharge. Look for puckering or dimpling.

2. Watching closely in the mirror, clasp the hands behind the head and press them against the head. This position helps make subtle changes caused by cancer more noticeable. Look for changes in the shape and contour of the breasts, especially in the lower part of the breasts.

3. Place the hands firmly on the hips and bend slightly toward the mirror, pressing the shoulders and elbows forward. Again, look for changes in shape and contour.

Many women perform the next part of the examination in the shower because the hand moves easily over wet, slippery skin.

4. Raise the left arm. Using three or four fingers of the right hand, probe the left breast thoroughly with the flat part of the fingers. Moving the fingers in small circles around the breast, begin at the outer edge and gradually move in toward the nipple. Press gently but firmly, feeling for any unusual lump or mass under the skin. Be sure to check the whole breast. Also, carefully probe the armpit and the area between the breast and armpit for lumps.

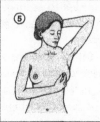

5. Squeeze the left nipple gently and look for a discharge. (See a doctor if a discharge appears at any time of the month, regardless of whether it happens during a breast self-examination.)

Repeat steps 4 and 5 for the right breast, raising the right arm and using the left hand.

6. Lie flat on the back with a pillow or folded towel under the left shoulder and with the left arm overhead. This position flattens the breast and makes it easier to examine. Examine the breast as in steps 4 and 5. Repeat for the right breast.

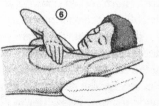

A woman should repeat this procedure at the same time each month. For menstruating women, 2 or 3 days after their period ends is a good time because the breasts are less likely to be tender and swollen. Postmenopausal women may choose any day of the month that is easy to remember, such as the first.

Adapted from a publication of the National Cancer Institute.

Routine self-examination enables a woman to detect lumps at an early stage. Self-examination does not reduce the death rate from breast cancer or detect as many early cancers as routine screening with mammography. With tumors detected by self-examination, the prognosis is usually better, and breast-conserving surgery can usually be performed rather than mastectomy.

A breast examination is a routine part of a physical examination. A doctor inspects the breasts for irregularities, dimpling, tightened skin, lumps, and a discharge. The doctor feels (palpates) each breast with a flat hand and checks for enlarged lymph nodes in the armpit—the area most breast cancers invade first—and also above the collarbone. Normal lymph nodes cannot be felt through the skin, so those that can be felt are considered enlarged. However, noncancerous conditions can also cause lymph nodes to enlarge. Lymph nodes that can be felt are checked to see if they adhere to the skin or chest wall and if they are matted together.

Mammography uses low-level x-rays to detect abnormal areas in the breast. It is one of the best ways to detect breast cancer early (see page 131). Mammography is designed to be sensitive enough to detect the possibility of cancer at an early stage. For this reason, the procedure may indicate cancer when none is present—a false-positive result. Typically, when the result is positive, more specific follow-up procedures, usually a breast biopsy, are scheduled to confirm the result. Mammography may miss up to 15% of breast cancers.

Having a mammogram every 1 to 2 years can reduce the rate of death due to breast cancer by 25 to 35% among women aged 50 and older. As yet, no study has shown that having mammograms regularly can reduce the death rate among women younger than 50. However, evidence may be harder to obtain because breast cancer is not common among younger women. Many experts recommend that women aged 40 to 49 have mammograms every 1 to 2 years. All experts recommend yearly mammograms for women aged 50 and older.

Diagnosis

When a lump or another suspicious change is detected in the breast during a physical examination or by a screening procedure, other procedures are necessary. Mammography is performed first if it was not the way the abnormality was detected.

Ultrasonography is sometimes used to help distinguish between a fluid-filled sac (cyst) and a solid lump. This distinction is important because cysts are usually not cancerous. Cysts may be monitored (with no treatment) or drained with a small needle and syringe. Rarely, when cancer is suspected, cysts are removed. If the abnormality is a solid lump, which is more likely to be cancerous, a biopsy is performed. Often, an aspiration biopsy is performed: Some cells are removed from the lump through a needle attached to a syringe. If this procedure detects cancer, the diagnosis is confirmed. If no cancer is detected, removal of an additional piece of tissue (incisional biopsy) or of the entire lump (excisional biopsy) is necessary to be sure that the aspiration biopsy did not miss the cancer. Most women do not need to be hospitalized for these procedures. Usually, only a local anesthetic is needed.

If Paget's disease of the nipple is suspected, a biopsy of nipple tissue is performed. Sometimes this cancer can be diagnosed by examining a sample of the nipple discharge under a microscope.

A pathologist examines the biopsy samples under the microscope to determine whether cancer cells are present. Generally, a biopsy confirms cancer in one of four women in whom mammography detects an abnormality. If cancer cells are detected, the sample is analyzed to determine the characteristics of the cancer cells, such as whether the cancer cells have estrogen or progesterone receptors, how many HER-2/*neu* receptors are present, and how quickly the cancer cells are dividing. This information helps doctors estimate how rapidly the cancer may spread and which treatments are more likely to be effective.

A chest x-ray is taken and blood tests to evaluate liver function are performed to determine whether the cancer has spread. If the tumor is large or if the lymph nodes are enlarged, x-rays of bones throughout the body (a bone scan) may be taken.

Treatment

Usually, treatment begins after the woman's condition has been thoroughly evaluated, about a week or more after the biopsy. Treatment options depend on the stage and type of breast cancer. However, treatment is complex because the different types of breast cancer differ greatly in growth rate, tendency to spread (metastasize), and response to treatment. Also, much is still unknown about breast cancer. Consequently, doctors may have different opinions about the most appropriate treatment for a particular woman.

The preferences of a woman and her doctor affect treatment decisions. A woman with breast cancer should ask for a clear explanation of what is known about the cancer and what is still unknown, as well as a complete description of treatment options. Then, a woman can consider the advantages and disadvantages of the different treatments and accept or reject the options offered. Losing some or all of a breast can be emotionally traumatic. A woman must consider how she feels about this treatment, which can deeply affect her sense of wholeness and sexuality.

Doctors may ask a woman with breast cancer to participate in research studies investigating a new treatment, which may improve her chances of survival or her quality of life. All women who participate in a research study are treated, because a new treatment is compared with other effective treatments. A woman should ask her doctor to explain the risks and possible benefits of participation, so that she can make a well-informed decision.

Treatment usually involves surgery and may include radiation therapy, chemotherapy, or hormone-blocking drugs. Often, a combination of these treatments is used.

Surgery for Breast Cancer

Surgery for breast cancer consists of two main options: Breast-conserving surgery (in which only the tumor and an area of normal tissue surrounding it is removed) and mastectomy (in which all breast tissue is removed). Breast-conserving surgery includes lumpectomy (in which a small amount of surrounding normal tissue is removed), wide excision or partial mastectomy (in which a somewhat larger amount of the surrounding normal tissue is removed), and quadrantectomy (in which one fourth of the breast is removed).

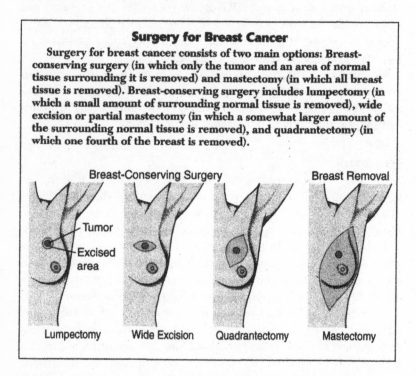

Breast-Conserving Surgery

Breast Removal

Tumor
Excised area

Lumpectomy · Wide Excision · Quadrantectomy · Mastectomy

Surgery: The cancerous tumor and varying amounts of the surrounding tissue are removed. There are two main options for removing the tumor: breast-conserving surgery and removal of the breast (mastectomy).

Breast-conserving surgery leaves as much of the breast intact as possible. There are several types:

- Lumpectomy is removal of the tumor with a small amount of surrounding normal tissue
- Wide excision or partial mastectomy is removal of the tumor and a somewhat larger amount of surrounding normal tissue
- Quadrantectomy is removal of one fourth of the breast

Removing the tumor with some normal tissue provides the best chance of preventing cancer from recurring within the breast. Breast-conserving surgery is usually combined with radiation therapy.

The major advantage of breast-conserving surgery is cosmetic: This surgery may help preserve body image. Thus, when the tumor is large in relation to the breast, this type of surgery is less likely to be useful. In such cases, removing the tumor plus some surrounding normal tissue means removing most of the breast. Breast-conserving surgery is usually more appropriate when tumors are small. In about 15% of women who undergo breast-conserving surgery, the amount of tissue removed is so small that little difference can be seen between the treated and untreated breasts. However, in most women, the treated breast shrinks somewhat and may change in contour.

Mastectomy is the other main surgical option. There are several types:

- Simple mastectomy consists of removing all breast tissue but leaving the muscle under the breast and enough skin to cover the wound. Reconstruction of the breast is much easier if these tissues are left. A simple mastectomy, rather than breast-conserving surgery, is usually performed when there is a substantial amount of cancer in the milk ducts.
- Modified radical mastectomy consists of removing all breast tissue and some lymph nodes in the armpit but leaving the muscle under the breast. This procedure is usually performed instead of a radical mastectomy.

- Radical mastectomy consists of removing all breast tissue plus the lymph nodes in the armpit and the muscle under the breast. This procedure is rarely performed now.

Lymph node surgery (lymph node dissection) is also performed if the cancer is or is suspected to be invasive. Nearby lymph nodes (usually about 10 to 20) are removed and examined to determine whether the cancer has spread to them. If cancer cells are detected in the lymph nodes, the likelihood that the cancer has spread to other parts of the body is increased. In such cases, additional treatment is needed. Removal of lymph nodes often causes problems, because it affects the drainage of fluids in tissues. As a result, fluids may accumulate, causing persistent swelling (lymphedema) of the arm or hand. Arm and shoulder movement may be limited. Other problems include temporary or persistent numbness, a persistent burning sensation, and infection.

A **sentinel lymph node biopsy** is an alternative approach that may minimize or avoid the problems of lymph node surgery. This procedure involves locating and removing the first lymph node (or nodes) into which the tumor drains. If this node contains cancer cells, the other lymph nodes are removed. If it does not, the other lymph nodes are not removed. Whether this procedure is as effective as standard lymph node surgery is being studied.

Breast reconstruction surgery may be performed at the same time as a mastectomy or later. A silicone or saline implant or tissue taken from other parts of the woman's body may be used. The safety of silicone implants, which sometimes leak, has been questioned. However, there is almost no evidence suggesting that silicone leakage has serious effects.

Radiation Therapy: This treatment is used to kill cancer cells at the site from which the tumor was removed and in the surrounding area, including nearby lymph nodes. Side effects include swelling in the breast, reddening and blistering of the skin in the treated area, and fatigue. These effects usually disappear within several months, up to about 12 months. Fewer than 5% of women treated with radiation therapy have rib fractures that cause minor discomfort. In about 1% of women, the lungs become mildly inflamed 6 to 18

What Is a Sentinel Lymph Node?

A network of lymphatic vessels and lymph nodes drain fluid from the tissue in the breast. The lymph nodes are designed to trap foreign or abnormal cells (such as bacteria or cancer cells) that may be contained in this fluid. Sometimes cancer cells pass through the nodes and spread to other parts of the body by moving through the lymphatic vessels. Usually, the fluid from breast tissue drains through a single nearby lymph node first, but it may drain through more than one. Such lymph nodes are called sentinel lymph nodes.

Doctors can identify the sentinel lymph node by injecting blue dye or a radioactive substance in the fluid surrounding the breast cells. The dye can be seen or the radioactive substance detected with a Geiger counter as it reaches the first lymph node. The sentinel lymph node is then removed and examined to determine whether it contains cancer cells. If it does, other nearby lymph nodes are removed. If the sentinel lymph node does not contain cancer cells, the other lymph nodes are not removed. In about 2 to 3% of women, cancer has spread to other lymph nodes when the sentinel lymph node is clear.

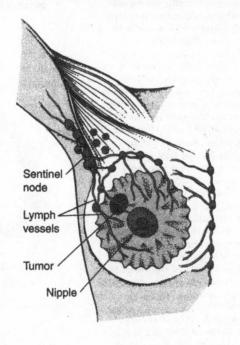

Sentinel node

Lymph vessels

Tumor

Nipple

Rebuilding a Breast

After a general surgeon removes a breast tumor and the surrounding breast tissue (mastectomy), a plastic surgeon may reconstruct the breast. A silicone or saline implant may be used. Or in a more complex operation, tissue may be taken from other parts of the woman's body, usually the abdomen. Reconstruction may be performed at the same time as the mastectomy—a choice that involves being under anesthesia for a longer time—or later—a choice that involves being under anesthesia a second time.

In many women, a reconstructed breast looks more natural than one that has been treated with radiation therapy, especially if the tumor was large. If a silicone or saline implant is used and enough skin was left to cover it, the sensation in the skin over the implant is relatively normal. However, neither type of implant feels like breast tissue to the touch. If tissue from other parts of the body is used, much of the sensation in the skin is lost since the skin is also from another part of the body. However, tissue from other parts of the body feels more like breast tissue than does a silicone or saline implant.

Silicone occasionally leaks out of its sack. As a result, an implant can become hard, cause discomfort, and appear less attractive. Also, silicone sometimes enters the bloodstream. Some women are concerned about whether the leaking silicone causes cancer in other parts of the body or rare diseases such as lupus (systemic lupus erythematosus). There is almost no evidence suggesting that silicone leakage has these serious effects, but because it might, the use of silicone implants has decreased, especially among women who have not had breast cancer.

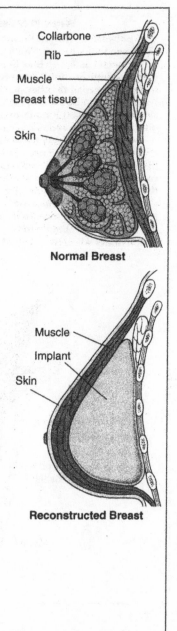

Normal Breast

Reconstructed Breast

months after radiation therapy is completed. Inflammation causes a dry cough and shortness of breath during physical activity that last for up to about 6 weeks.

To improve radiation therapy, doctors are studying several experimental procedures. In one procedure, tiny radioactive seeds are inserted through a catheter to the tumor site. Radiation therapy can be completed in only 5 days. In another procedure, a tiny coil that emits radiation is implanted in the space left by the tumor. Radiation therapy can be completed in 25 minutes.

Drugs: Chemotherapy and hormone-blocking drugs are used to suppress the growth of cancer cells throughout the body. Chemotherapy and sometimes hormone-blocking drugs are used in addition to surgery and radiation therapy if cancer cells are detected in the lymph nodes and often if they are not. These drugs are often started soon after breast surgery and are continued for several months. Some, such as tamoxifen, may be continued for up to 5 years. These drugs delay the recurrence of cancer and prolong survival in most women.

Chemotherapy is used to kill rapidly multiplying cells or slow their multiplication. Chemotherapy alone cannot cure breast cancer; it must be used with surgery or radiation therapy. Chemotherapy drugs are usually given intravenously in cycles. Sometimes they are given by mouth. Typically, a day of treatment is followed by several weeks of recovery. Using several chemotherapy drugs together is more effective than using a single drug. The choice of drugs depends partly on whether cancer cells are detected in nearby lymph nodes. Commonly used drugs include cyclophosphamide, doxorubicin, epirubicin, fluorouracil, methotrexate, and paclitaxel. Side effects (such as vomiting and nausea, hair loss, and fatigue) vary depending on which drugs are used. Chemotherapy can also cause infertility and early menopause by destroying the eggs in the ovaries.

Hormone-blocking drugs interfere with the actions of estrogen or progesterone, which stimulate the growth of cancer cells that have estrogen or progesterone receptors. These drugs may be used when cancer cells have these receptors. Tamoxifen, given by mouth, is the most commonly used estrogen-blocking drug. In women who have estrogen receptor-positive cancer, use of tamoxifen increases the likelihood of survival during the first 10 years after diagnosis by about 20 to 25%. Tamoxifen, which is related to estrogen, has some of the benefits and risks of estrogen therapy taken after menopause (see page 138). For example, it may decrease the risk of developing osteoporosis and it may increase the risk of developing cancer of the uterus (endometrial cancer). However, unlike estrogen therapy, tamoxifen may worsen the vaginal dryness or hot flashes that occur after menopause.

Biologic response modifiers are natural substances or slightly modified versions of natural substances that are part of the body's immune system. These drugs enhance the immune system's ability to fight cancer. They include interferons, interleukin-2, lymphocyte-activated killer cells, tumor necrosis factor, and monoclonal antibodies. Trastuzumab, a monoclonal antibody, is used to treat metastatic breast cancer only when the cancer cells have too many HER-2/*neu* receptors. This drug binds with HER-2/*neu* and thus prevents it from promoting the growth of cancer cells. Herceptin can cause heart problems by weakening the heart muscle. Other biologic response modifiers are sometimes tried experimentally as treatment for breast cancer, but their role has not been established.

Tumor Ablation

In an experimental procedure called tumor ablation, doctors insert a multipronged probe into the tumor. Then a highly focused beam of light (laser), high-energy radio waves, or cold is used to destroy only the cancer cells.

Treatment of Noninvasive Cancer (Stage 0)

For **ductal carcinoma in situ**, treatment usually consists of a simple mastectomy or lumpectomy and sometimes radiation therapy.

For **lobular carcinoma in situ**, treatment is less clear-cut. For most women, the preferred treatment is close observation with no treatment. Observation consists of a physical examination every 6 to 12 months for 5 years and once a year thereafter plus mammography once a year. No treatment is usually needed.

How Lymph Node Status Influences Survival

LYMPH NODE STATUS	CHANCES OF SURVIVING 5 YEARS	CHANCES OF SURVIVING 10 YEARS	CHANCES OF SURVIVING 10 YEARS WITHOUT RECURRENCE
No cancer in any node	Better than 90%	Better than 80%	Better than 70%
Cancer in one to three nodes	About 60 to 70%	About 40 to 50%	About 25 to 40%
Cancer in four or more nodes	About 40 to 50%	About 25 to 40%	About 15 to 35%

Although invasive breast cancer may develop (the risk is 1.3% per year or 26% for 20 years), the invasive cancers that develop are usually not fast growing and can usually be treated effectively. Furthermore, because invasive cancer is equally likely to develop in either breast, the only way to eliminate the risk of breast cancer for women with lobular carcinoma in situ is removal of both breasts (bilateral mastectomy). Some women, particularly those who are at high risk of developing invasive breast cancer, choose this option.

Alternatively, tamoxifen, a hormone-blocking drug, may be given for 5 years. It reduces but does not eliminate the risk of developing invasive cancer.

Treatment of Localized or Regional Invasive Cancer (Stages I through III)

For cancers that have not spread beyond nearby lymph nodes, treatment almost always includes surgery to remove as much of the tumor as possible and nearby lymph nodes or the sentinel lymph node.

A simple mastectomy is commonly used to treat invasive cancer that has spread extensively within the milk ducts (invasive ductal carcinoma), because this type of cancer often recurs when breast-conserving surgery is used. A modified radical mastectomy may also be used. A radical mastectomy, in which the underlying chest muscles and other tissues are also removed, does not improve life expectancy. Women who have had a simple or a modified radical mastectomy live as long as women who have had a radical mastectomy.

Whether radiation therapy, chemotherapy, or both are used after surgery depends on how large the tumor is and how many lymph nodes contain cancer cells. Sometimes, when the tumor is large, chemotherapy is given before surgery to reduce the size of the tumor. If chemotherapy reduces the size of the tumor, doctors can sometimes perform breast-conserving surgery rather than a mastectomy. After surgery and radiation therapy, additional chemotherapy is usually given, and women who have estrogen receptor-positive cancer are usually given tamoxifen.

Treatment of Cancer That Has Spread (Stage IV)

Breast cancer that has spread beyond the lymph nodes is rarely cured, but most women who have it live at least 2 years and a few live 10 to 20 years. Treatment extends life only slightly but may relieve symptoms and improve quality of life.

Initial treatment almost always includes surgery to remove the primary tumor, even though such removal is unlikely to cure cancer that has spread. If the cancer recurs in the breast after initial treatment, breast surgery is not usually repeated. Instead, radiation may be tried. However, surgery to remove tumors in other parts of the body (such as the brain) may be recommended, because such surgery can relieve symptoms.

Other treatments, such as chemotherapy, especially if they have uncomfortable side effects, are often postponed until a woman develops symptoms (pain or other discomfort) or the cancer starts to worsen quickly. Pain is usually treated with analgesics. Other drugs may be given to relieve other symptoms. Chemotherapy or hormone-blocking drugs are given to relieve symptoms and improve quality of life rather than to prolong life. The most effective chemotherapy regimens for breast cancer that has spread include capecitabine, cyclophosphamide, docetaxel, doxorubicin, epirubicin, gemcitabine, paclitaxel, and vinorelbine.

Hormone-blocking drugs are preferred to chemotherapy in certain situations. For example, these drugs may be preferred when the cancer is estrogen receptor-positive, when cancer has not recurred for more than 2 years after diagnosis and initial treatment, or when cancer is not immediately life threatening. Hormone-blocking drugs are especially effective for women in their 40s who are still menstruating and producing a lot of estrogen, as well as for those who are at least 5 years past menopause. However, these guidelines are not absolute. For women who are still menstruating, tamoxifen is usually the first hormone-blocking drug used because it has few side effects. For postmenopausal women who have estrogen receptor-positive breast cancer, aromatase inhibitors (such as anastrozole, letrozole, and exemestane) may be more effective as a first treatment than tamoxifen. These drugs inhibit the enzyme aromatase (which converts some hormones to estrogen), possibly reducing estrogen production. Progestins, such as medroxyprogesterone or megestrol, may be used instead of aromatase inhibitors and tamoxifen and have almost as few side effects. Fulvestrant, a new drug, may be used when tamoxifen is no longer effective. It destroys the estrogen receptors in cancer cells. The most common side effect is stomach upset. Alternatively, for women who are still menstruating, surgery to remove the ovaries, radiation to destroy them, or drugs to inhibit their activity may be used to stop estrogen production.

The monoclonal antibody trastuzumab can be combined with paclitaxel as initial treatment for breast cancer that has spread throughout the body. Trastuzumab can be combined with hormone-blocking drugs to treat women who have estrogen receptor-positive breast cancer. Sometimes trastuzumab can be used to treat women who do not respond to chemotherapy.

In some situations, radiation therapy may be used instead of or before drugs. For example, if only one area of cancer is detected in a bone, without any other evidence of recurrences, radiation to that bone might be the only treatment used. Radiation therapy is usually the most effective treatment for cancer that has spread to bone, sometimes keeping it in check for years. It is also often the most effective treatment for cancer that has spread to the brain.

Treatment of Specific Types of Breast Cancer

For inflammatory breast cancer, treatment usually consists of both chemotherapy and radiation therapy. Mastectomy is usually performed.

For Paget's disease of the nipple, treatment usually consists of a simple mastectomy and removal of the lymph nodes. Less commonly, the nipple with some surrounding normal tissue is removed.

For cystosarcoma phyllodes, treatment usually consists of wide excision mastectomy, in which the tumor and a large amount of surrounding normal tissue are removed. If the tumor is large in relation to the breast, a simple mastectomy may be performed. After surgical removal, about 20 to 35% of cancers recur near the same site.

Follow-up Care

After treatment is completed, follow-up physical examinations, including examination of the breasts, chest, neck, and armpit, are performed every 3 months for 2 years, then every 6 months for 5 years from the date the cancer was diagnosed. Regular mammograms and breast self-examinations are also important. A woman should report any changes in her breasts to her doctor immediately. Other symptoms should also be reported. They include pain, loss of appetite or weight, changes in menstruation, bleeding from the vagina (if not associated with the menstrual period), and blurred vision. Any symptoms that seem unusual or that persist should also be reported. Diagnostic procedures, such as chest x-rays, blood tests, bone scans, and computed tomography (CT), are not needed unless a woman has symptoms suggesting recurrence of the cancer.

The effects of treatment for breast cancer cause many changes in a woman's life. Support from family members and friends can help, as can support groups. Counseling may be helpful.

End-of-Life Issues

For a woman with metastatic breast cancer, quality of life may deteriorate and the possibilities for further treatment may become limited. Staying comfortable may eventually become more important than trying to prolong life. Cancer pain can be adequately controlled with appropriate drugs. So if a woman is having pain, she should ask her doctor for treatment to relieve it. Psychologic and spiritual counseling may also help.

A woman with metastatic breast cancer should prepare advance directives indicating the type of care she desires in case she is no longer able to make such decisions. Also, making or updating a will is important.

CHAPTER 18

Cancers of the Female Reproductive System

Cancers can occur in any part of the female reproductive system—the vulva, vagina, cervix, uterus, fallopian tubes, or ovaries. These cancers are called gynecologic cancers.

Gynecologic cancers can directly invade nearby tissues and organs or spread (metastasize) through the lymphatic vessels and lymph nodes (lymphatic system) or bloodstream to distant parts of the body.

DID YOU KNOW?

- Having regular pelvic examinations and Papanicolaou (Pap) tests can help prevent cancer.
- A vaccine is available to prevent cervical cancer.
- The main treatment for cancers of the female reproductive system is surgical removal of the tumor.

Diagnosis

Regular pelvic examinations and Papanicolaou (Pap) tests or other similar tests (see page 125) can lead to the early detection of certain gynecologic cancers, especially cancer of the cervix and uterus. Such examinations can sometimes prevent cancer by detecting abnormalities (precancerous conditions) before they develop into cancer.

If cancer is suspected, a biopsy can usually confirm or rule out the diagnosis. If cancer is diagnosed, one or more procedures may be performed to determine the stage of the cancer. The stage is based on how large the cancer is and how far it has spread. Some commonly used procedures include ultrasonography, computed tomography (CT), magnetic resonance imaging (MRI), chest x-rays, and bone and liver scans using radioactive substances.

Staging a cancer helps doctors choose the best treatment. Doctors often determine the stage of cancer after they remove the cancer and perform biopsies of the surrounding tissues, including lymph nodes. For cancers of the uterus and ovaries, stages range from I (the earliest) to IV (advanced). For the other gynecologic cancers, stage 0 is the earliest stage, when the cancer is confined to a surface of the affected organ. For some cancers, further distinctions, designated by letters of the alphabet, are made within stages.

Staging Cancers of the Female Reproductive System*

TYPE	STAGE 0	STAGE I	STAGE II	STAGE III	STAGE IV
Endo-metrial cancer	–	Only in the upper part of the uterus (not the cervix)	Spread to the cervix	Spread to nearby tissues but still within the pelvic area	A: Spread to the bladder or rectum B: Spread to distant organs
Ova-rian cancer	–	Only in one or both ovaries	Spread to the uterus, fallopian tubes, and/or nearby tissues within the pelvis	Spread outside the pelvis to the lymph nodes or other organs in the abdomen (such as the surface of the liver or intestine)	Spread outside the abdomen or to the inside of the liver

(Continued)

Staging Cancers of the Female Reproductive System* (Continued)

TYPE	STAGE 0	STAGE I	STAGE II	STAGE III	STAGE IV
Cervical cancer	Only on the surface of the cervix	Only in the cervix	Spread to nearby tissues but still within the pelvic area	Spread throughout the pelvic area, sometimes blocking the ureters	A: Spread to the bladder or rectum B: Spread to distant organs
Vulvar cancer	Only on the surface of the vulva	Only in the vulva and/or the area between the opening of the rectum and vagina (perineum); ³/₄ inch (2 centimeters) or smaller	In the vulva and/or perineum, but larger than ³/₄ inch	In the vulva and/or perineum and spread to nearby tissues and/or lymph nodes	Spread beyond nearby tissues to the bladder, to the intestine, or to more distant lymph nodes
Vaginal cancer	Only in the lining of the vagina	Only in the vagina but deeper (in the wall)	Spread to nearby tissues but still within the pelvic area	Spread throughout the pelvic area and possibly to nearby organs and lymph nodes	A: Spread to the bladder or rectum B: Spread to distant organs
Fallopian tube cancer	Only in the lining of the fallopian tubes	Only in the fallopian tubes but deeper (in the wall)	Spread to nearby tissues but still within the pelvic area	Spread throughout the pelvic area and possibly to nearby organs and lymph nodes	Spread to distant organs

*Simplified from the International Federation of Gynecology and Obstetrics staging system.

Treatment

The main treatment of gynecologic cancer is surgical removal of the tumor. Surgery may be followed by radiation therapy or chemotherapy. Radiation therapy may be external (using a large machine) or internal (using radioactive implants placed directly on the cancer). External radiation therapy is usually given several days a week for several weeks. Internal radiation therapy involves staying in the hospital for several days while the implants are in place.

Chemotherapy may be given by injection or by mouth. Chemotherapy is given for 5 days to 6 weeks (depending on the drugs) followed by a recovery period of several weeks without chemotherapy. The cycle may be repeated several times. A woman may have to remain at the hospital while she receives chemotherapy.

When a gynecologic cancer is very advanced and a cure is not possible, radiation therapy or chemotherapy may still be recommended to reduce the size of the cancer or its metastases and to relieve pain and other symptoms. Women with incurable cancer should establish advance directives. Because end-of-life care has improved, more and more women with incurable cancer are able to die comfortably at home. Appropriate drugs can be used to relieve the anxiety and pain commonly experienced by people with incurable cancer.

Cancer of the Uterus

- Cancer of the uterus begins in the uterine lining (endometrium) and is called endometrial cancer.
- Abnormal vaginal bleeding is the main symptom.
- A biopsy and sometimes dilation and curettage is done to make the diagnosis.
- If the cancer is detected early, nearly 90% of women survive at least 5 years, and most are cured.
- Surgery is required, sometimes with chemotherapy, radiation therapy, a progestin, or a combination.

Cancer of the uterus begins in the lining of the uterus (endometrium) and is more precisely termed endometrial cancer (carcinoma). It is the most common gynecologic cancer and the fourth most common cancer among women. This cancer usually develops after menopause, most often in women aged 50 to 60.

Risk factors for endometrial cancer include the following:

- Early menarche (the start of menstrual periods), menopause after age 52, or both
- Menstrual problems (such as excessive bleeding, spotting between menstrual periods, or long intervals without periods)
- Never having had children
- Tumors that produce estrogen
- High doses of drugs that contain estrogen, such as estrogen therapy without a progestin (synthetic drugs similar to the hormone progesterone), taken after menopause
- Use of tamoxifen
- Obesity
- High blood pressure
- Diabetes
- Family history of cancer of the breast, ovaries, large intestine (colon), or lining of the uterus.

Many of these conditions increase the risk of endometrial cancer because they result in a high level of estrogen but not progesterone. Estrogen promotes the growth of tissue and rapid cell division in the lining of the uterus (endometrium). Progesterone helps balance the effects of estrogen. Levels of estrogen are high during part of the menstrual cycle. Thus, having more menstrual periods during a lifetime may increase the risk of endometrial cancer. Tamoxifen, a drug used to treat breast cancer, blocks the effects of estrogen in the breast, but it has the same effects as estrogen in the uterus. Thus, this drug may increase the risk of endometrial cancer. Taking oral contraceptives that contain estrogen and a progestin appears to reduce the risk of endometrial cancer.

More than 80% of endometrial cancers are adenocarcinomas, which develop from gland cells. About 5% are sarcomas, which develop from connective tissue and tend to be more aggressive.

Symptoms and Diagnosis

Abnormal bleeding from the vagina is the most common early symptom. Abnormal bleeding includes bleeding after menopause or between menstrual periods and periods that are irregular, heavy, or longer than normal. One of three women with vaginal bleeding after menopause has endometrial cancer. Women who have vaginal bleeding after menopause should see a doctor promptly. A watery, blood-tinged discharge may also occur. Post-menopausal women may have a vaginal discharge for several weeks or months, followed by vaginal bleeding.

If doctors suspect endometrial cancer or if Papanicolaou (Pap) test results are abnormal, doctors perform an endometrial biopsy in their office. This test accurately detects endometrial cancer more than 90% of the time. If the diagnosis is still uncertain, doctors perform dilation and curettage (D and C—see page 129), in which tissue is scraped from the uterine lining. At the same time, doctors may view the interior of the uterus using a thin, flexible viewing tube inserted through the vagina and cervix into the uterus in a procedure called hysteroscopy.

If endometrial cancer is diagnosed, some or all of the following procedures may be performed to determine whether the cancer has spread beyond the uterus: blood tests, liver function tests, a chest x-ray, and computed tomography (CT) or magnetic resonance imaging (MRI). Other procedures are sometimes required. Staging is based on information obtained from these procedures and during surgery to remove the cancer.

DID YOU KNOW?

- Endometrial cancer is the most common cancer of the female reproductive organs.
- Taking oral contraceptives that contain estrogen and a progestin appears to reduce the risk of endometrial cancer.
- One of three women with vaginal bleeding after menopause has endometrial cancer.

Prognosis and Treatment

If endometrial cancer is detected early, nearly 90% of women who have it survive at least 5 years, and most are cured. The prognosis is better for women whose cancer has not spread beyond the uterus. If the cancer grows relatively slowly, the prognosis is also better. Fewer than one third of women who have this cancer die of it.

Hysterectomy, the surgical removal of the uterus, is the mainstay of treatment for women who have endometrial cancer. If the cancer has not spread beyond the uterus, removal of the uterus plus removal of the fallopian tubes and ovaries (salpingo-oophorectomy) almost always cures the cancer. Nearby lymph nodes are usually removed at the same time. These tissues are examined by a pathologist to determine whether the cancer has

---

UNDERSTANDING HYSTERECTOMY

A hysterectomy is the removal of the uterus. Usually, the uterus is removed through an incision in the lower abdomen. Sometimes the uterus can be removed through the vagina. Either method usually takes about 1 to 2 hours and requires a general anesthetic. Afterward, vaginal bleeding and pain may occur. The hospital stay is usually 2 to 3 days, and recovery may take up to 6 weeks. When the uterus is removed through the vagina, less bleeding occurs, recovery is faster, and there is no visible scar.

In addition to treatment of certain gynecologic cancers, a hysterectomy may be performed to treat prolapse of the uterus, endometriosis, or fibroids (if causing severe symptoms). Sometimes it is performed to treat cancer of the colon, rectum, or bladder.

There are several types of hysterectomy. The type used depends on the disorder being treated. For a subtotal hysterectomy, only the upper part of the uterus is removed, but the cervix is not. The fallopian tubes and ovaries may or may not be removed. For a total hysterectomy, the entire uterus including the cervix is removed. For a radical hysterectomy, the entire uterus plus the surrounding tissues, ligaments, and lymph nodes are removed. Both fallopian tubes and ovaries are usually also removed in women older than 45.

After a hysterectomy, menstruation stops. However, a hysterectomy does not cause menopause unless the ovaries are also removed. Removal of the ovaries has the same effects as menopause, so hormone therapy may be recommended (see page 138). Many women anticipate feeling depressed or losing interest in sex after a hysterectomy. However, hysterectomy rarely has these effects unless the ovaries are also removed.

spread and, if so, how far it has spread. With this information, doctors can determine whether additional treatment (chemotherapy, radiation therapy, or a progestin) is needed after surgery.

Chemotherapy may be given after surgery, even when the cancer does not appear to have spread, in case some undetected cancer cells remain. More than half of women with cancer limited to the uterus do not need radiation therapy. However, if the cancer has spread, radiation therapy is usually needed after surgery.

A progestin is often effective. (Progestins are synthetic drugs similar to the hormone progesterone, which blocks the effects of estrogen on the uterus.) If the cancer has spread beyond the uterus, higher doses may be needed. In 15 to 30% of women who have cancer that has spread, a progestin reduces the cancer's size and controls its spread for 2 to 3 years or longer. A progestin may be continued as long as it seems to be working well. Side effects may include mood changes and weight gain due to water retention.

If the cancer has spread, is not responding to a progestin, or recurs, chemotherapy drugs (such as cisplatin, cyclophosphamide, doxorubicin, and paclitaxel) may be used instead of or sometimes with radiation therapy. These drugs are much more toxic than progestins and cause many side effects. However, they reduce the cancer's size and control its spread in more than half of women treated.

Cancer of the Ovaries

- Women have symptoms only after ovarian cancer is advanced and then often experience only vague discomfort in the lower abdomen, bloating, and loss of appetite.
- When an enlarged ovary is detected during a physical examination, ultrasonography, computed tomography, magnetic resonance imaging, or sometimes laparoscopy is done.
- Ovarian cancer is often fatal because it is advanced when diagnosed.
- Surgery to remove as much of the cancer as possible is done, usually followed by chemotherapy.

Cancer of the ovaries (ovarian carcinoma) develops most often in women aged 50 to 70. This cancer eventually develops in about

1 of 70 women. It is the second most common gynecologic cancer. However, more women die of ovarian cancer than of any other gynecologic cancer.

The risk of this cancer is higher in industrialized countries because the diet tends to be high in fat. Risk is increased for women who were unable to become pregnant, who had their first child late in life, who started menstruating early, or who reached menopause late. Risk is also increased for women who have a family history of cancer of the uterus, breast, or large intestine (colon). Less than 5% of ovarian cancer cases are related to the BRCA1 gene, which is also related to breast cancer. Use of oral contraceptives significantly decreases risk.

There are many types of ovarian cancer. They develop from the many different types of cells in the ovaries. Cancers that start on the surface of the ovaries (epithelial carcinomas) account for more than 80%. Most other ovarian cancers are germ cell tumors (which start from the cells that produce eggs) and stromal cell tumors (which start in connective tissue). Germ cell tumors are much more common among women younger than 30. Sometimes cancers from other parts of the body spread to the ovaries.

Ovarian cancer can spread directly to the surrounding area and through the lymphatic system to other parts of the pelvis and abdomen. It can also spread through the bloodstream, eventually appearing in distant parts of the body, mainly the liver and lungs.

DID YOU KNOW?

- More women die of ovarian cancer than any other cancer of the female reproductive organs.
- Ovarian cancer is more common in industrialized countries.
- An enlarged ovary may indicate cancer in postmenopausal women but is likely to result from cysts in younger women.

Symptoms and Diagnosis

Ovarian cancer causes the affected ovary to enlarge. In young women, enlargement of an ovary is likely to be caused by a non-cancerous fluid-filled sac (cyst). However, after menopause, an enlarged ovary is often a sign of ovarian cancer.

Many women have no symptoms until the cancer is advanced. The first symptom may be vague discomfort in the lower abdomen, similar to indigestion. Other symptoms may include bloating, loss of appetite (because the stomach is compressed), gas pains, and backache. Ovarian cancer rarely causes vaginal bleeding.

Eventually, the abdomen may swell because the ovary enlarges or fluid accumulates in the abdomen. At this stage, pain in the pelvic area, anemia, and weight loss are common. Rarely, germ cell or stromal cell tumors produce estrogens, which can cause tissue in the uterine lining to grow excessively and breasts to enlarge. Or these tumors may produce male hormones (androgens), which can cause body hair to grow excessively, or hormones that resemble thyroid hormones, which can cause hyperthyroidism.

Diagnosing ovarian cancer in its early stages is difficult, because symptoms usually do not appear until the cancer is quite large or has spread beyond the ovaries and because many less serious disorders cause similar symptoms.

If doctors detect an enlarged ovary during a physical examination, they order ultrasonography, computed tomography (CT), or magnetic resonance imaging (MRI) to help distinguish an ovarian cyst from a cancerous mass. If cancer seems unlikely, doctors reexamine the woman every few months. If doctors suspect cancer or test results are unclear, the ovaries are examined using a thin, flexible viewing tube (laparoscope) inserted through a small incision just below the navel. Also, tissue samples are removed using instruments threaded through the laparoscope. In addition, blood tests are usually performed to measure levels of substances that may indicate the presence of cancer (tumor markers), such as cancer antigen 125 (CA 125). Abnormal marker levels alone do not confirm the diagnosis of cancer, but when combined with other information, they can help confirm it.

If fluid has accumulated in the abdomen, it can be drawn out (aspirated) through a needle and tested to see whether cancer cells are present.

Prognosis and Treatment

If ovarian cancer is suspected or confirmed, surgery is performed to remove the mass and to determine how far the cancer has spread (its stage). The prognosis is based on the stage (see page 237). With treatment, 70 to 100% of women with stage I cancer and 50 to 70% of those with stage II cancer are alive 5 years after diagnosis. Only 5 to 40% of women with stage III or IV cancer are alive after 5 years.

The extent of surgery depends on the type of ovarian cancer and the stage. If the cancer has not spread beyond the ovary, removal of only the affected ovary and the adjoining fallopian tube may be sufficient. When cancer has spread beyond the ovary, both ovaries and fallopian tubes and the uterus are removed, as are nearby lymph nodes and surrounding structures that the cancer typically spreads through. If a woman has stage I cancer that affects only one ovary and she wishes to become pregnant, doctors may remove only the

---

WHAT IS AN OVARIAN CYST?

An ovarian cyst is a fluid-filled sac in or on an ovary. Such cysts are relatively common. Most are noncancerous and disappear on their own. Cancerous cysts are more likely to occur in women older than 40.

Most noncancerous ovarian cysts do not cause symptoms. However, some cause pressure, aching, or a feeling of heaviness in the abdomen. Pain may be felt during sexual intercourse. If a cyst ruptures or becomes twisted, severe stabbing pain is felt in the abdomen. The pain may be accompanied by nausea and fever. Some cysts produce hormones that affect menstrual periods. As a result, periods may be irregular or heavier than normal. In postmenopausal women, such cysts may cause vaginal bleeding. Women who have any of these symptoms should see a doctor.

Diagnosis begins with a pelvic examination. Ultrasonography or computed tomography (CT) may be performed to confirm the diagnosis. If the cyst appears to be noncancerous, a woman may be asked to return periodically for pelvic examinations as long as the cyst remains. If the cyst could be cancerous, the ovaries may be examined through a laparoscope, inserted through a small incision just below the navel. Blood tests can help confirm or rule out cancer.

For noncancerous cysts, no treatment is necessary. But if a cyst is larger than about 2 inches (5 centimeters) and persists or if cancer cannot be ruled out, the cyst may be removed. Sometimes the affected ovary is also removed. Cancerous cysts plus the affected ovary and fallopian tube are removed.

affected ovary and fallopian tube. For more advanced cancers that have spread to other parts of the body, removing as much of the cancer as possible improves the prognosis.

After surgery, women with stage I epithelial carcinomas usually require no further treatment. For other stage I cancers or for more advanced cancers, chemotherapy may be used to destroy any small areas of cancer that may remain. Chemotherapy consists of paclitaxel combined with cisplatin or carboplatin. Most women with advanced germ cell tumors can be cured with combination chemotherapy, usually with bleomycin, etoposide, and cisplatin. Radiation therapy is rarely used.

Advanced ovarian cancer usually recurs. So after chemotherapy, doctors typically measure levels of cancer markers. If the cancer recurs, chemotherapy (using such drugs as topotecan, hexamethylmelamine, ifosfamide, doxorubicin, or etoposide) is given.

Cancer of the Cervix

- Cervical cancer is caused by the human papillomavirus, which is transmitted through sexual intercourse.
- Most women have no symptoms at first, but later, abnormal vaginal bleeding is common.
- A Papanicolaou (Pap) test can detect most cervical cancers.
- A new vaccine against human papillomavirus can help prevent cervical cancer.
- Surgery, radiation therapy, chemotherapy, or a combination is required.

The cervix is the lower part of the uterus. It extends into the vagina. Of gynecologic cancers, cervical cancer (cervical carcinoma) is the third most common among all women and the most common among younger women. It usually affects women aged 35 to 55, but it can affect women as young as 20.

This cancer is caused by the human papillomavirus which is transmitted during sexual intercourse. This virus also causes genital warts (see page 80). The younger a woman was the first time she had sexual intercourse and the more sex partners she has had, the higher her risk of cervical cancer.

About 85% of cervical cancers are squamous cell carcinomas, which develop in the scaly, flat, skinlike cells covering the cervix. Most other cervical cancers are adenocarcinomas, which develop from gland cells, or adenosquamous carcinomas, which develop from a combination of cell types.

Cervical cancer begins on the surface of the cervix and can penetrate deep beneath the surface. The cancer can spread directly to nearby tissues, including the vagina. Or it can enter the rich network of small blood and lymphatic vessels inside the cervix, then spread to other parts of the body.

Symptoms and Diagnosis

In the early stages, cervical cancer usually causes no symptoms. It may cause spotting or heavier bleeding between periods, bleeding after intercourse, or unusually heavy periods. In later stages, such abnormal bleeding is common. Other symptoms may include a foul-smelling discharge from the vagina, pain in the pelvic area or lower back, and swelling of the legs. The urinary tract may be blocked; without treatment, kidney failure and death can result.

Routine Papanicolaou (Pap) tests or other similar tests can detect the beginnings of cervical cancer (see page 125). Cervical cancer begins with slow, progressive changes in normal cells on the surface of the cervix. These changes are called dysplasia. Untreated, these cells may become cancerous with time, sometimes after years. When performing a Pap test, doctors look for these changes as well as for cancer. Women with dysplasia should be checked again in 3 to 4 months.

DID YOU KNOW?

- Among young women, cervical cancer is the most common cancer of the female reproductive organs.
- If all women had regular Pap tests, deaths from this cancer could be virtually eliminated.
- About half of women in the United States do not have regular Pap tests.

A Pap test can accurately and inexpensively detect up to 90% of cervical cancers, even before symptoms develop. Consequently, the number of deaths due to cervical cancer has been reduced by more than 50% since Pap tests were introduced. Doctors often recommend that women have their first Pap test when they become sexually active or reach the age of 18 and that a Pap test be performed annually. If test results are normal for 3 consecutive years, women may schedule Pap tests every 2 or 3 years as long as they do not change their sexual lifestyle. Any woman who has had cervical cancer or dysplasia should continue to have Pap tests at least annually. If all women had Pap tests on a regular basis, deaths from this cancer could be virtually eliminated. However, about 50% of American women are not tested regularly.

If a growth, a sore, or another abnormal area is seen on the cervix during a pelvic examination or if a Pap test detects an abnormality or cancer, a biopsy is performed. Usually, doctors use an instrument with a binocular magnifying lens (colposcope) to examine the cervix and to choose the best biopsy site. Two different types of biopsy are performed. In a punch biopsy, a tiny piece of the cervix, selected using the colposcope, is removed. In endocervical curettage, tissue that cannot be viewed is scraped from inside the cervix. These biopsies cause little pain and a small amount of bleeding. The two together usually provide enough tissue for pathologists to make a diagnosis.

If the diagnosis is not clear, doctors perform a cone biopsy to remove a larger cone-shaped piece of tissue. Usually, a thin wire loop with an electrical current running through it is used. This procedure is called the loop electrosurgical excision procedure (LEEP). Alternatively, a laser (using a highly focused beam of light) can be used. Either procedure requires only a local anesthetic and can be performed in the doctor's office. A cold (nonelectric) knife is sometimes used, but this procedure requires an operating room and an anesthetic.

If cervical cancer is diagnosed, its exact size and locations (its stage) are determined. Staging begins with a physical examination of the pelvis and various procedures (such as cystoscopy, a chest x-ray, intravenous urography, and sigmoidoscopy) to determine whether the cancer has spread to nearby tissues or to distant parts of the body. Other procedures, such as computed tomography

(CT), magnetic resonance imaging (MRI), a barium enema, and bone and liver scans, may be performed.

Prognosis and Treatment

Vaccination against most of the human papillomaviruses that cause cervical cancer and genital warts is available in the US for girls and women 9 to 26 years old. The vaccine should be administered before the onset of sexual activity, but girls and women who are sexually active should still be vaccinated. The vaccine is highly effective and an important preventive measure against the development of cervical cancer.

Prognosis depends on the stage of the cancer (see page 238). With treatment, 80 to 90% of women with stage I cancer and 50 to 65% of those with stage II cancer are alive 5 years after diagnosis. Only 25 to 35% of women with stage III cancer and 15% or fewer of those with stage IV cancer are alive after 5 years.

Treatment also depends on the stage. If only the surface of the cervix is involved, doctors can often completely remove the cancer by removing part of the cervix using the loop electrosurgical excision procedure, a laser, or a cold knife. Or cryotherapy may be used to destroy the cancer by freezing it. These treatments preserve a woman's ability to have children. Because cancer can recur, doctors advise women to return for examinations and Pap tests every 3 months for the first year and every 6 months after that. Rarely, removal of the uterus (hysterectomy) is necessary.

If the cancer has begun to spread within the pelvic area, hysterectomy plus removal of surrounding tissues, ligaments, and lymph nodes (radical hysterectomy) is necessary. The ovaries may be removed. Normal, functioning ovaries in younger women are not removed. Alternatively, radiation therapy may be used. It usually causes few or no immediate side effects, but it may irritate the bladder or rectum. Later, as a result, the intestine may become blocked, and the bladder and rectum may be damaged. Also, the ovaries usually stop functioning. With either radical hysterectomy or radiation therapy, about 85 to 90% of women are cured.

If the cancer has spread further within the pelvis or to other organs, radiation therapy is preferred. This treatment is ineffective in about 40% of women with large or extensive cancers.

When the cancer has spread extensively or recurs, chemotherapy, usually with cisplatin and ifosfamide, is sometimes recommended. However, chemotherapy reduces the cancer's size and controls its spread in only 25 to 30% of women treated, and this effect is usually temporary.

Cancer of the Vulva

- Vulvar cancer is usually a skin cancer that develops near the opening of the vagina.
- Unusual lumps or flat, red sores, often accompanied by itching, appear and do not heal.
- A biopsy is needed to confirm the diagnosis.
- Surgery is required, sometimes with radiation therapy, chemotherapy, or both.

The vulva refers to the area that contains the external female reproductive organs. Cancer of the vulva (vulvar carcinoma) is the fourth most common gynecologic cancer, accounting for only 3 to 4% of these cancers. Vulvar cancer usually occurs after menopause. The average age at diagnosis is 70 years. As more women live longer, this cancer is likely to become more common.

The risk of developing vulvar cancer is increased for women who have persistent itching of the vulva, have genital warts due to human papillomavirus (HPV), or have had cancer of the vagina or cervix.

Most vulvar cancers are skin cancers that develop near or at the opening of the vagina. About 90% of vulvar cancers are squamous cell carcinomas, and 5% are melanomas. The remaining 5% include basal cell carcinomas and rare cancers such as Paget's disease and cancer of Bartholin's gland.

Vulvar cancer begins on the surface of the vulva. Most of these cancers grow slowly, remaining on the surface for years. However, some grow quickly. Untreated, vulvar cancer can eventually invade the vagina, the urethra, or the anus and spread into lymph nodes in the area.

Symptoms and Diagnosis

White, brown, or red patches on the vulva are precancerous; that is, they may indicate that cancer is likely to eventually develop. Vulvar cancer is usually seen and felt as unusual lumps or flat, red sores that do not heal. Sometimes scaly patches develop or the area becomes discolored. The surrounding tissue may contract and pucker. Usually, vulvar cancer causes little discomfort, but itching is common. Eventually, the lump or sore may bleed or produce a watery discharge (weep). These symptoms should be evaluated promptly by a doctor. About one fifth of women have no symptoms, at least at first.

Doctors diagnose vulvar cancer by performing a biopsy of the abnormal skin. The biopsy can identify whether the abnormal skin is cancerous or just infected or irritated. It also identifies the type of cancer, if present, so that doctors can develop a treatment plan. Sometimes doctors apply stains to the sores to help determine where to take a sample of tissue for a biopsy. Sometimes an instrument with a binocular magnifying lens (colposcope) is used to examine the surface of the vulva.

DID YOU KNOW?

- White, blue, brown, or red patches on the vulva may be an early sign of cancer.

Prognosis and Treatment

If vulvar cancer is detected early, about 3 of 4 women have no sign of cancer 5 years after diagnosis. If the lymph nodes are involved, less than one third of women survive for 5 years.

Because most vulvar cancers can spread quickly, surgical removal of the vulva (vulvectomy) is usually necessary. Depending on the extent of the cancer, all or part of the vulva is removed. Sometimes nearby lymph nodes are also removed. Treatment with radiation therapy, chemotherapy, or both may be used to shrink very large cancers so that they can be surgically removed. Sometimes the clitoris must be removed. Doctors work closely with the woman to develop a treatment plan that is best suited to her and takes into account her age, sexual lifestyle, and any other medical problems. Sexual intercourse is usually possible after vulvectomy.

For some small vulvar cancers that do not extend below the skin, treatment consists of removal with a highly focused beam of light (laser surgery), surgical removal of only the skin, or use of an ointment containing a chemotherapy drug (such as fluorouracil). Some small cancers are treated with radiation therapy alone.

Because basal cell carcinoma of the vulva does not tend to spread (metastasize) to distant sites, surgery usually involves removing only the cancer. The whole vulva is removed only if the cancer is extensive.

Cancer of the Vagina

- Vaginal cancer is often caused by the same virus that causes cervical cancer.
- The main symptom is abnormal vaginal bleeding.
- Evaluation of cells scraped from the vaginal wall or biopsy is needed to confirm the diagnosis.
- Surgery, sometimes with radiation therapy, or radiation therapy plus chemotherapy is required.

Only about 1% of gynecologic cancers occur in the vagina. Cancer of the vagina (vaginal carcinoma) usually affects women older than 45. The average age at diagnosis is 60 to 65.

More than 95% of vaginal cancers are squamous cell carcinomas. Vaginal squamous cell carcinoma may be caused by human papillomavirus (HPV), the same virus that causes genital warts and cervical cancer. Most other vaginal cancers are adenocarcinomas. One rare type, clear cell carcinoma, occurs almost exclusively in women whose mothers took the drug diethylstilbestrol (DES), prescribed to prevent miscarriage during pregnancy. (In 1971, the drug was banned in the United States.)

Depending on the type, vaginal cancer may begin on the surface of the vaginal lining. If untreated, it continues to grow and invades surrounding tissue. Eventually, it may spread to other parts of the body.

Symptoms and Diagnosis

The most common symptom is bleeding from the vagina, which may occur during or after sexual intercourse, between menstrual periods, or after menopause. Sores may form on the lining of the vagina. They may bleed and become infected. Other symptoms include a watery discharge and pain during sexual intercourse. A few women have no symptoms. Large cancers can also affect the bladder, causing a frequent urge to urinate and pain during urination. In advanced cancer, abnormal connections (fistulas) may form between the vagina and the bladder or rectum.

Doctors may suspect vaginal cancer on the basis of symptoms, abnormal areas seen during a routine pelvic examination, or an abnormal Papanicolaou (Pap) test result. Doctors may use an instrument with a binocular magnifying lens (colposcope) to examine the vagina. To confirm the diagnosis, doctors scrape cells from the vaginal wall to examine under a microscope. They also perform a biopsy on any growth, sore, or other abnormal area seen during the examination.

Prognosis and Treatment

The prognosis depends on the stage of the cancer (see page 238). If the cancer is limited to the vagina, about 65 to 70% of women survive at least 5 years after diagnosis. If the cancer has spread beyond the pelvis or to the bladder or rectum, only about 15 to 20% survive.

Treatment also depends on the stage. For most vaginal cancers, surgery is the treatment of choice, with or without radiation therapy. Radiation therapy may be internal (using radioactive implants placed inside the vagina) or external (directed at the pelvis from outside the body). Radiation therapy is often combined with or followed by surgical removal of the cancer. For cancer in the upper third of the vagina, a hysterectomy with removal of lymph nodes in the pelvis and the upper part of the vagina may be needed. For very advanced cancer, surgery is often not possible. In such cases, radiation therapy and chemotherapy are usually used.

Intercourse may be difficult or impossible after treatment for vaginal cancer, although sometimes a new vagina can be constructed with skin grafts or part of the intestine.

Cancer of the Fallopian Tubes

- Fallopian tube cancer causes vague abdominal or pelvic discomfort or pain and an enlarged mass in the pelvis.

- Doctors use a laparoscope to view the tubes, and if they see a mass, they remove it for biopsy.
- Surgery and chemotherapy are usually needed, and radiation therapy is sometimes useful.

The fallopian tubes lead from the ovaries to the uterus. Less than 1% of gynecologic cancers are fallopian tube cancers. Most often, cancer that affects the fallopian tubes is cancer that has spread from the ovaries rather than started in the fallopian tubes. Fallopian tube cancer usually affects women aged 50 to 60. Occasionally, it appears to be associated with having been infertile.

More than 95% of fallopian tube cancers are adenocarcinomas, which develop from gland cells. A few are sarcomas, which develop from connective tissue. Fallopian tube cancer spreads in much the same way as ovarian cancer.

Symptoms and Diagnosis

Symptoms include vague abdominal discomfort, bloating, and pain in the pelvic area or abdomen. Some women have a watery or blood-tinged discharge from the vagina. Usually, an enlarged mass is found in the pelvis.

The diagnosis is made by viewing the fallopian tubes and surrounding tissues through a thin viewing tube (laparoscope) inserted through a small incision just below the navel or by performing surgery to remove the mass. Biopsies of the surrounding tissues are performed.

Prognosis and Treatment

The prognosis is similar to that for women who have ovarian cancer. Treatment almost always consists of removal of the uterus (hysterectomy) and removal of the ovaries and fallopian tubes (salpingo-oophorectomy), adjacent lymph nodes, and surrounding tissues. Chemotherapy (as for ovarian cancer) is usually necessary after surgery. For some cancers, radiation therapy is useful. For cancer that has spread to other parts of the body, removing as much of the cancer as possible improves the prognosis.

Hydatidiform Mole

A hydatidiform mole is growth of an abnormal fertilized egg or an overgrowth of tissue from the placenta.

- A hydatidiform mole usually develops from an abnormal fertilized egg.
- Most moles are not cancerous and disappear spontaneously.
- A mole causes the abdomen to enlarge much faster than a normal uterus does during pregnancy and may cause severe nausea, vomiting, and vaginal bleeding.
- Ultrasonography and blood tests can distinguish a hydatidiform mole from a fetus.
- Usually, dilation and curettage with suction is effective, but cancerous moles require chemotherapy.

Most often, a hydatidiform mole is an abnormal fertilized egg. The abnormal egg develops into a hydatidiform mole rather than a fetus (a condition called molar pregnancy). However, a hydatidiform mole can develop from cells that remain in the uterus after a miscarriage or a full-term pregnancy. Rarely, a hydatidiform mole develops when the fetus is normal.

About 80% of hydatidiform moles are not cancerous and disappear spontaneously. About 15 to 20% invade the surrounding tissue and tend to persist. Of these invasive moles, 2 to 3% become cancerous and spread throughout the body; they are then called choriocarcinomas. Choriocarcinomas can spread quickly through the lymphatic vessels or bloodstream.

The risk of hydatidiform moles is highest for women who become pregnant before age 17 or in their late 30s or later. Hydatidiform moles occur in about 1 of 2,000 pregnancies in the United States and, for unknown reasons, are nearly 10 times more common among Asian women.

Symptoms and Diagnosis

Women who have a hydatidiform mole feel as if they are pregnant. But because hydatidiform moles grow much faster than a fetus, the abdomen becomes larger much faster than it does in a normal pregnancy. Severe nausea and vomiting are common, and vaginal bleeding may occur. These symptoms indicate the need for prompt evaluation by a doctor. Hydatidiform moles can cause serious complications, including infections, bleeding, and pre-eclampsia or eclampsia (see page 318).

Often, doctors can diagnose a hydatidiform mole shortly after conception. No fetal movement and no fetal heartbeat are detected. As parts of the mole decay, small amounts of tissue that resemble a bunch of grapes may pass through the vagina. After examining this tissue under a microscope, a pathologist can confirm the diagnosis.

Ultrasonography may be performed to be sure that the growth is a hydatidiform mole and not a fetus or amniotic sac (which contains the fetus and fluid around it). Blood tests to measure the level of human chorionic gonadotropin (HCG—a hormone normally produced early in pregnancy) may be performed. If a hydatidiform mole is present, the level is usually very high because the mole produces a large amount of this hormone.

DID YOU KNOW?

- Having a hydatidiform mole does not interfere with later childbearing.

Treatment

The cure rate for a hydatidiform mole is virtually 100% if the mole has not spread. The cure rate is 60 to 80% if the hydatidiform mole has spread widely. Most women can have children afterward and do not have a higher risk of having complications, a miscarriage, or children with birth defects. About 1% of women who have had a hydatidiform mole have another one. So for women who have had a hydatidiform mole, ultrasonography is performed early during subsequent pregnancies.

A hydatidiform mole that does not disappear spontaneously is completely removed usually by dilation and curettage (D and C) with suction (see page 129). Only rarely is removal of the uterus (hysterectomy) necessary.

If the hydatidiform mole is detected, a chest x-ray is performed after surgery to make sure that it has not become cancerous (that is, a choriocarcinoma) and spread to the lungs. After surgery, the level of human chorionic gonadotropin in the blood is measured to determine whether the hydatidiform mole was completely removed. When removal is complete, the level returns to normal, usually within 8 weeks, and remains normal. Women who have had a mole removed are advised not to become pregnant for 1 year.

Hydatidiform moles do not require chemotherapy, but choriocarcinomas do. Usually, only one drug (methotrexate or dactinomycin) is needed. Sometimes both or another combination of chemotherapy drugs is needed.

CHAPTER 19

Violence Against Women

Violence against women is broadly defined as any act that is likely to cause physical, sexual, or psychologic harm or extreme suffering to a woman. Violence can occur in the home, workplace, or community. Two common forms of violence against women are domestic violence and rape.

Domestic Violence

- Domestic violence includes physical, sexual, and psychologic abuse between intimate partners.
- The victim is usually a woman.
- Physical injuries, psychologic problems, social isolation, loss of a job, financial difficulties, and even death can result.
- Keeping safe—for example, having a plan of escape—is the most important consideration.

Domestic violence includes physical, sexual, and psychologic abuse between intimate partners. It occurs among people of all cultures, races, occupations, income levels, and ages. In the United States, as many as 30% of marriages are considered physically aggressive.

Women are more commonly victims of domestic violence than are men. About 95% of people who seek medical attention as a result of domestic violence are women. Women are more likely to be severely assaulted or killed by a male partner than by anyone else. Each year in the United States, about 2 million women are severely beaten by their partner.

Physical abuse is the most obvious form of domestic violence. It may include hitting, slapping, kicking, punching, breaking bones, pulling hair, pushing, and twisting arms. The victim may be deprived of food or sleep. Weapons, such as a gun or knife, may be used to threaten or cause injury.

Sexual assault is also common: 33 to 50% of women who are physically assaulted by their partner are also sexually assaulted by their partner. Sexual assault involves the use of threats or force to obtain unwanted sexual contact.

Psychologic abuse may be even more common than physical abuse and may precede it. Psychologic abuse involves any non-physical behavior that undermines or belittles the victim or that enables the perpetrator to control the victim. Psychologic abuse can include abusive language, social isolation, and financial control. Usually, the perpetrator uses language to demean, degrade, humiliate, intimidate, or threaten the victim in private or in public. The perpetrator may make the victim think she is crazy or make her feel guilty or responsible, blaming her for the abusive relationship. The perpetrator may also humiliate the victim in terms of her sexual performance, physical appearance, or both.

The perpetrator may try to partly or completely isolate the victim by controlling the victim's access to friends, relatives, and other people. Control may include forbidding direct, written, telephone, or e-mail contact with others. The perpetrator may use jealousy to justify his actions.

Often, the perpetrator withholds money to control the victim. The victim may depend on the perpetrator for most or all of her money. The perpetrator may maintain control by preventing the victim from getting a job, by keeping information about their finances from her, and by taking money from her.

DID YOU KNOW?

- In the United States, about 2 million women are severely beaten by their partners each year.
- The abusing partner may try to control the victim by limiting her access to other people, even by telephone or e-mail, and money.
- Victims of domestic violence may develop depression, anxiety, or drug or alcohol abuse.
- Women are in greatest danger of serious harm after their partner knows they have decided to leave.

Effects

A victim of domestic violence may be physically injured. Physical injuries can include bruises, black eyes, cuts, scratches, broken bones, lost teeth, and burns. Injuries may prevent the victim from going to work regularly, causing her to lose her job. Injuries, as well as the abusive situation, may embarrass the victim, causing her to isolate herself from family and friends. The victim may also have to move often—a financial burden—to escape the perpetrator. Sometimes the perpetrator kills the victim.

As a result of domestic violence, many victims have psychologic problems. Such problems include posttraumatic stress disorder, substance abuse, anxiety, and depression. About 60% of battered women are depressed. Women who are more severely battered are more likely to develop psychologic problems. Even when physical abuse decreases, psychologic abuse often continues, reminding the woman that she can be physically abused at any time. Abused women may feel that psychologic abuse is more damaging than physical abuse. Psychologic abuse increases the risk of depression and substance abuse.

Management

In cases of domestic violence, the most important consideration is safety. During a violent incident, the victim should try to move away from areas in which she can be trapped or in which

---

CHILDREN WHO WITNESS DOMESTIC VIOLENCE

Each year, at least 3.3 million children are estimated to witness physical or verbal abuse in their homes. These children may develop problems such as excessive anxiety or crying, fearfulness, difficulty sleeping, depression, social withdrawal, and difficulty in school. Also, children may blame themselves for the situation. Older children may run away from home. Boys who see their father abuse their mother may be more likely to become abusive adults. Girls who see their father abuse their mother may be more likely to tolerate abuse as adults. The perpetrator may also physically hurt the children. In homes where domestic violence is present, children are much more likely to be physically mistreated.

---

the perpetrator can obtain weapons, such as the kitchen. If she can, the victim should promptly call 911 or the police and leave the house. The victim should have any injuries treated and documented with photographs.

Developing a safety plan is important. It should include where to go for help, how to get away, and how to access money. The victim should also make and hide copies of official documents (such as children's birth certificates, social security cards, insurance cards, and bank account numbers). She should keep an overnight bag packed in case she needs to leave quickly.

Sometimes the only solution is to leave the abusive relationship permanently, because domestic violence tends to continue, especially among very aggressive men. Also, even when physical abuse decreases, psychologic abuse may persist. The decision to leave is not simple. After the perpetrator knows the victim has decided to leave, the victim's risk of serious harm may be greatest. At this time, the victim should take additional steps (such as obtaining a restraining or protection order) to protect herself and her children. Help is available through shelters for battered women, support groups, and the courts.

Rape

- Rape refers to unwanted penetration of the vagina, anus, or mouth.

- Victims may have tears in the vagina, cuts and bruises, upsetting emotions, and difficulty sleeping.
- Sexual transmitted diseases, including HIV (human immunodeficiency virus) infection, and pregnancy are risks.
- Women who are raped should be thoroughly evaluated in a center staffed by specially trained people (rape center).
- Treatment of physical injuries, antibiotics to prevent infections, emergency contraception, and counseling or psychotherapy may be needed.
- If possible, family members and close friends should meet with a member of the rape crisis team to discuss how to support a rape victim.

Rape is typically considered to be unwanted penetration of the victim's vagina, anus, or mouth. In victims younger than the age of consent, such penetration—whether wanted or not—is considered rape (statutory rape). Sexual assault is a broader term, including the use of force and threats to coerce sexual contact. The reported percentage of women who have been raped during their lifetime varies widely: from 2% to almost 30%. The reported percentage of children who are sexually abused is similarly high. Reported percentages are probably lower than the actual percentages, because rape and sexual abuse are less likely to be reported to the police than are other crimes.

Men are also raped. For men as for women, injuries may occur and the psychologic effects can be devastating.

Symptoms

Physical injuries resulting from a rape may include tears in the upper part of the vagina and injuries to other parts of the body, such as bruises, black eyes, cuts, and scratches.

The psychologic effects of a rape are often more devastating than the physical. Shortly after a rape occurs, almost all women have symptoms of posttraumatic stress disorder (which can occur after any stressful event. Women feel fearful, anxious, and irritable. They may feel angry, depressed, or guilty (wondering whether they may have done something to provoke the rape or could have done something to avoid it). They may have intrusive, upsetting thoughts about or mental images of the assault, and they may relive the rape. Or they may stifle thoughts and feelings about the rape. They may avoid situations that remind them of the rape. Difficulty sleeping and nightmares are common. These symptoms may last for months, interfering with social activities and work. However, for most women, symptoms lessen substantially over a period of months.

In addition to her own feelings, the rape victim may have to handle negative, sometimes judgmental or derisive reactions of friends, family members, and officials. These reactions can interfere with the victim's recovery.

After a rape, there is a risk of infection with sexually transmitted diseases (such as gonorrhea, chlamydial infection, and syphilis) and hepatitis B and C. Infection with the human immunodeficiency virus (HIV) is a particular concern, even though the chances of acquiring it in a single encounter are low. Rarely, a woman becomes pregnant.

DID YOU KNOW?

- The psychologic effects of being raped may last for months.
- Women who are raped often feel guilty about it.
- Family members and friends of rape victims sometimes react negatively to the victim.
- The best evidence of rape is obtained when the victim goes to the hospital as soon as possible, without showering, without changing clothes, and, if possible, without urinating.

Evaluation

Having a thorough medical evaluation after a rape is important. Whenever possible, women who have been raped or sexually assaulted are taken to a sexual assault evaluation treatment center that is separate from the emergency department and that is staffed by trained, concerned support personnel.

After a rape, doctors are required by law to notify the police and to examine the victim. The examination provides evidence for prosecution of the rapist and is necessary before medical care of the victim can begin. The best evidence is obtained when the rape victim goes to the hospital as soon as possible, without showering, without changing clothes, and, if possible, without even urinating. The medical record resulting from this examination is sometimes admissible in court as evidence. However, the medical record cannot be released unless the victim gives her consent in writing or a subpoena is issued. The record may also help the victim recall details of the rape if her testimony is required later.

Immediately after a rape, a woman may be afraid of undergoing a physical examination. If possible, a female doctor examines the woman. If not, a female nurse or volunteer is present to help allay any anxiety the woman may be feeling. Before beginning the examination, the doctor should ask the woman's permission to proceed. The woman should feel no pressure to consent, although consent is generally in her best interest. The woman can ask the doctor to explain what will happen during the examination so that she knows what to expect.

The doctor asks the woman to describe the events to help guide the examination and treatment. However, talking about the rape is often frightening for the woman. She may request to give a complete description later, after her immediate needs have been met. She may first need to be treated for injuries, to clean up, and to have some time for calming down. The woman, if she wishes, is provided with bathroom facilities so that she can wash.

To help determine the likelihood of pregnancy, the doctor asks the woman when her last menstrual period was and whether she uses a contraceptive. To help interpret the analysis of any sperm samples, the doctor asks the woman if she recently had sex before the rape and, if so, when.

The doctor notes physical injuries, such as cuts and scrapes, and may examine the vagina for injuries. Photographs of injuries are taken. Because some injuries such as bruises become apparent later, a second set of photographs may be taken later. A swab is used to take samples of semen and other body fluids for evidence. Other samples, such as samples of the perpetrator's hair, blood, or skin (sometimes found under the woman's nails), are collected. Sometimes DNA testing of the samples is performed to identify the perpetrator.

If the woman consents, blood tests are performed to check for infections, including HIV infection. If the initial test results for gonorrhea, chlamydial infection, syphilis, and hepatitis are negative, the woman is tested again within 6 weeks. If results for syphilis and hepatitis are still negative, tests are repeated at 6 months. Blood tests for HIV infection may be repeated after 90 and 120 days.

Usually, a pregnancy test (to measure the level of human chorionic gonadotropin in the urine—see page 268) is performed within a few days and again within 6 weeks. If the woman may have been pregnant before the rape, the urine test is performed during the initial examination. The test cannot detect a pregnancy that has just occurred. Thus, performed at this time, the test would detect a preexisting pregnancy, but not one that resulted from the rape.

Treatment

Most physical injuries are easily treated. Severe injuries may require surgery. For preventing infections, the woman is given antibiotics, typically one dose of ceftriaxone injected into a muscle, one dose of metronidazole given by mouth, and doxycycline given by mouth for 7 days. If test results for HIV were positive, treatment for HIV is started immediately (see page 95).

If pregnancy is a concern, emergency contraception may be used. A high dose of an oral contraceptive is given immediately, then repeated 12 hours later (see page 38). This treatment is 99% effective if given within 72 hours of the rape. If the woman may have been pregnant before the rape, the oral contraceptive is given only if results from the pregnancy test do not detect pregnancy. If pregnancy results from the rape, abortion can be considered.

Common psychologic reactions to the rape (such as excessive anxiety or fear) are explained to the woman. As soon as feasible, a person trained in rape crisis intervention meets with her. The woman is referred to a rape crisis team if one is located in the area. This team can provide helpful medical, psychologic, and legal support. For the woman, talking about the rape and her feelings about it can help her recover. If symptoms of posttraumatic stress disorder persist, psychotherapy or antidepressants can be effective. If necessary, the woman can be referred to a psychologist, social worker, or psychiatrist.

Family members and friends may have some of the same feelings as the victim: anxiety, anger, or guilt. They may irrationally blame the victim. Family members or close friends may benefit from meeting with a member of the rape crisis team or sexual assault evaluation unit to discuss their feelings and how they can help the victim. Usually, listening supportively to the victim and not expressing strong feelings about the rape are most helpful. Blaming or criticizing the victim may interfere with her recovery. A support network of health care workers, friends, and family members can be very helpful to the victim.

CHAPTER 20

Normal Pregnancy

Pregnancy begins when an egg is fertilized by a sperm. For about 9 months, a pregnant woman's body provides a protective, nourishing environment in which the fertilized egg can develop into a fetus. Pregnancy ends at delivery, when a baby is born.

Detecting and Dating a Pregnancy

- When a woman's menstrual period is late, doctors test a urine sample to determine whether she is pregnant.
- Ultrasonography is usually done during the first 12 weeks to help establish an accurate due date.

If a menstrual period is a week or more late in a woman who usually has regular menstrual periods, she may be pregnant. Sometimes a woman may guess she is pregnant because she has typical symptoms. They include enlarged and tender breasts, nausea with occasional vomiting, a need to urinate frequently, unusual fatigue, and changes in appetite.

When a menstrual period is late, a woman may wish to use a home pregnancy test to determine whether she is pregnant. Home pregnancy tests detect human chorionic gonadotropin (HCG) in the urine. Human chorionic gonadotropin is a hormone produced by the placenta. Results of home pregnancy tests are accurate about 97% of the time. If results are negative but the woman still suspects she is pregnant, she should repeat the home pregnancy test a few days later. The first test may have been performed too early (before the next menstrual period is expected to start). If results are positive, the woman should contact her doctor, who may perform another pregnancy test to confirm the results.

Doctors test a sample of blood or urine from the woman to determine whether she is pregnant. These tests are very accurate. One of these tests, called an enzyme-linked immunosorbent assay (ELISA), can quickly and easily detect a low level of human chorionic gonadotropin in the urine. Some tests can detect the very low level that is present about 1½ weeks after fertilization (before a menstrual period is missed). Results may be available in about half an hour. During the first 60 days of a normal pregnancy with one fetus, the level of human chorionic gonadotropin in the blood approximately doubles about every 2 days. Measurement of these levels during the pregnancy can be used to determine whether the pregnancy is progressing normally.

After pregnancy is confirmed, the doctor asks the woman when her last menstrual period was. Pregnancies are conventionally dated in weeks, starting from the first day of the last menstrual period. The doctor calculates the approximate date of delivery by counting back 3 calendar months from the first day of the last menstrual period and adding 1 year and 7 days. Only 10% or fewer of pregnant women give birth on the calculated date, but 50% give birth within 1 week and almost 90% give birth within 2 weeks (before or after the date). Delivery between 3 weeks before and 2 weeks after the calculated date is considered normal.

Ovulation usually occurs about 2 weeks after a woman's menstrual period starts, and fertilization usually occurs shortly after ovulation. Consequently, the embryo is about 2 weeks younger than the number of weeks traditionally assigned to the pregnancy. In other words, a woman who is 4 weeks pregnant is carrying a 2-week-old embryo. If a woman's periods are irregular, the actual difference may be more or less than 2 weeks. Pregnancy lasts an average of 266 days (38 weeks) from the date of fertilization (conception) or 280 days (40 weeks) from the first day of the last menstrual period if the woman has regular 28-day periods. Pregnancy is divided into three 3-month periods, based on the date of the last menstrual period. They are called the 1st trimester (0 to 12 weeks of pregnancy), 2nd trimester (13 to 24 weeks), and 3rd trimester (25 weeks to delivery).

If a woman and her doctor cannot confidently calculate when she became pregnant based on her menstrual period, ultrasonography may be performed to measure the fetus and thus establish the date. For the most accurate measurements, ultrasonography is performed during the first 12 weeks of a pregnancy. An accurate date helps doctors determine whether the pregnancy is progressing normally.

Stages of Development

- The egg is fertilized in a fallopian tube, then implants in the uterus, where it develops into an embryo, then a fetus.

A baby goes through several stages of development, beginning as a fertilized egg. The egg develops into a blastocyst, an embryo, then a fetus.

Fertilization

During each normal menstrual cycle, one egg (ovum) is usually released from one of the ovaries, about 14 days before the next menstrual period. Release of the egg is called ovulation. The egg is swept into the funnel-shaped end of one of the fallopian tubes.

At ovulation, the mucus in the cervix becomes more fluid and more elastic, allowing sperm to enter the uterus rapidly. Within 5 minutes, sperm may move from the vagina, through the cervix into the uterus, and to the funnel-shaped end of a fallopian tube—the usual site of fertilization. The cells lining the fallopian tube facilitate fertilization.

If a sperm penetrates the egg, fertilization results. Tiny hairlike cilia lining the fallopian tube propel the fertilized egg (zygote) through the tube toward the uterus. The cells of the zygote divide repeatedly as the zygote moves down the fallopian tube. The zygote enters the uterus in 3 to 5 days. In the uterus, the cells continue to divide, becoming a hollow ball of cells called a blastocyst. If fertilization does not occur, the egg degenerates and passes through the uterus with the next menstrual period.

If more than one egg is released and fertilized, the pregnancy involves more than one fetus, usually two (twins). Such twins are fraternal. Identical twins result when one fertilized egg separates into two embryos after it has begun to divide.

Development of the Blastocyst

Between 5 and 8 days after fertilization, the blastocyst attaches to the lining of the uterus, usually near the top. This process, called implantation, is completed by day 9 or 10.

The wall of the blastocyst is one cell thick except in one area, where it is three to four cells thick. The inner cells in the thickened area develop into the embryo, and the outer cells burrow into the wall of the uterus and develop into the placenta. The placenta produces several hormones that help maintain the pregnancy. For example, the placenta produces human chorionic gonadotropin, which prevents the ovaries from releasing eggs and stimulates the ovaries to produce estrogen and progesterone continuously. The placenta also carries oxygen and nutrients from mother to fetus and waste materials from fetus to mother.

The wall of the blastocyst becomes the outer layer of membranes (chorion) surrounding the embryo. An inner layer of membranes (amnion) develops by about day 10 to 12, forming the amniotic sac. The amniotic sac fills with a clear liquid (amniotic fluid) and expands to envelop the developing embryo, which floats within it.

As the placenta develops, it extends tiny hairlike projections (villi) into the wall of the uterus. The projections branch and rebranch in a complicated treelike arrangement. This arrangement greatly increases the area of contact between the wall of the uterus and the placenta, so that more nutrients and waste materials can be exchanged. The placenta is fully formed by 18 to 20 weeks but continues to grow throughout pregnancy. At delivery, it weighs about 1 pound.

Development of the Embryo

The next stage in development is the embryo, which develops under the lining of the uterus on one side. This stage is characterized

DID YOU KNOW?

- By about 10 weeks of pregnancy (8 weeks after the egg is fertilized), almost all of the fetus's organs are formed.
- Most malformations occur before 10 weeks of pregnancy.
- By about 14 weeks of pregnancy, the fetus's sex can be identified.
- By 16 to 20 weeks, the woman can feel the fetus moving.

by the formation of most internal organs and external body structures. Organ formation begins about 3 weeks after fertilization, when the embryo is first recognizable as having a human shape. Shortly thereafter, the area that will become the brain and spinal cord (neural tube) begins to develop. The heart and major blood vessels begin to develop by about day 16 or 17. The heart begins to pump fluid through blood vessels by day 20, and the first red blood cells appear the next day. Blood vessels continue to develop in the embryo and placenta.

Almost all organs are completely formed by about 8 weeks after fertilization (which equals 10 weeks of pregnancy). The excep-

From Egg to Embryo

Once a month, an egg is released from an ovary into a fallopian tube. After sexual intercourse, sperm move from the vagina through the cervix and uterus to the fallopian tubes, where one sperm fertilizes the egg. The fertilized egg (zygote) divides repeatedly as it moves down the fallopian tube to the uterus. First, the zygote becomes a solid ball of cells. Then it becomes a hollow ball of cells called a blastocyst. Inside the uterus, the blastocyst implants in the wall of the uterus, where it develops into an embryo attached to a placenta and surrounded by fluid-filled membranes.

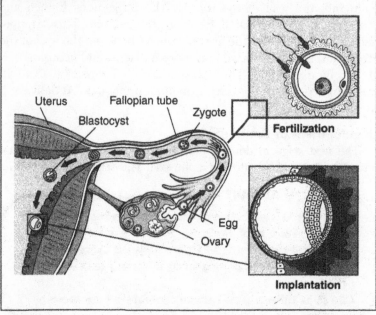

tions are the brain and spinal cord, which continue to mature throughout pregnancy. Most malformations occur during the period when organs are forming. During this period, the embryo is most vulnerable to the effects of drugs, radiation, and viruses. Therefore, a pregnant woman should not be given any live-virus vaccinations or take any drugs during this period unless they are considered essential to protect her health (see page 331).

Development of the Fetus

At the end of the 8th week after fertilization (10 weeks of pregnancy), the embryo is considered a fetus. During this stage, the structures that have already formed grow and develop. By 12 weeks of pregnancy, the fetus fills the entire uterus. By about 14 weeks, the sex can be identified. Typically, the pregnant woman can feel the fetus moving at about 16 to 20 weeks. Women who have been pregnant before typically feel movements about 2 weeks earlier than women who are pregnant for the first time. By about 23 to 24 weeks, the fetus has a chance of survival outside the uterus.

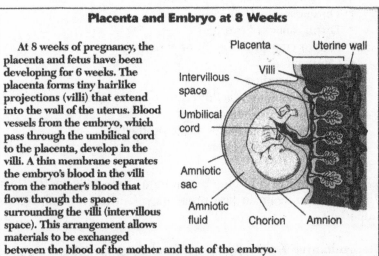

Placenta and Embryo at 8 Weeks

At 8 weeks of pregnancy, the placenta and fetus have been developing for 6 weeks. The placenta forms tiny hairlike projections (villi) that extend into the wall of the uterus. Blood vessels from the embryo, which pass through the umbilical cord to the placenta, develop in the villi. A thin membrane separates the embryo's blood in the villi from the mother's blood that flows through the space surrounding the villi (intervillous space). This arrangement allows materials to be exchanged between the blood of the mother and that of the embryo.

The embryo floats in fluid (amniotic fluid), which is contained in a sac (amniotic sac). The amniotic fluid provides a space in which the embryo can grow freely. The fluid also helps protect the embryo from injury. The amniotic sac is strong and resilient.

Labels: Placenta, Uterine wall, Villi, Intervillous space, Umbilical cord, Amniotic sac, Amniotic fluid, Chorion, Amnion

The lungs continue to mature until near the time of delivery. The brain accumulates new cells throughout pregnancy and the first year of life after birth.

Physical Changes in a Pregnant Woman

- Pregnancy temporarily affects most body systems.
- Being able to distinguish between normal changes and symptoms that should be immediately reported to a doctor is important.

Pregnancy causes many changes in a woman's body. Most of them disappear after delivery. In some women, certain disorders, such as a skin rash or gestational diabetes (see page 321), develop during pregnancy. Some symptoms should be immediately reported to a doctor if they occur during pregnancy. They include the following:

- Persistent headaches
- Persistent nausea and vomiting
- Dizziness
- Disturbances of eyesight
- Pain or cramps in the lower abdomen
- Contractions
- Vaginal bleeding
- Leakage of amniotic fluid (described as "the water breaks")
- Swelling of the hands or feet
- Decreased or increased urine production
- Any illness or infection.

General Health: Fatigue is common, especially in the first 12 weeks and again in late pregnancy. Getting enough rest is important.

Reproductive Tract: By 12 weeks of pregnancy, the enlarging uterus may cause the woman's abdomen to protrude slightly. The uterus continues to enlarge throughout pregnancy. The enlarging uterus extends to the level of the navel by 20 weeks and to the lower edge of the rib cage by 36 weeks.

The amount of normal vaginal discharge, which is clear or whitish, commonly increases. This increase is usually normal. However, if the discharge has an unusual color or smell or is accompanied by vaginal itching and burning, a woman should see her doctor. Such symptoms may indicate a vaginal infection. Some vaginal infections, such as trichomoniasis (a protozoan infection) and candidiasis (a yeast infection), are common during pregnancy and can be easily treated (see page 178).

Breasts: The breasts tend to enlarge because hormones (mainly estrogen) are preparing the breasts for milk production. The breasts enlarge because the glands that produce milk gradually increase in number and become able to produce milk. The breasts may feel firm and tender. Wearing a bra that fits properly and provides support may help.

During the last weeks of pregnancy, the breasts may produce a thin, yellowish or milky discharge (colostrum). Colostrum is also produced during the first few days after delivery, before breast milk is produced. This fluid, which is rich in minerals and antibodies, is the breastfed baby's first food.

DID YOU KNOW?

- The uterus reaches the navel by 20 weeks of pregnancy and the lower rib cage by 36 weeks.
- The amount of blood in the body increases by 50%.
- The ankles swell because the enlarging uterus interferes with blood returning from the legs to the heart.
- Lying on the left side improves blood flow to the kidneys, contributing to frequent urination at night.
- Pregnancy may result in anemia, varicose veins, morning sickness, belching and heartburn, skin and joint changes, diabetes, and excess thyroid gland activity.

Heart and Blood Flow: During pregnancy, the woman's heart must work harder because as the fetus grows, the heart must pump more blood to the uterus. By the end of pregnancy, the uterus is receiving one fifth of the woman's blood supply. During pregnancy, the amount of blood pumped by the heart (cardiac output) increases by 30 to 50%. As cardiac output increases, the heart rate at rest speeds up from a normal prepregnancy rate of about 70 beats per minute to 80 or 90 beats per minute. During exercise, cardiac output and heart rate increase more when a woman is pregnant than when she is not. During labor, cardiac output increases by an additional 10%. After delivery, cardiac output decreases rapidly at first, then more slowly. It returns to the prepregnancy level about 6 weeks after delivery.

Certain heart murmurs and irregularities in heart rhythm may appear because the heart is working harder. Sometimes a pregnant woman may feel these irregularities. Such changes are normal during pregnancy. However, certain abnormal heart rhythms, which occur more often in pregnant women, may require treatment.

Blood pressure usually decreases during the 2nd trimester but may return to a normal prepregnancy level in the 3rd trimester.

The volume of blood increases by 50% during pregnancy. The amount of fluid in the blood increases more than the number of red blood cells (which carry oxygen). The result is mild anemia, which is normal. For reasons not clearly understood, the number of white blood cells (which fight infection) increases slightly during pregnancy and markedly during labor and the first few days after delivery.

The enlarging uterus interferes with the return of blood from the legs and the pelvic area to the heart. As a result, swelling (edema) is common, especially in the legs. Varicose veins commonly develop in the legs and in the area around the vaginal opening (vulva), sometimes causing discomfort. Clothing that is loose around the waist and legs is more comfortable and does not restrict blood flow. Wearing elastic support hose, resting frequently with the legs elevated, or lying on the left side usually reduces leg swelling and may ease the discomfort caused by varicose veins. Varicose veins may disappear after delivery.

Urinary Tract: Like the heart, the kidneys work harder throughout pregnancy. They filter the increasing volume of blood. The volume of blood filtered by the kidneys reaches a maximum between 16 and 24 weeks and remains at the maximum until immediately before delivery. Then, pressure from the enlarging uterus may slightly decrease the blood supply to the kidneys.

The activity of the kidneys normally increases when a person lies down and decreases when a person stands. This difference is amplified during pregnancy—one reason a pregnant woman needs to urinate frequently while trying to sleep. Late in pregnancy, lying on the side, particularly the left side, increases kidney activity more than lying on the back. Lying on the left side relieves the pressure that the enlarged uterus puts on the main vein that carries blood from the legs. As a result, blood flow improves and kidney activity increases.

The uterus presses on the bladder, reducing its size so that it fills with urine more quickly than usual. This pressure also makes a pregnant woman need to urinate more often and more urgently.

Respiratory Tract: The increased production of the hormone progesterone signals the brain to lower the level of carbon dioxide in the blood. As a result, a pregnant woman breathes faster and more deeply to exhale more carbon dioxide and keep the carbon dioxide level low. The circumference of the woman's chest enlarges slightly.

Virtually every pregnant woman becomes somewhat more out of breath when she exerts herself, especially toward the end of pregnancy. During exercise, the breathing rate increases more when a woman is pregnant than when she is not.

Because more blood is being pumped, the lining of the airways receives more blood and swells somewhat, narrowing the airways. As a result, the nose occasionally feels stuffy, and the eustachian tubes (which connect the middle ear and back of the nose) may become blocked. The tone and quality of the woman's voice may change slightly.

Digestive Tract: Nausea and vomiting, particularly in the mornings (morning sickness), are common. They may be caused by the high levels of estrogen and human chorionic gonadotropin (HCG), two hormones that help maintain the pregnancy. Nausea and vomiting may be relieved by changing the diet or patterns of eating. For example, drinking and eating small portions frequently, eating before getting hungry, and eating bland foods (such as bouillon, consommé, rice, and pasta) may help. Eating plain soda crackers and sipping a carbonated drink may relieve nausea. Keeping crackers by the bed and eating one or two before getting up may relieve morning sickness. No drugs specifically designed to treat morning sickness are currently available. If nausea and vomiting are so intense or persistent that dehydration, weight loss, or other problems develop, a woman may need to be treated with antiemetic drugs or be hospitalized temporarily and given fluids intravenously (see page 318).

Heartburn and belching are common, possibly because food remains in the stomach longer and because the ringlike muscle (sphincter) at the lower end of the esophagus tends to relax, allowing the stomach's contents to flow backward into the esophagus. Heartburn can be relieved by eating smaller meals, by not bending or lying flat for several hours after eating, and by taking antacids. However, the antacid sodium bicarbonate should not be used because it contains so much salt (sodium). Heartburn during the night can be relieved by not eating for several hours before going to bed and by raising the head of the bed or using pillows to raise the head and shoulders.

The stomach produces less acid during pregnancy. Consequently, stomach ulcers rarely develop during pregnancy, and those that already exist often start to heal.

As pregnancy progresses, pressure from the enlarging uterus on the rectum and the lower part of the intestine may cause constipation. Constipation may be worsened because the high level of progesterone during pregnancy slows the automatic waves of muscular contractions in the intestine, which normally move food along. Eating a high-fiber diet, drinking plenty of fluids, and exercising regularly can help prevent constipation.

Hemorrhoids, a common problem, may result from the pressure of the enlarging uterus or from constipation. Stool softeners, an anesthetic gel, or warm soaks can be used if hemorrhoids hurt.

Pica, a craving for strange foods or nonfoods (such as starch or clay), may develop. Occasionally, pregnant women, usually those who also have morning sickness, have excess saliva. This symptom may be distressing but is harmless.

Skin: Mask of pregnancy (melasma) is a blotchy, brownish pigment that may appear on the skin of the forehead and cheeks. The skin surrounding the nipples (areolae) may also darken. A dark line commonly appears down the middle of the abdomen. These changes may occur because the placenta produces a hormone that stimulates melanocytes, the cells that make a dark brown skin pigment (melanin).

Pink stretch marks sometimes appear on the abdomen. This change probably results from rapid growth of the uterus and an increase in levels of adrenal hormones.

SKIN RASHES DURING PREGNANCY

Two intensely itchy rashes, urticaria of pregnancy and herpes gestationis, occur only during pregnancy.

Urticaria of pregnancy is common. The cause is unknown. Red, irregularly shaped, flat or slightly raised patches appear on the abdomen. The patches sometimes have tiny fluid-filled blisters in the center. Often, the skin around them is pale. The rash spreads to the thighs, buttocks, and occasionally the arms. Hundreds of itchy patches may develop. Typically, the rash appears during the last 2 to 3 weeks of pregnancy and occasionally during the last few days. However, it may occur at any time after the 24th week. Itching is bothersome enough to keep the woman awake at night. Usually, the rash clears up promptly after delivery and does not recur during subsequent pregnancies. Doctors may have difficulty making a definite diagnosis.

Herpes gestationis is thought to be caused by abnormal antibodies that attack the body's own tissues—an autoimmune reaction. Blisters often form on the abdomen first, then spread. The blisters are small or large, irregularly shaped, and fluid-filled. The rash can appear any time after the 12th week of pregnancy or immediately after delivery. Typically, the rash worsens soon after delivery and disappears within a few weeks or months. It often reappears during subsequent pregnancies. The baby may be born with a similar rash, which usually disappears without treatment within a few weeks. This rash is diagnosed by removing a tiny piece of affected skin and testing it for abnormal antibodies.

For either rash, applying a corticosteroid cream (such as triamcinolone acetonide) directly to the skin often helps. For more widespread rashes, a corticosteroid (such as prednisone) is given by mouth.

Small blood vessels may form a red spiderlike pattern on the skin, usually above the waist. These formations are called spider angiomas. Thin-walled, dilated capillaries may become visible, especially in the lower legs.

Hormones: Pregnancy affects virtually all hormones in the body, mostly because of the effects of hormones produced by the placenta. For example, the placenta produces a hormone that stimulates the woman's thyroid gland to become more active and produce larger amounts of thyroid hormones. When the thyroid gland becomes more active, the heart may beat faster, causing the woman to become aware of her heartbeat (have palpitations). Perspiration may increase, mood swings may occur, and the thyroid gland may enlarge. The disorder hyperthyroidism, in which the thyroid gland is truly overactive, develops in fewer than 1% of pregnancies.

Levels of estrogen and progesterone increase early in pregnancy because human chorionic gonadotropin, the main hormone the placenta produces, stimulates the ovaries to continuously produce them. After 9 to 10 weeks of pregnancy, the placenta itself produces large amounts of estrogen and progesterone. Estrogen and progesterone help maintain the pregnancy.

During pregnancy, changes in hormone levels affect how the body handles sugar. Early in pregnancy, the sugar (glucose) level in the blood may decrease slightly. But in the last half of pregnancy, the level may increase. More insulin (which controls the sugar level in the blood) is needed and is produced by the pancreas. Consequently, diabetes, if already present, may worsen during pregnancy. Diabetes can also begin during pregnancy. This disorder is called gestational diabetes (see page 321).

Joints and Muscles: The joints and ligaments (fibrous cords and cartilage that connect bones) in the woman's pelvis loosen and become more flexible. This change helps make room for the enlarging uterus and prepare the woman for delivery of the baby. As a result, the woman's posture changes somewhat.

Backache in varying degrees is common, because the spine curves more to balance the weight of the enlarging uterus. Avoiding heavy lifting, bending the knees (not the waist) to pick things up, and maintaining good posture can help. Wearing flat shoes with good support or a lightweight maternity girdle may reduce strain on the back.

Stages of Pregnancy		
Although pregnancy involves a continuous process, it is divided into three 3-month periods called trimesters (weeks 0 to 12, 13 to 24, and 25 to delivery).		
EVENTS	**WEEKS OF PREGNANCY**	
1st Trimester		
The woman's last period before fertilization occurs.	0	
Fertilization occurs.	2	
The fertilized egg (zygote) develops into a hollow ball of cells called the blastocyst.		
The blastocyst implants in the wall of uterus.	3	
The amniotic sac forms.		
The area that will become the brain and spinal cord (neural tube) begins to develop.	5	
The heart and major blood vessels are developing. The beating heart can be seen during ultrasonography.	6	3 months
The beginnings of arms and legs appear.	7	
Bones and muscles form. The face and neck develop.	9	
Most organs are formed. Brain waves can be detected.		
The skeleton is formed. Fingers and toes are fully defined.		
The kidneys begin to function.	10	
The fetus can move and respond to touch (when prodded through the woman's abdomen).		
The woman has gained some weight, and her abdomen may be slightly enlarged.		

2nd Trimester

The fetus's sex can be identified.	14
The fetus can hear.	

The fetus's fingers can grasp. 16
The fetus moves more
vigorously, so that the mother
can feel it.

The fetus's body begins
to fill out as fat is deposited
beneath the skin. Hair appears
on the head and skin.
Eyebrows and eyelashes
are present.

The placenta is fully formed.

The fetus has a chance of 23-24
survival outside the uterus.

The woman begins to gain
weight more rapidly.

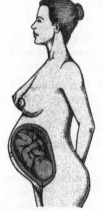

6 months

3rd Trimester

The fetus is active, changing 25
positions often.

The lungs continue to mature.

The fetus's head moves into
position for delivery.

On average, the fetus is about 20
inches long and weighs about 7
pounds. The woman's enlarged
abdomen causes the navel to
bulge.

9 months

DELIVERY 37-42

Medical Care During Pregnancy

- Regular visits to a health care practitioner during pregnancy make having a safe delivery and healthy baby more likely.
- The first visit includes a thorough physical examination, pelvic examination, and testing.
- Later visits include measuring weight and blood pressure, testing a urine sample for sugar and protein, determining the size of the uterus, and checking the ankles for swelling.
- Pregnant women should not use tobacco or alcohol and should avoid exposure to secondhand smoke and cat feces.

Ideally, a couple who is thinking of having a baby should see a doctor or other health care practitioner to discuss steps that they can take to help make the pregnancy as healthy as possible. The woman should ask the doctor about factors that could impair her health or the health of the developing fetus. Knowing about and dealing with such factors before pregnancy may help reduce the risk of problems during pregnancy (see page 301). These factors include the use of tobacco or alcohol and exposure to possibly harmful substances. For example, a pregnant woman should avoid exposure to secondhand smoke because it may harm the fetus. A pregnant woman should avoid contact with cats or cat feces unless the cats are strictly confined to the home and are not exposed to other cats. Such contact can transmit toxoplasmosis, an infection by a protozoan that can damage the fetus's brain. Rubella (German measles) can cause birth defects. In addition, the woman can discuss her diet and her social, emotional, and medical concerns with the doctor.

When a woman sees a doctor or other health care practitioner before she is pregnant, she can be given any needed vaccines, such as the rubella vaccine. She can also start taking prenatal multivitamins containing folic acid. If needed, genetic screening can be performed to determine whether the woman and her partner are at increased risk of having a baby with a hereditary genetic disorder (see page 289).

After pregnancy is confirmed, the woman should have a physical examination, preferably between 6 and 8 weeks of pregnancy.

At this time, the length of the pregnancy can be estimated and the date of delivery can be predicted as accurately as possible.

The first physical examination during pregnancy is very thorough. Weight, height, and blood pressure are measured. The doctor performs a pelvic examination, noting the size and position of the uterus.

A sample of blood is taken and analyzed. Analysis includes a complete blood cell count, tests for infectious diseases (such as syphilis and hepatitis), and tests for evidence of immunity to rubella. Blood type, including Rh factor status (positive or negative), is determined. A test for the human immunodeficiency virus (HIV) is recommended. Other routine tests include an extensive analysis of a sample of the woman's urine and a Papanicolaou (Pap) test for cancer of the cervix. A sample from the cervix may be obtained to test for sexually transmitted diseases, such as gonorrhea and chlamydial infection.

Other tests may be performed, depending on the woman's situation. If the woman has Rh-negative blood, it is tested for antibodies to the Rh factor (see page 322). Having Rh antibodies can cause severe problems (even death) for a fetus who has Rh-positive blood. If antibodies in a pregnant woman's blood are detected early, the doctor can take measures to protect the fetus.

Women of African descent are tested for sickle cell trait or disease if they have not been tested previously. Skin tests for tuberculosis are advisable for all women. X-rays are not routinely taken early in pregnancy, but they can be taken safely when necessary. If an x-ray is required, the fetus is shielded by placing a lead-filled garment over the woman's lower abdomen to cover the uterus.

DID YOU KNOW?

- Ultrasonography can show the fetus's beating heart at 6 weeks and can identify fetal sex at 14 weeks of pregnancy.
- Pregnant women should receive influenza vaccination during flu season.

After the first examination, a pregnant woman should see her doctor every 4 weeks until 32 weeks of pregnancy, then every 2 weeks until 36 weeks, then once a week until delivery. At each examination, the woman's weight and blood pressure are usually recorded, and the size of the uterus is noted to determine whether the fetus is growing normally. The ankles are examined for swelling.

At each visit, urine is tested for sugar. Sugar in the urine may indicate diabetes. Women who have sugar in the urine should be screened for diabetes at 24 to 28 weeks of pregnancy, as should women who have had large babies or unexplained stillbirths, who are overweight, who are older than 25, who have a close relative with diabetes, or who have polycystic ovary syndrome. At each visit, the urine is also tested for protein. Protein in the urine may indicate preeclampsia (a type of high blood pressure that develops during pregnancy—see page 318).

For women who have a high risk of conceiving a baby with a genetic disorder, prenatal diagnostic testing is performed (see page 291).

Many doctors believe that ultrasonography, the safest imaging procedure, should be performed at least once during a pregnancy to make sure the fetus is normally formed and to verify the expected date of delivery. For the procedure, a device that produces sound waves (transducer) is placed on the woman's abdomen. The sound waves are processed to form an image that is displayed on a monitor. Sometimes doctors use an ultrasound device that can be inserted in the vagina. Ultrasonography produces high-quality images, including live-action images that show the fetus in motion. These images provide the doctor with useful information and can reassure a pregnant woman.

Before ultrasonography of the abdomen is performed, especially early in pregnancy, a woman must drink a lot of water. A full bladder pushes the uterus out of the pelvis so that a clearer image of the fetus can be obtained. When a vaginal ultrasound device is used, the bladder does not have to be full, and a doctor can detect pregnancy even earlier.

Ultrasonography can show the fetus's beating heart at 6 weeks of pregnancy and thus can confirm that the fetus is alive. Doctors may periodically use an ultrasound device to listen to the fetus's heartbeat. Or they may use a stethoscope designed to listen to a fetus's heartbeat (fetoscope). The fetoscope can detect the heartbeat as early as 18 to 20 weeks of pregnancy.

Ultrasonography can identify the sex of the fetus at 14 weeks of pregnancy. Ultrasonography is also used to see whether a woman is carrying more than one fetus and to identify abnormalities, such as a mislocated placenta (placenta previa) or an abnormal position of the fetus. Ultrasonography is used for guidance during certain procedures, such as prenatal diagnostic testing.

Toward the end of pregnancy, ultrasonography may be used to identify premature rupture of the fluid-filled membranes containing the fetus. Ultrasonography can provide information that helps doctors decide whether to perform a cesarean section.

Experts recommend that all pregnant women be vaccinated against the influenza virus during the influenza (flu) season.

Self-Care During Pregnancy

- Most women should gain about 25 to 30 pounds during pregnancy.
- Women should avoid taking drugs during pregnancy if possible.
- Women should take a prenatal multivitamin containing iron and folic acid daily.
- Women who plan to breastfeed do not need to do anything to prepare their nipples.

There is much a pregnant woman can do to take care of herself during pregnancy. If she has any questions about diet, the use of drugs or nutritional supplements, physical activity, and sexual intercourse during pregnancy, she can talk with her doctor.

Diet and Weight: During pregnancy, the woman's diet should be adequate and nutritious. Most women should add about 250 calories to their daily diet to provide nourishment for the developing fetus. The diet should be well balanced, including fresh fruits, grains, and vegetables. High-fiber, sugar-free cereals are a good choice. The fetus has first choice of nutrients, but the pregnant woman must make sure that the fetus has something worthwhile to choose from. In the United States, most women get enough salt in their diet, without adding salt to their food at the table. Commercially prepared foods often contain excessive amounts of salt and should be consumed sparingly. Dieting to lose weight during pregnancy is not recommended, even for obese women, because some weight gain is essential for the fetus to develop normally. Dieting reduces the supply of nutrients to the fetus.

An average-size woman should gain about 25 to 30 pounds during pregnancy. Gaining more than 30 to 35 pounds puts fat on the woman and the fetus. Because controlling weight gain is more difficult later in pregnancy, a woman should try to avoid gaining most of the weight during the first months. On the other hand, not gaining weight is an ominous sign, especially if the total weight gain is less than 10 pounds. Growth of the fetus may be slowed or inadequate.

Sometimes a pregnant woman gains weight because she is retaining fluid. Fluid may be retained because when she stands, the enlarging uterus interferes with blood flow from the legs back to the heart. Lying on one side, preferably the left side, for 30 to 45 minutes 2 or 3 times a day may relieve this problem.

DID YOU KNOW?

- Pregnancy is not the time for dieting to lose weight.
- A pregnant woman should check with her doctor before taking any drug, even medicinal herbs, aspirin, or other over-the-counter drugs.
- Most pregnant women can continue their usual physical activities and exercise, as well as sexual intercourse.

Drugs and Dietary Supplements: Generally, avoiding drugs during pregnancy is best. However, drugs must sometimes be used (see page 331). A pregnant woman should check with her doctor before taking any drug—including nonprescription (over-the-counter) drugs, such as aspirin, or medicinal herbs—particularly during the first 3 months.

Pregnancy doubles the amount of iron needed. Most pregnant women need an iron supplement, because the average woman does not absorb enough iron from food to meet the requirements of pregnancy, even when iron from food is combined with iron already stored in her body. If a woman has anemia or develops anemia during pregnancy, she may need to take a larger dose of iron than other pregnant women. Iron supplements may cause mild stomach upset and constipation.

All pregnant women should take a folic acid supplement (usually included in prenatal vitamins) daily. Ideally, the folic acid supplement is begun before pregnancy. A deficiency of folic acid increases the risk of having a baby with a birth defect of the brain or spinal cord, such as spina bifida. Women who have had a baby with spina bifida should start taking a high dose of folic acid before they become pregnant. Excessive ultraviolet (UV) light exposure, particularly in fair-skinned women, can decrease folic acid levels. Women who have taken oral contraceptives are more likely to develop a folic acid deficiency, but there is no proof that they are more likely to have a baby with spina bifida.

If the diet is adequate, other vitamin supplements may not be needed, although most doctors recommend that pregnant women take a prenatal multivitamin containing iron and folic acid daily.

Physical Activity: Many pregnant women are concerned about moderating their activities. However, most women can continue their usual activities and exercises throughout pregnancy. Mildly strenuous sports, such as swimming and brisk walking, are good choices. Vigorous activities, such as running and horseback riding, are also possible if performed cautiously. But contact sports should be avoided.

Sexual Intercourse: Sexual desire may increase or decrease during pregnancy. Sexual intercourse is safe throughout pregnancy unless a woman has vaginal bleeding, pain, leakage of amniotic fluid, or uterine contractions. In such cases, sexual intercourse should be avoided.

Preparing for Breastfeeding: Women who are planning to breastfeed do not need to do anything to prepare their nipples for breastfeeding during pregnancy. Expressing fluids from the breast manually before delivery may lead to an infection of the breast (mastitis) or even early labor. The body prepares the areola and nipple for breastfeeding by secreting a lubricant to protect the surface. This lubricant should not be rubbed off. Observing and talking with women who have breastfed successfully may be instructive and encouraging.

CHAPTER 21

Detection of Genetic Disorders

A big concern of prospective parents is whether their baby will be healthy. Some problems that occur in babies are due to genetic disorders. These disorders may result from abnormalities in one or more genes or in chromosomes. Abnormalities may be hereditary or may occur spontaneously. A spontaneous abnormality may result from exposure before birth to drugs, chemicals, or other damaging substances (such as x-rays) or may occur by chance.

To determine whether the risk of having a baby with a hereditary genetic disorder is increased, a couple who is thinking of having a baby can undergo genetic screening. If a couple is considered at increased risk, procedures to test the fetus during the pregnancy (prenatal diagnostic testing) can be performed.

Genetic Screening

- Doctors evaluate a couple's family history to determine whether their risk of having a baby with a hereditary genetic disorder is increased.
- If the family history suggests increased risk and if certain other conditions are met, blood tests are done to check for the gene for the disorder.

Genetic screening is used to determine whether a couple is at increased risk of having a baby with a hereditary genetic disorder. Genetic screening is not for everyone. Counseling is recommended when one or both partners know they have a genetic disorder or have family members who have or may have a genetic disorder. Genetic screening involves assessing the couple's family history and may involve determining whether a prospective parent who does not have symptoms of a particular disorder has a gene for that disorder (carrier screening).

Family History Assessment

To determine whether having a baby with a genetic disorder is likely, doctors ask the couple about disorders that family members have had and about the cause of death in family members. Information about three generations is usually needed. Doctors also ask about the health of all living first-degree relatives (parents, siblings, and children) and second-degree relatives (aunts, uncles, and grandparents). Information about miscarriages, stillborn babies, or babies who have died soon after birth is also helpful, as is information about intermarriages among relatives and ethnic background. If the family history is complicated, information about more distant relatives may be needed. Sometimes doctors review the medical records of relatives who may have had a genetic disorder.

DID YOU KNOW?

- Some hereditary genetic disorders are more likely to occur in certain ethnic, racial, or geographic groups.

Carrier Screening

Carrier screening involves testing people who do not have symptoms of a particular disorder but may have one nonsex (autosomal) recessive gene for that disorder and one normal gene. (If a disorder results from an abnormal autosomal recessive gene, a person must have two of the abnormal genes to develop the disorder and have symptoms.) Prospective parents are screened if they have a family history of certain disorders or characteristics (such as ethnic background) that increase the risk of having certain disorders.

Screening is performed only if the following criteria are met:

- The disorder is very debilitating or lethal.
- A reliable screening test is available.
- One or both parents are likely to be a carrier because the disorder runs in the family or is common in their ethnic, racial, or geographic group.
- The fetus can be treated, or reproductive options (such as abortion or elective sterilization) are available and acceptable to the parents.

In the United States, sickle cell anemia, the thalassemias, Tay-Sachs disease, and cystic fibrosis meet these criteria.

Screening usually consists of analyzing a blood sample. But sometimes a sample of cells from the inside of the cheek is analyzed. The person provides the sample by swishing a special fluid in the mouth, then spitting it into a specimen container. If both parents carry one abnormal autosomal recessive gene for the same disorder, their baby may be born with the disorder. In such cases, the chance of a baby receiving an abnormal recessive gene from each parent is 1 in 4 for each pregnancy.

If carrier screening indicates that both parents have an autosomal recessive gene for the same disorder, the parents may decide to have prenatal diagnostic testing. That is, the fetus may be tested for the disorder before birth. If the fetus has the disorder, treatment of the fetus may be possible, or termination of the pregnancy may be considered.

Prenatal Diagnostic Testing

- Before birth, the fetus can be tested for certain genetic disorders.
- Most commonly, tests are offered when the risk of having a baby with a neural tube defect or chromosomal abnormality is increased.

- In the United States, ultrasonography, which can detect obvious structural defects, is often done routinely during pregnancy.
- Chorionic villus sampling, amniocentesis, or percutaneous umbilical blood sampling can provide more information, but these tests have some risks.

Prenatal diagnostic testing involves testing the fetus before birth (prenatally) to determine whether it has a certain hereditary or spontaneous genetic disorder. The most common tests used to detect abnormalities in a fetus include ultrasonography, chorionic villus sampling, amniocentesis, and percutaneous umbilical blood sampling. Most of these tests are offered primarily to couples with an increased risk of having a baby with a genetic abnormality (particularly neural tube defects) or a chromosomal abnormality (particularly when the woman is aged 35 or older). In the United States, ultrasonography is often performed as part of routine prenatal care.

Some Genetic Disorders That Can Be Detected Before Birth

DISORDER	INCIDENCE	INHERITANCE PATTERN
Cystic fibrosis	1 of 3,300 white people	Autosomal recessive
Congenital adrenal hyperplasia	1 of 10,000	Autosomal recessive
Duchenne's muscular dystrophy	1 of 3,500 male births	X-linked recessive
Hemophilia A	1 of 8,500 male births	X-linked recessive
Alpha- and beta-thalassemia	Varies widely by ethnic and racial group	Autosomal recessive
Huntington's disease	4 to 7 of 100,000	Autosomal dominant
Polycystic kidney disease (adult type)	1 of 3,000	Autosomal dominant
Sickle cell anemia	1 of 400 black people in the United States	Autosomal recessive
Tay-Sachs disease (GM$_2$ gangliosidosis)	1 of 3,600 Ashkenazi Jews and French Canadians; 1 of 400,000 in other groups	Autosomal recessive

Neural Tube Defects: Prenatal diagnostic testing is commonly used to detect neural tube defects, which are birth defects of the brain or spinal cord. Examples are spina bifida (in which the spine does not completely enclose the spinal cord) and anencephaly (in which a large part of the brain and skull is missing). In the United States, neural tube defects occur in 1 of 500 to 1,000 births. Most of these defects are caused by abnormalities in several genes. A few result from abnormalities in a single gene, chromosomal abnormalities, or exposure to drugs. Prenatal diagnosis by amniocentesis and ultrasonography is recommended for couples who have at least a 1% risk of having a baby with a neural tube defect.

The risk of having a baby with a neural tube defect is increased by having a family history (including the couple's own children) of such defects. For couples who have had a baby with spina bifida or anencephaly, the risk of having another baby with one of these defects is 2 to 3%. For couples who have had two children with these defects, the risk is 5 to 10%. However, about 95% of neural tube defects occur in families without a history of the defects.

Risk also depends on where a person lives. For example, the risk is higher in the United Kingdom than in the United States. Risk may also be increased by a diet that is low in folic acid. Therefore, folic acid supplements are now routinely recommended for all women of childbearing age.

DID YOU KNOW?

- Chromosomal abnormalities account for at least half of all 1st-trimester miscarriages.
- Blood tests in pregnant women help detect some birth defects and chromosomal abnormalities in the fetus.
- Down syndrome is the most common chromosomal abnormality among live-born babies.
- For some couples, risks of tests such as amniocentesis and chorionic villus sampling outweigh their benefits.
- Chorionic villus sampling provides results much earlier in pregnancy than amniocentesis does.

Chromosomal Abnormalities: Chromosomal abnormalities occur in about 1 of 200 live births and account for at least half of all miscarriages that occur during the 1st trimester. Most fetuses that have chromosomal abnormalities die before birth. Tests to diagnose chromosomal abnormalities before birth are considered if a couple has an increased risk of having a baby with a chromosomal abnormality. However, diagnostic tests can have risks, although very small, particularly for the fetus. For some couples, the risks outweigh the benefits of knowing whether their baby has a chromosomal abnormality, so they choose not to be tested.

Several factors increase the risk of having a baby with a chromosomal abnormality. The risk of having a baby with Down syndrome increases with a woman's age—steeply after age 35. (Down syndrome is the most common chromosomal abnormality among live-born babies.) Testing for chromosomal abnormalities in the fetus is usually offered to women who will be 35 or older when they give birth and may be offered to younger women, such as those who have already had a child with Down syndrome. The couple's anxiety, regardless of the woman's age, often justifies prenatal diagnostic testing.

Having a family history (including the couple's own children) of a chromosomal abnormality also increases the risk. If a couple has had one baby with the most common form of Down syndrome (trisomy 21) and the woman is younger than 30, the risk of having another baby with a chromosomal abnormality is increased to about 1%.

Having had a live-born or stillborn baby with a birth defect—even when no one knows whether the baby had a chromosomal abnormality—increases the risk of having a baby with a chromosomal abnormality. About 30% of babies born with a birth defect and 5% of apparently normal stillborn babies have a chromosomal abnormality.

A chromosomal abnormality in one or both parents increases the risk, even if the parent is only a carrier, is healthy, and has no physical sign of the abnormality.

Having had several miscarriages may increase the risk of having a baby with a chromosomal abnormality. If the fetus in a first miscarriage has a chromosomal abnormality, a fetus in subsequent miscarriages is also likely to have one, although not necessarily the same one. If a woman has had several miscarriages, the couple's chromosomes should be analyzed before they try to have another baby. If abnormalities are identified, the couple may choose to have prenatal diagnostic testing early in the next pregnancy.

Abnormal levels of certain substances in a pregnant woman's blood indicate that a chromosomal abnormality in the fetus is more likely. Such substances are called markers. An important marker is alpha-fetoprotein (a protein produced by the fetus). Other markers include estriol (an estrogen) and human chorionic gonadotropin (a hormone produced by the placenta). For pregnant women, measuring marker levels is part of routine prenatal care.

A Woman's Age and Her Risk of Having a Baby With a Chromosomal Abnormality

AGE OF WOMAN	RISK OF DOWN SYNDROME	RISK OF ANY CHROMOSOMAL ABNORMALITY
20	1 in 1,667	1 in 526
22	1 in 1,429	1 in 500
24	1 in 1,250	1 in 476
26	1 in 1,176	1 in 476
28	1 in 1,053	1 in 435
30	1 in 952	1 in 384
32	1 in 769	1 in 323
34	1 in 500	1 in 238
36	1 in 294	1 in 156
38	1 in 175	1 in 102
40	1 in 106	1 in 66
42	1 in 64	1 in 42
44	1 in 38	1 in 26
46	1 in 23	1 in 16
48	1 in 14	1 in 10

Data based on information in Hook EB: "Rates of chromosome abnormalities at different maternal ages." *Obstetrics and Gynecology* 58:282-285, 1981; and Hook EB, Cross PK, Schreinemachers DM: "Chromosomal abnormality rates at amniocentesis and in live-born infants." *Journal of the American Medical Association* 249(15):2034-2038, 1983.

INTERPRETING ABNORMAL ALPHA-FETOPROTEIN LEVELS

Doctors routinely offer pregnant women blood tests to screen for various birth defects. Certain substances (called markers) in the blood indicate that a chromosomal abnormality in the fetus is more likely. Results are most accurate when the blood sample is taken between 16 and 18 weeks of pregnancy. Normal levels of these substances do not guarantee a normal fetus, and abnormal levels can have different meanings.

A high level of alpha-fetoprotein in a pregnant woman's blood indicates that the risk of having a baby with a brain defect (anencephaly) or spinal cord defect (spina bifida) is increased. A high level may also indicate that more than one fetus is present, a miscarriage is likely, or the fetus has died. A low level of alpha-fetoprotein in a pregnant woman's blood suggests other chromosomal abnormalities, including Down syndrome.

If a woman has a high alpha-fetoprotein level, ultrasonography is performed to determine whether an abnormality is present. If ultrasonography cannot determine the cause, amniocentesis is usually performed to measure the alpha-fetoprotein level in the fluid that surrounds the fetus (amniotic fluid), and chromosomes may be analyzed. If the alpha-fetoprotein level in the amniotic fluid is high, the level of an enzyme called acetylcholinesterase is also measured. In most cases of anencephaly and spina bifida, the alpha-fetoprotein level is high and acetylcholinesterase is detected in the amniotic fluid. A high level of alpha-fetoprotein in the amniotic fluid, with or without acetylcholinesterase, may indicate abnormalities in other organs, such as the esophagus and stomach. A high alpha-fetoprotein level in the amniotic fluid also indicates an increased risk of complications during pregnancy, such as slowed growth or death of the fetus and early detachment of the placenta (placental abruption).

PROCEDURES

Several procedures can be used to detect genetic and chromosomal abnormalities.

Ultrasonography

Ultrasonography is commonly performed during pregnancy (see page 130). It has no known risks for the woman or fetus. After the third month, ultrasonography can be used to detect whether the fetus has certain obvious structural birth defects. Ultrasonography is often used to check for abnormalities in the fetus when a pregnant woman has a high or low alpha-fetoprotein level or a family history of birth defects. However, normal results do not guarantee a normal baby, because no test is completely accurate.

Ultrasonography is performed before chorionic villus sampling and amniocentesis to confirm the length of the pregnancy. Chorionic villus sampling and amniocentesis can then be performed at the appropriate time during the pregnancy. Ultrasonography can also locate the placenta and indicate whether the fetus is alive. Ultrasonography is used to monitor the fetus and to guide placement of instruments during chorionic villus sampling or amniocentesis.

Chorionic Villus Sampling

In chorionic villus sampling, a doctor removes a small sample of the chorionic villi, which are tiny projections that make up part of the placenta (see page 273). This procedure is used to diagnose some disorders in the fetus, usually between 10 and 12 weeks of pregnancy. Chorionic villus sampling may be used instead of amniocentesis unless a sample of amniotic fluid is needed. For example, a sample is needed when the alpha-fetoprotein level in amniotic fluid must be measured.

The main advantage of chorionic villus sampling is that its results are available much earlier in the pregnancy than those of amniocentesis. Thus, if no abnormality is detected, the couple's anxiety can be relieved earlier. If an abnormality is detected earlier, simpler, safer methods can be used to terminate the pregnancy. Also, early detection of an abnormality may be necessary for appropriate treatment of the fetus before birth. For example, a pregnant woman may be given a corticosteroid to prevent male characteristics from developing in a female fetus that has congenital adrenal hyperplasia. In this hereditary disorder, the adrenal glands are enlarged and produce excessive amounts of male hormones (androgens).

Before the procedure, ultrasonography is performed to determine whether the fetus is alive, to confirm the fetus's age, to check for obvious abnormalities, and to locate the placenta.

A sample of the chorionic villi can be removed through the cervix (transcervically) or the abdominal wall (transabdominally). With both methods, ultrasonography is used for guidance and the tissue sample is suctioned into a catheter with a syringe and then analyzed.

To remove tissue through the cervix, a doctor inserts a thin flexible tube (catheter) through the vagina and the cervix into the placenta. The woman lies on her back with her hips and knees bent, usually supported by heel or knee stirrups, as for a pelvic examination. For most women, the procedure feels very similar to a Papanicolaou (Pap) test, but a few women find it more uncomfortable. This method cannot be used in women who have a certain abnormality of the cervix or an active genital infection, such as genital herpes, gonorrhea, or chronic inflammation of the cervix.

To remove tissue through the abdominal wall, a doctor anesthetizes an area of skin over the abdomen and inserts a needle through the abdominal wall into the placenta. Most women do not find this procedure painful. But for some women, the area over the abdomen feels slightly sore for an hour or two afterward.

After chorionic villus sampling, most women who have Rh-negative blood and who do not have antibodies to Rh factor are given an injection of $Rh_0(D)$ immune globulin to prevent them from producing antibodies to Rh factor (see page 322). A woman with Rh-negative blood may produce these antibodies if the fetus has Rh-positive blood that comes into contact with her blood, as it may during chorionic villus sampling. These antibodies can cause problems in the fetus. The injection is not needed if the father also has Rh-negative blood, because the fetus will have Rh-negative blood.

The risks of chorionic villus sampling are comparable to those of amniocentesis, except the risk of injuring the fetus's hands or feet may be slightly higher. Such injury occurs in 1 of 3,000 fetuses. Rarely, the diagnosis is unclear after chorionic villus sampling, and amniocentesis may be necessary. In general, the accuracy of the two procedures is comparable.

Amniocentesis

One of the most common procedures for detecting abnormalities before birth is amniocentesis. In this procedure, a sample of the fluid that surrounds the fetus (amniotic fluid) is removed. Amniocentesis is usually performed at 14 weeks of pregnancy or later. If the reason for performing amniocentesis is a high alpha-fetoprotein level in the woman's blood, the procedure is best performed between 15 and 17 weeks of pregnancy. Amniocentesis enables doctors to measure the alpha-fetoprotein level in the

Detecting Abnormalities Before Birth

Chorionic villus sampling and amniocentesis are used to detect abnormalities in a fetus. During both procedures, ultrasonography is used for guidance.

In chorionic villus sampling, a sample of chorionic villi (part of the placenta) is removed by one of two methods. In the transcervical method, a doctor inserts a flexible tube (catheter) through the vagina and cervix into the placenta. In the transabdominal method, a doctor inserts a needle through the abdominal wall into the placenta. In both methods, a sample of the placenta is suctioned out with a syringe and analyzed.

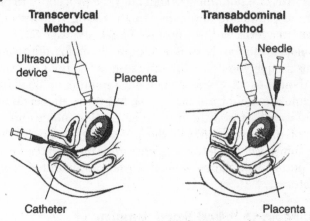

Transcervical Method

Ultrasound device

Placenta

Catheter

Transabdominal Method

Needle

Placenta

Chorionic Villus Sampling

In amniocentesis, a doctor inserts a needle through the abdominal wall into the amniotic fluid. A sample of fluid is withdrawn for analysis.

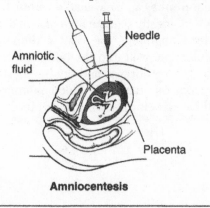

Needle

Amniotic fluid

Placenta

Amniocentesis

amniotic fluid. This measurement more reliably indicates whether the fetus has a brain or spinal cord defect than measurement of this level in the woman's blood.

After anesthetizing an area of skin over the abdomen, a doctor inserts a needle through the abdominal wall into the amniotic fluid. During the procedure, ultrasonography is performed so that the fetus can be monitored and the needle guided into place. Fluid is withdrawn, and the needle is removed. Results are usually available in 1 to 3 weeks. Women who have Rh-negative blood are given $Rh_0(D)$ immune globulin after the procedure to prevent them from producing antibodies to Rh factor, which can cause problems in a fetus with Rh-positive blood (see page 322).

Amniocentesis rarely causes any problems for the woman or the fetus. Some women feel slightly sore for an hour or two afterward. About 1 to 2% of the women have spotting of blood or leakage of amniotic fluid from the vagina, but these effects do not last long and usually stop without treatment. After amniocentesis, the chance of miscarriage due to the procedure is about 1 in 200. Needle injuries to the fetus are very rare. Amniocentesis can usually be performed when a woman is pregnant with twins or even more fetuses.

Percutaneous Umbilical Blood Sampling

Percutaneous umbilical blood sampling is used when rapid chromosome analysis is needed, particularly toward the end of pregnancy when ultrasonography has detected abnormalities in the fetus. Often, results can be available within 48 hours.

The doctor first anesthetizes an area of skin over the abdomen. Guided by ultrasonography, the doctor then inserts a needle through the abdominal wall into the umbilical cord. A sample of the fetus's blood is withdrawn and analyzed, and the needle is removed. Percutaneous umbilical blood sampling is an invasive procedure and has risks for the woman and fetus.

CHAPTER 22

High-Risk Pregnancy

- Factors that increase the risk of harm to the woman or baby may be present before the pregnancy or may develop during the pregnancy.
- As a result, a baby may be underweight, be too big to pass through the birth canal, have a birth defect, be born too soon, or be born dead.
- All of the risk factors have a chance of causing miscarriage.

There is no formal or universally accepted definition of a "high-risk" pregnancy. Generally, however, a high-risk pregnancy involves at least one of the following: The woman or baby is more likely to become ill or die than usual, or complications before or after delivery are more likely to occur than usual.

Certain conditions or characteristics, called risk factors, make a pregnancy high risk. Doctors identify these factors and use a scoring system to determine the degree of risk for a particular woman. Identifying high-risk pregnancies ensures that women who most need medical care receive it.

Risk Factors Present Before Pregnancy

- Women may have physical or social characteristics, habits (such as smoking or alcohol consumption), problems in previous pregnancies, or disorders (such as diabetes) that increase their risk of having problems during pregnancy.

Some risk factors are present before women become pregnant. These risk factors include certain physical and social characteristics of women, problems that have occurred in previous pregnancies, and certain disorders women already have.

Physical Characteristics

The age, weight, and height of women affect risk during pregnancy. Girls aged 15 and younger are at increased risk of preeclampsia (a type of high blood pressure that develops during pregnancy). Young girls are also at increased risk of having underweight (small-for-gestational-age) or undernourished babies. Women aged 35 and older are at increased risk of problems such as high blood pressure, gestational diabetes (diabetes that develops during pregnancy), and complications during labor.

Women who weigh less than 100 pounds before becoming pregnant are more likely to have small, underweight babies. Obese women are more likely to have very large babies, which may be difficult to deliver. Also, obese women are more likely to develop gestational diabetes and preeclampsia.

Women shorter than 5 feet are more likely to have a small pelvis, which may make movement of the fetus through the pelvis and vagina (birth canal) difficult during labor. For example, the fetus's shoulder is more likely to lodge against the pubic bone. This complication is called shoulder dystocia (see page 362). Also, short women are more likely to have preterm labor and a baby who has not grown as much as expected.

Structural abnormalities in the reproductive organs increase the risk of a miscarriage. Examples are a double uterus or a weak (incompetent) cervix that tends to open (dilate) as the fetus grows.

Social Characteristics

Being unmarried or in a lower socioeconomic group increases the risk of problems during pregnancy. The reason these characteristics increase risk is unclear but is probably related to other characteristics that are more common among these women. For example, these women are more likely to smoke and less likely to consume a healthy diet and to obtain appropriate medical care.

DID YOU KNOW?

- During pregnancy, risks can be reduced by good management of disorders (such as diabetes, asthma, and seizures) that are already present.
- Women with diabetes are more likely to have large babies.
- Most women with heart disease can give birth to healthy babies with no ill effects to their own health.
- Chronic high blood pressure may become worse during pregnancy, may cause the fetus to grow less than expected, and may increase the risk of a stillbirth.
- Drug treatment of HIV infection in the mother greatly reduces the risk of transmitting it to the baby.

Problems in a Previous Pregnancy

When women have had a problem in one pregnancy, they are more likely to have a problem, often the same one, in subsequent pregnancies. Such problems include having had a premature baby, an underweight baby, a baby that weighed more than 10 pounds, a baby with birth defects, a previous miscarriage, a late (postterm) delivery (after 42 weeks of pregnancy), Rh incompatibility that required a blood transfusion to the fetus, or a delivery that required a cesarean section. If women have had a baby who died shortly after birth, they are also more likely to have problems in subsequent pregnancies.

Women may have a condition that tends to make the same problem recur. For example, women with diabetes are more likely to have babies that weigh more than 10 pounds at birth.

Women who had a baby with a genetic disorder or birth defect are more likely to have another baby with a similar problem. Genetic testing of the baby, even if stillborn, and of both parents may be appropriate before another pregnancy is attempted (see page 289). If these women become pregnant again, tests such as ultrasonography, chorionic villus sampling, and amniocentesis may help determine whether the fetus has a genetic disorder or birth defect.

Having had six or more pregnancies increases the risks of very rapid labor and excessive bleeding after delivery. It also increases the risk of a mislocated placenta (placenta previa—see page 324).

Disorders Present Before Pregnancy

Before becoming pregnant, women may have a disorder that can increase the risk of problems during pregnancy. These women should talk with a doctor and try to get in the best physical condition possible before they become pregnant. After they become pregnant, they may need special care, often from an interdisciplinary team. The team may include an obstetrician (who may also be a specialist in the disorder), a specialist in the disorder, and other health care practitioners (such as nutritionists).

Heart Disease: Most women who have heart disease—including heart valve disorders (such as mitral valve prolapse) and some birth defects of the heart—can safely give birth to healthy children, without any permanent ill effects on heart function or life span. However, women who have heart failure before pregnancy are at considerable risk of problems.

Pregnancy requires the heart to work harder. Consequently, pregnancy may worsen heart disease or cause heart disease to produce symptoms for the first time. Usually, serious problems, including death of the woman or fetus, occur only when heart disease is severe before the woman becomes pregnant. About 1% of women who have severe heart disease before becoming pregnant die as a result of the pregnancy, usually because of heart failure.

The risk of problems increases throughout pregnancy as demands on the heart increase. Pregnant women with heart disease may become unusually tired and may need to limit their activities. Rarely, women with severe heart disease are advised to have an abortion early in pregnancy. Risk is also increased during labor and delivery. After delivery, women with severe heart disease may not be out of danger for at least 6 months, depending on the type of heart disease.

Heart disease in pregnant women may affect the fetus. The fetus may be born prematurely. Women with birth defects of the heart are more likely to have children with similar birth defects. Ultrasonography can detect some of these defects before the fetus is born. If severe heart disease in a pregnant woman suddenly worsens, the fetus may die.

During labor, women who have severe heart disease may be given an epidural anesthetic, which blocks sensation in the lower spinal cord and prevents women from pushing. Pushing during labor strains the heart, because it increases the amount of blood returning to the heart. Because pushing is not possible, the baby may have to be delivered with forceps.

For women with some types of heart disease, pregnancy is inadvisable because it so increases their risk of death. Primary pulmonary hypertension and Eisenmenger's syndrome are examples. If women who have one of these disorders become pregnant, doctors advise them to terminate the pregnancy as early as possible.

High Blood Pressure: Women who have high blood pressure (chronic hypertension) before they become pregnant are more likely to have potentially serious problems during pregnancy. These problems include preeclampsia (a type of high blood pressure that develops during pregnancy—see page 318), worsening of high blood pressure, a fetus that does not grow as much as expected, premature detachment of the placenta from the uterus (placental abruption), and stillbirth.

For most women with moderately high blood pressure (140/90 to 150/100 millimeters of mercury [mm Hg]), treatment with antihypertensive drugs is not recommended. Such treatment does not seem to reduce the risk of preeclampsia, premature detachment of the placenta, or a stillbirth nor to improve the growth of the fetus. However, some women are treated to prevent pregnancy from causing episodes of even higher blood pressure (which require hospitalization).

For women whose blood pressure is higher than 150/100 mm Hg, treatment with anti-hypertensive drugs is recommended. Treatment can reduce the risk of stroke and other complications due to very high blood pressure. Treatment is also recommended for women who have high blood pressure and a kidney disorder because if high blood pressure is not controlled well, the kidneys may be damaged further.

Most antihypertensive drugs used to treat high blood pressure can be used safely during pregnancy. However, angiotensin-converting enzyme (ACE) inhibitors are discontinued during pregnancy, particularly during the last two trimesters. These drugs can cause severe kidney damage in the fetus. As a result, the baby may die shortly after birth.

During pregnancy, women with high blood pressure are monitored closely to make sure blood pressure is well controlled, the kidneys are functioning normally, and the fetus is growing normally. However, premature detachment of the placenta cannot be prevented or anticipated. Often, a baby must be delivered early to prevent stillbirth or complications due to high blood pressure (such as stroke) in the woman.

Anemia: Having a hereditary anemia, such as sickle cell disease, hemoglobin S-C disease, and some thalassemias, increases the risk of problems during pregnancy. Before delivery, blood tests are routinely performed to check for hemoglobin abnormalities in women who are at increased risk of having these abnormalities because of race, ethnic background, or family history. Chorionic villus sampling or amniocentesis may be performed to detect a hemoglobin abnormality in the fetus.

Women who have sickle cell disease are particularly at risk of developing infections during pregnancy. Pneumonia, urinary tract infections, and infections of the uterus are the most common. About one third of pregnant women who have sickle cell disease develop high blood pressure during pregnancy. A sudden, severe attack of pain, called sickle cell crisis, may occur during pregnancy as at any other time. Heart failure and blockage of arteries of the lungs by blood clots (pulmonary embolism), which may be life threatening, may also occur. Bleeding during labor or after delivery may be more severe. The fetus may grow slowly or not as much as expected. The fetus may even die. The more severe sickle cell disease was before pregnancy, the higher the risk of health problems for pregnant women and the fetus and the higher the risk of death for the fetus during pregnancy. With regular blood transfusions, women are less likely to have sickle cell crises but are more likely to reject the transfused blood. This condition, called alloimmunization, can be life threatening. Also, transfusions to pregnant women do not reduce risks for the fetus.

Kidney Disorders: Women with a severe kidney disorder before pregnancy are more likely to have problems during pregnancy. Kidney function may rapidly worsen during pregnancy. High blood pressure, which often accompanies a kidney disorder, may also worsen, and preeclampsia (a type of high blood pressure that develops during pregnancy) may develop. The fetus may not grow as much as expected or may be stillborn. In pregnant women who have a kidney disorder, kidney function and blood pressure are monitored closely as is the growth of the fetus. Often, the baby must be delivered early.

Women who have had a kidney transplant that has been in place for 2 or more years are usually able to safely give birth to healthy babies if their kidneys are functioning normally, if they have had no episodes of rejection, and if their blood pressure is normal. Many women who have a kidney disorder and who undergo hemodialysis regularly can also give birth to healthy babies.

Seizure Disorders: For most women who take anticonvulsants to treat a seizure disorder, the frequency of seizures does not change during pregnancy. However, sometimes the dose of the anticonvulsant must be increased.

Taking anticonvulsants increases the risk of birth defects (see page 336). Women who take anticonvulsants should discuss the risk of birth defects with an expert in the field, preferably before they become pregnant. Some women may be able to safely discontinue anticonvulsants during pregnancy, but most women should continue to take the drugs. The risks resulting from not taking the drugs (resulting in more frequent seizures, which can harm the fetus and the woman) usually outweigh the risks resulting from taking them during pregnancy.

Sexually Transmitted Diseases: Women who have a sexually transmitted disease may have problems during pregnancy. Chlamydial infection may cause preterm labor and premature rupture of the membranes containing the fetus. It can also cause conjunctivitis in newborns, as can gonorrhea. Syphilis in pregnant women may be transmitted to the fetus through the placenta. Syphilis can cause several birth defects.

About one fourth of pregnant women who have untreated human immunodeficiency virus (HIV) infection, which causes AIDS, transmit it to their baby. Experts recommend that women with HIV infection take antiretroviral drugs during pregnancy. When pregnant women take these drugs, the risk of transmitting HIV to their baby is reduced to less than 2%. For some women with HIV infection, delivery by cesarean section, planned in advance, may further reduce the risk of transmitting HIV to the baby. Pregnancy does not seem to accelerate the progress of HIV infection in women.

Genital herpes can be transmitted to a baby during a vaginal delivery. A baby who is infected with herpes can develop a life-threatening brain infection called herpes encephalitis. If herpes produces sores in the genital area late in pregnancy, women are usually advised to give birth by cesarean section, so that the virus is not transmitted to the baby. If no sores are present, the risk of transmission is very low.

Diabetes: For women who have diabetes before they become pregnant, the risks of complications during pregnancy depend on how long diabetes has been present and whether complications of diabetes, such as high blood pressure and kidney damage, are present. (In some women, diabetes develops during pregnancy; this disorder is called gestational diabetes—see page 321.)

The risk of complications during pregnancy can be reduced by controlling the level of sugar (glucose) in the blood. The level should be kept as nearly normal as possible throughout pregnancy. Measures to control the blood sugar level (such as diet, exercise, and insulin) should be started before pregnancy. Most pregnant women are asked to measure their blood sugar level several times a day at home. Controlling diabetes is particularly important late in pregnancy. Then, the blood sugar level tends to increase because the body becomes less responsive to insulin. A higher dose of insulin is usually needed.

If diabetes is poorly controlled very early in the pregnancy, the risks of early miscarriage and significant birth defects are increased. When diabetes is poorly controlled later in pregnancy, the fetus is large and the risk of stillbirth is increased. A large fetus is less likely to pass easily through the vagina and is more likely to be injured during vaginal delivery. Consequently, delivery by cesarean section is often necessary. The risk of preeclampsia (a type of high blood pressure that occurs during pregnancy) is also increased for women with diabetes.

The fetus's lungs tend to mature slowly. If an early delivery is being considered (for example, because the fetus is large), the doctor may remove and analyze a sample of the fluid that surrounds the fetus (amniotic fluid). This procedure, called amniocentesis, helps the doctor determine whether the fetus's lungs are mature enough for the newborn to breathe air.

Newborns of women with diabetes are at increased risk of having low sugar, low calcium, and high bilirubin levels in the blood. Hospital staff members measure the levels of these substances and observe the newborns for symptoms of these abnormalities.

For women with diabetes, the requirement for insulin drops dramatically immediately after delivery. But the requirement usually returns to what it was before pregnancy within about 1 week.

Liver and Gallbladder Disorders: Women who have chronic viral hepatitis or cirrhosis (scarring of the liver) are more likely to miscarry or to give birth prematurely. Cirrhosis can cause varicose veins to develop around the esophagus (esophageal varices). Pregnancy slightly increases the risk of massive bleeding from these veins, especially during the last 3 months of pregnancy.

Pregnant women who develop gallstones are closely monitored. If a gallstone blocks the gallbladder or causes an infection, surgery may be necessary. This surgery is usually safe for pregnant women and the fetus.

Asthma: In about half of the women who have asthma and become pregnant, the frequency or severity of asthma attacks does not change during pregnancy. About one fourth of the women improve during pregnancy, and about one fourth get worse. If pregnant women with severe asthma are treated with prednisone, the risk that the fetus will not grow as much as expected or will be born prematurely is increased.

Because asthma can change during pregnancy, doctors may ask women with asthma to use a peak flow meter to monitor their breathing more often. Pregnant women with asthma should see their doctor regularly so that treatment can be adjusted as needed. Maintaining good control of asthma is important. Inadequate treatment can result in serious problems. Cromolyn, bronchodilators (such as albuterol), and corticosteroids (such as beclomethasone) can be taken during pregnancy. Inhalation is the preferred way for taking these drugs. When inhaled, the drugs affect mainly the lungs and affect the whole body and the fetus less. Aminophylline (taken by mouth or given intravenously) and theophylline (taken by mouth) are occasionally used during pregnancy. Corticosteroids are taken by mouth only when other treatments are ineffective. Being vaccinated against the influenza virus during the influenza (flu) season is particularly important for pregnant women with asthma.

Autoimmune Disorders: The abnormal antibodies produced in autoimmune disorders can cross the placenta and cause problems in the fetus. Pregnancy affects different autoimmune disorders in different ways.

Systemic lupus erythematosus (lupus) may appear for the first time, worsen, or become less severe during pregnancy. How a pregnancy affects the course of lupus cannot be predicted, but the most common time for flare-ups is immediately after delivery.

Women who develop lupus often have a history of repeated miscarriages, fetuses that do not grow as much as expected, and preterm delivery. If women have complications due to lupus (such as kidney damage or high blood pressure), the risk of death for the fetus or newborn is increased.

In pregnant women, lupus antibodies may cross the placenta to the fetus. As a result, the fetus may have a very slow heart rate, anemia, a low platelet count, or a low white blood cell count. However, these antibodies gradually disappear over several weeks after the baby is born, and the problems they cause resolve except for the slow heart rate.

In **Graves' disease,** antibodies stimulate the thyroid gland to produce excess thyroid hormone. These antibodies can cross the placenta and stimulate the thyroid gland in the fetus. As a result, the fetus may have a rapid heart rate and may not grow as much as expected. The fetus's thyroid gland may enlarge, forming a goiter. Very rarely, a goiter may be so large that it interferes with delivery through the vagina.

Usually, women with Graves' disease take the lowest possible effective dose of propylthiouracil, which slows the activity of the thyroid gland. Physical examinations and measurements of thyroid hormone levels are performed regularly because propylthiouracil crosses the placenta and may prevent the fetus from producing enough thyroid hormone. Often, Graves' disease becomes less severe during the 3rd trimester, so the dose of propylthiouracil can be reduced or stopped. If necessary, the thyroid gland of pregnant women may be removed during the 2nd trimester. These women must begin taking thyroid hormone 24 hours after surgery. Taking this hormone causes no problems for the fetus.

Myasthenia gravis, which causes muscle weakness, does not usually cause serious or permanent complications during pregnancy. However, very rarely during labor, women who have myasthenia gravis may need help with breathing (assisted ventilation). The antibodies that cause this disorder can cross the placenta. So about one of five babies born to women with myasthenia gravis is born with the disorder. However, the resulting muscle weakness in the baby is usually temporary, because the antibodies from the mother gradually disappear and the baby does not produce antibodies of this type.

Idiopathic thrombocytopenic purpura can cause bleeding problems in pregnant women and their babies. If not treated during pregnancy, the disorder tends to become more severe. Corticosteroids, usually prednisone given by mouth, can increase the platelet count and improve blood clotting in pregnant women with this disorder. However, prednisone increases the risk that the fetus will not grow as much as expected or will be born prematurely. High doses of gamma globulin may be given intravenously shortly before delivery. This treatment temporarily increases the platelet count and improves blood clotting. As a result, labor can proceed safely, and women can have a vaginal delivery without uncontrolled bleeding. Pregnant women are given platelet transfusions only when delivery by a cesarean section is needed or when the platelet count is so low that severe bleeding may occur. Rarely, when the platelet count remains dangerously low despite treatment, the spleen, which normally traps and destroys old blood cells and platelets, is removed. The best time for this surgery is during the 2nd trimester.

The antibodies that cause the disorder may cross the placenta to the fetus, resulting rarely in a dangerously low platelet count before and immediately after birth. The baby may then bleed during labor and delivery and may, as a result, be injured or die, especially if bleeding occurs in the brain. The antibodies disappear within several weeks, and the baby's blood then clots normally.

Rheumatoid arthritis does not affect the fetus, but delivery may be difficult for women if arthritis has damaged their hip joints or lower (lumbar) spine. The symptoms of rheumatoid arthritis may lessen during pregnancy, but they usually return to their original level after pregnancy.

Fibroids: Fibroids in the uterus (see page 171), which are relatively common noncancerous tumors, may increase the risk of preterm labor, abnormal presentation of the fetus, a mislocated placenta (placenta previa), and repeated miscarriages. Rarely, fibroids interfere with the movement of the fetus through the vagina during labor.

Cancer: Because cancer tends to be life threatening and because delays in treatment may reduce the likelihood of successful treatment, cancer is usually treated the same way whether women are pregnant or not. Some of the usual treatments (surgery, chemotherapy drugs, and radiation therapy) may harm the fetus. Thus, some women may consider abortion. However, treatments can sometimes be timed so that risk to the fetus is reduced.

Risk Factors That Develop During Pregnancy

• Some drugs taken during pregnancy can cause birth defects.
• Certain disorders, including blood clots, anemia, diabetes, heart failure, and urinary tract infections, are more likely to develop during pregnancy.

- Pregnancy may cause certain disorders, such as excessive vomiting.
- Problems with the placenta may occur.
- Common serious complications of pregnancy include Rh incompatibility and preeclampsia.
- Sometimes a fertilized egg remains in the fallopian tubes (ectopic pregnancy), resulting in death of the fetus and threatening the life of the woman.

During pregnancy, a problem may occur or a condition may develop to make the pregnancy high risk. For example, pregnant women may be exposed to something that can produce birth defects (teratogens), such as radiation, certain chemicals, drugs, or infections. Or a disorder may develop. Some disorders are related to (are complications of) pregnancy.

Drugs

Some drugs taken during pregnancy cause birth defects (see page 335). Examples are alcohol, isotretinoin (used to treat severe acne), some anticonvulsants, lithium, some antibiotics (such as streptomycin, kanamycin, and tetracycline), thalidomide, warfarin, and angiotensin-converting enzyme (ACE) inhibitors (taken during the last two trimesters). Taking drugs that block the actions of folic acid (such as the immunosuppressant methotrexate or the antibiotic trimethoprim) can also cause birth defects (a deficiency of folic acid increases the risk of having a baby with a birth defect). Using cocaine may cause birth defects, premature detachment of the placenta (placental abruption), and premature birth. Smoking cigarettes increases the risk of having a baby with a low birth weight. Early in pregnancy, women are asked if they are using any of these drugs. Of particular concern are alcohol, cocaine, and cigarette smoking.

Disorders That Develop During Pregnancy

During pregnancy, women may develop disorders that are not directly related to pregnancy. Some disorders increase the risk of problems for pregnant women or the fetus. They include disorders that cause a high fever, infections, and disorders that require abdominal surgery. Certain disorders are more likely to occur during pregnancy because of the many changes pregnancy causes in a woman's body. Examples are thromboembolic disease, anemia, and urinary tract infections.

Fevers: A disorder that causes a temperature greater than 103°F (39.5°C) during the 1st trimester increases the risk of a miscarriage and defects of the brain or spinal cord in the baby. Fever late in pregnancy increases the risk of preterm labor.

Infections: Some infections that occur coincidentally during a pregnancy can cause birth defects. German measles (rubella) can cause birth defects, particularly of the heart and inner ear. Cytomegalovirus infection can cross the placenta and damage the fetus's liver and brain. Other viral infections that may harm the fetus or cause birth defects include herpes simplex and chickenpox (varicella). Toxoplasmosis, a protozoal infection, may cause miscarriage, death of the fetus, and serious birth defects. Listeriosis, a bacterial infection, can also harm the fetus. Bacterial infections of the vagina (such as bacterial vaginosis) during pregnancy may lead to preterm labor or premature rupture of the membranes containing the fetus. Treatment of infections with antibiotics may reduce the likelihood of these problems.

DID YOU KNOW?

- Urinary tract infections are more common during pregnancy because the enlarging uterus slows urine flow.
- In the United States, thromboembolic disease (blood clots) is a leading cause of death in pregnant women.
- Pregnancy itself can cause temporary but potentially dangerous high blood pressure (preeclampsia).
- Pregnancy itself can cause a type of temporary diabetes.
- Destruction of the fetus's red blood cells by antibodies from the mother is a potentially severe complication of pregnancy that can be prevented.

Disorders That Require Surgery: During pregnancy, a disorder that requires emergency surgery involving the abdomen may develop. This type of surgery increases the risk of preterm labor and can cause a miscarriage, especially early in pregnancy. Thus, surgery is usually delayed as long as possible unless the woman's long-term health may be affected.

If appendicitis develops during pregnancy, surgery to remove the appendix (appendectomy) is performed immediately because a ruptured appendix may be fatal. An appendectomy is not likely to harm the fetus or cause a miscarriage. However, appendicitis may be difficult to recognize during pregnancy. The cramping pain of appendicitis resembles uterine contractions, which are common during pregnancy. The appendix is pushed higher in the abdomen as the pregnancy progresses, so the location of pain due to appendicitis may not be what is expected.

If an ovarian cyst persists during pregnancy, surgery is usually postponed until after the 12th week of pregnancy. The cyst may be producing hormones that are supporting the pregnancy and often disappears without treatment. However, if a cyst or another mass is enlarging, surgery may be necessary before the 12th week. Such a mass may be cancerous.

Obstruction of the intestine during pregnancy can be very serious. If obstruction leads to gangrene of the intestine and peritonitis (inflammation of the membrane that lines the abdominal cavity), a woman may miscarry and her life is endangered. Exploratory surgery is usually performed promptly when pregnant women have symptoms of intestinal obstruction, particularly if they have had abdominal surgery or an abdominal infection.

Thromboembolic Disease: In the United States, thromboembolic disease is the leading cause of death in pregnant women. In thromboembolic disease, blood clots form in blood vessels. They may travel through the bloodstream and block an artery. The risk of developing thromboembolic disease is increased for about 6 to 8 weeks after delivery. Most complications due to blood clots result from injuries that occur during delivery. The risk is much greater after a cesarean section than after vaginal delivery.

Blood clots usually form in the superficial veins of the legs as thrombophlebitis or in the deep veins as deep vein thrombosis.

Symptoms include swelling, pain in the calves, and tenderness. The severity of the symptoms does not correlate with the severity of the disease. A clot can move from the legs to the lungs, where it may block one or more arteries in the lungs. This blockage, called pulmonary embolism, can be life threatening. If a clot blocks an artery supplying the brain, a stroke can result. Blood clots can also develop in the pelvis.

Women who have had a blood clot during a previous pregnancy may be given heparin (an anticoagulant) during subsequent pregnancies to prevent blood clots from forming. If women have symptoms suggesting a blood clot, Doppler ultrasonography may be performed to check for clots. If a blood clot is detected, heparin is started without delay. Heparin may be injected into a vein (intravenously) or under the skin (subcutaneously). Heparin does not cross the placenta and cannot harm the fetus. Treatment is continued for 6 to 8 weeks after delivery, when the risk of blood clots is high. After delivery, warfarin may be used instead of heparin. Warfarin can be taken by mouth, has a lower risk of complications than heparin, and can be taken by women who are breastfeeding.

If pulmonary embolism is suspected, a lung ventilation and perfusion scan may be performed to confirm the diagnosis. This procedure involves injecting a tiny amount of a radioactive substance into a vein. The procedure is safe during pregnancy because the dose of the radioactive substance is so small. If the diagnosis of pulmonary embolism is still uncertain, pulmonary angiography is required.

Anemia: Most pregnant women develop some degree of anemia because they have an iron deficiency. The need for iron doubles during pregnancy, because iron is needed to make red blood cells in the fetus. Anemia may also develop during pregnancy because of a folic acid deficiency. Anemia can usually be prevented or treated by taking iron and folic acid supplements during pregnancy. However, if anemia becomes severe and persists, the blood's capacity to carry oxygen is decreased. As a result, the fetus may not receive enough oxygen, which is needed for normal growth and development, especially of the brain. Pregnant women who have severe anemia may become excessively tired, short of breath, and light-headed. The risk of preterm labor is increased. A normal amount of bleeding during labor and delivery can cause the anemia in these women to become dangerously severe. Women with anemia are more likely to develop infections after delivery. Also, if folic acid is deficient, the risk of having a baby with a birth defect of the brain or spinal cord, such as spina bifida, is increased.

Urinary Tract Infections: Urinary tract infections are common during pregnancy, probably because the enlarging uterus slows the flow of urine by pressing against the tubes that connect the kidneys to the bladder (ureters). When urine flow is slow, bacteria may not be flushed out of the urinary tract, increasing the risk of an infection. These infections increase the risk of preterm labor and premature rupture of the membranes containing the fetus. Sometimes an infection in the bladder or ureters spreads up the urinary tract and reaches a kidney, causing an infection there (see page 375). Treatment consists of antibiotic therapy.

Pregnancy Complications

Pregnancy complications are problems that occur only during pregnancy. They may affect the woman, the fetus, or both and may occur at different times during the pregnancy. For example, complications such as a mislocated placenta (placenta previa) or premature detachment of the placenta from the uterus (placental abruption) can cause bleeding from the vagina during the last 3 months of pregnancy. Women who bleed at this time are at risk of losing the baby or of bleeding excessively (hemorrhaging) or dying during labor and delivery. However, most pregnancy complications can be effectively treated.

Some problems that result from hormonal changes during pregnancy cause only minor, transient symptoms in pregnant women. For example, the normal hormonal effects of pregnancy can slow the movement of bile through the bile ducts. Cholestasis of pregnancy may result. The most obvious symptom is itching all over the body (usually in the last few months of pregnancy). No rash develops. If itching is intense, cholestyramine may be given. The disorder usually resolves after delivery but tends to recur in subsequent pregnancies.

Hyperemesis Gravidarum: Hyperemesis gravidarum is extremely severe nausea and excessive vomiting during pregnancy. Hyperemesis gravidarum differs from ordinary morning sickness. If women vomit often and have nausea to such an extent that they lose weight and become dehydrated, they have hyperemesis gravidarum. If women vomit occasionally but gain weight and are not dehydrated, they do not have hyperemesis gravidarum. The cause of hyperemesis gravidarum is unknown.

Because hyperemesis gravidarum can be life threatening to pregnant women and the fetus, women who have it are hospitalized. An intravenous line is inserted into a vein to give fluids, sugar (glucose), electrolytes, and occasionally vitamins. Women who have this complication are not allowed to eat or drink anything for at least 24 hours. Sedatives, antiemetics, and other drugs are given as needed. After women are rehydrated and vomiting has subsided, they can begin eating frequent, small portions of bland foods. The size of the portions is increased if they can tolerate more food. Usually, vomiting stops within a few days. If symptoms recur, the treatment is repeated. Rarely, if weight loss continues and symptoms persist despite treatment, women are fed via a tube passed through the nose and down the throat to the small intestine for as long as necessary.

Preeclampsia: About 5% of pregnant women develop preeclampsia (toxemia of pregnancy). In this complication, an increase in blood pressure is accompanied by protein in the urine (proteinuria). Preeclampsia usually develops between the 20th week of pregnancy and the end of the first week after delivery. The cause of preeclampsia is unknown. But it is more common among women who are pregnant for the first time, who are carrying two or more

---

Ectopic Pregnancy: A Mislocated Pregnancy

Normally, an egg is fertilized in the fallopian tube and becomes implanted in the uterus. However, if the tube is narrowed or blocked, the egg may move slowly or become stuck. The fertilized egg may never reach the uterus, resulting in an ectopic pregnancy. Ectopic pregnancies usually develop in one of the fallopian tubes (as a tubal pregnancy) but may develop in other locations. A fetus in an ectopic pregnancy cannot survive.

One of 100 to 200 pregnancies is an ectopic pregnancy. Risk factors for an ectopic pregnancy include having had a disorder of the fallopian tubes, pelvic inflammatory disease, a previous ectopic pregnancy, exposure to diethylstilbestrol as a fetus, or a tubal ligation (a sterilization procedure) that was unsuccessful or has been surgically reversed.

Symptoms include unexpected vaginal bleeding and cramping. The fetus may grow enough to rupture the structure containing it. If the fallopian tube ruptures (typically after about 6 to 8 weeks), a woman usually feels severe pain in the lower abdomen and may faint. If the tube ruptures later (after about 12 to 16 weeks), the risk of death for the woman is increased, because the fetus and placenta are larger and more blood is lost. If a woman is unsure she is pregnant, a pregnancy test is performed. If she is pregnant, ultrasonography is performed to determine the location of the fetus. If the uterus is empty, doctors may suspect an ectopic pregnancy. If ultrasonography shows the fetus in a location other than the uterus, the diagnosis is confirmed. Doctors may use a viewing tube called a laparoscope, inserted through a small incision just below the navel, to view the ectopic pregnancy directly.

An ectopic pregnancy must be ended as soon as possible to save the life of the woman. In most women, the fetus and placenta in an ectopic pregnancy must be removed surgically, usually with a laparoscope but sometimes through an incision in the abdomen (in a procedure called laparotomy). Rarely, the uterus is so damaged that a hysterectomy is required. Sometimes, the drug methotrexate, usually given in a single injection, can be used instead of surgery. The drug causes the ectopic pregnancy to shrink and disappear. Occasionally, surgery is needed in addition to methotrexate.

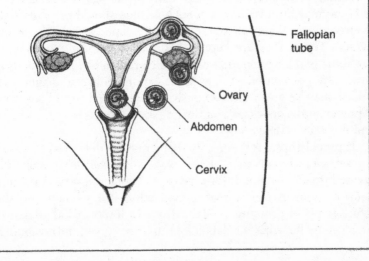

Fallopian tube

Ovary

Abdomen

Cervix

fetuses, who have had preeclampsia in a previous pregnancy, who already have high blood pressure or a blood vessel disorder, or who have sickle cell disease. It is also more common among girls aged 15 and younger and among women aged 35 and older.

A variation of severe preeclampsia, called the HELLP syndrome, occurs in some women. It consists of the following:

- *H*emolysis (the breakdown of red blood cells)
- *E*levated levels of *l*iver enzymes, indicating liver damage
- *L*ow *p*latelet count, making blood less able to clot and increasing the risk of bleeding during and after labor.

In 1 of 200 women who have preeclampsia, blood pressure becomes high enough to cause seizures; this condition is called **eclampsia.** One fourth of the cases of eclampsia occur after delivery, usually in the first 2 to 4 days. If not treated promptly, eclampsia may be fatal.

Preeclampsia may lead to premature detachment of the placenta from the uterus (placental abruption). Babies of women who have preeclampsia are 4 or 5 times more likely to have problems soon after birth than babies of women who do not have this complication. Babies may be small because the placenta malfunctions or because they are born prematurely.

If mild preeclampsia develops early in the pregnancy, bed rest at home may be sufficient, but such women should see their doctor frequently. If preeclampsia worsens, women are usually hospitalized. There, they are kept in bed and monitored closely until the fetus is mature enough to be delivered safely. Antihypertensives may be needed. A few hours before delivery, magnesium sulfate may be given intravenously to reduce the risk of seizures. If preeclampsia develops near the due date, labor is usually induced and the baby is delivered.

If preeclampsia is severe, the baby may be delivered by cesarean section, which is the quickest way, unless the cervix is already opened (dilated) enough for a prompt vaginal delivery. A prompt delivery reduces the risk of complications for women and the fetus. If blood pressure is high, drugs to lower blood pressure, such as hydralazine or labetalol, may be given intravenously before delivery is attempted. Treatment of the HELLP syndrome is usually the same as that of severe preeclampsia.

After delivery, women who have had preeclampsia or eclampsia are closely monitored for 2 to 4 days because they are at increased risk of seizures. As their condition gradually improves, they are encouraged to walk. They may remain in the hospital for a few days, depending on the severity of the preeclampsia and its complications. After returning home, these women may need to take drugs to lower blood pressure. Typically, they have a checkup at least every 2 weeks for the first few months after delivery. Their blood pressure may remain high for 6 to 8 weeks. If it remains high longer, the cause may be unrelated to preeclampsia.

Gestational Diabetes: About 1 to 3% of pregnant women develop diabetes during pregnancy. This disorder is called gestational diabetes. Unrecognized and untreated, gestational diabetes can increase the risk of health problems for pregnant women and the fetus and the risk of death for the fetus. Gestational diabetes is more common among obese women and among certain ethnic groups, particularly Native Americans, Pacific Islanders, and women of Mexican, Indian, and Asian descent.

Most women with gestational diabetes develop it because they cannot produce enough insulin as the need for insulin increases late in the pregnancy. More insulin is needed to control the increasing level of sugar (glucose) in the blood. Some women may have had diabetes before becoming pregnant, but it was not recognized until they became pregnant.

Some doctors routinely screen all pregnant women for gestational diabetes. Other doctors screen only women who have risk factors for diabetes, such as obesity and certain ethnic backgrounds. A blood test is used to measure the blood sugar level. Women who have gestational diabetes are usually taught to measure their blood sugar levels with a home blood sugar monitoring device.

Treatment consists of eliminating high-sugar foods from the diet, eating to avoid excess weight gain during the pregnancy, and, if the blood sugar level is high, taking insulin. After delivery, gestational diabetes usually disappears. However, many women who have gestational diabetes develop type 2 diabetes as they become older.

Rh Incompatibility: Rh incompatibility occurs when a pregnant woman has Rh-negative blood and the fetus has Rh-positive blood, inherited from a father who has Rh-positive blood. In about 13% of marriages in the United States, the man has Rh-positive blood and the woman has Rh-negative blood.

The Rh factor is a molecule that occurs on the surface of red blood cells of some people. Blood is Rh-positive if red blood cells have the Rh factor and Rh-negative if they do not. Problems can occur if the fetus's Rh-positive blood enters the woman's bloodstream. The woman's immune system may recognize the fetus's red blood cells as foreign and produce antibodies, called Rh antibodies, to destroy the fetus's red blood cells. The production of these antibodies is called Rh sensitization.

During a first pregnancy, Rh sensitization is unlikely, because no significant amount of the fetus's blood is likely to enter the woman's bloodstream until delivery. So the fetus or newborn rarely has problems. However, once a woman is sensitized, problems are more likely with each subsequent pregnancy in which the fetus's blood is Rh-positive. In each pregnancy, the woman produces Rh antibodies earlier and in larger amounts.

If Rh antibodies cross the placenta to the fetus, they may destroy some of the fetus's red blood cells. If red blood cells are destroyed faster than the fetus can produce new ones, the fetus can develop anemia. Such destruction is called hemolytic disease of the fetus (erythroblastosis fetalis) or of the newborn (erythroblastosis neonatorum. In severe cases, the fetus may die.

At the first visit to a doctor during a pregnancy, women are screened to determine whether they have Rh-positive or Rh-negative blood. If they have Rh-negative blood, their blood is checked for Rh antibodies and the father's blood type is determined. If he has Rh-positive blood, Rh sensitization is a risk. In such cases, the blood of pregnant women is checked for Rh antibodies periodically during the pregnancy. The pregnancy can proceed as usual as long as no antibodies are detected.

If antibodies are detected, steps may be taken to protect the fetus, depending on how high the antibody level is. If the level becomes too high, amniocentesis may be performed. In this procedure, a needle is inserted through the skin to withdraw fluid from the amniotic sac. The level of bilirubin (a yellow pigment resulting from the normal breakdown of red blood cells) is measured in the fluid sample. If this level is too high, the fetus is given a blood transfusion. Usually, additional transfusions are given until the fetus is mature enough to be safely delivered. Then labor is induced. The baby may need additional transfusions after birth. Sometimes no transfusions are needed until after birth.

As a precaution, women who have Rh-negative blood are given an injection of Rh antibodies at 28 weeks of pregnancy and within 72 hours after delivery of a baby who has Rh-positive blood, even after a miscarriage or an abortion. The antibodies given are called $Rh_0(D)$ immune globulin. This treatment destroys any red blood cells from the baby that may have entered the bloodstream of the women. Thus, there are no red blood cells from the baby to trigger the production of antibodies by these women, and subsequent pregnancies are usually not endangered.

Fatty Liver of Pregnancy: This rare disorder occurs toward the end of pregnancy. The cause is unknown. Symptoms include nausea, vomiting, abdominal discomfort, and jaundice. The disorder may rapidly worsen, and liver failure may develop. Diagnosis is based on results of liver function tests and may be confirmed by a liver biopsy. The doctor may advise immediate termination of the pregnancy. The risk of death for pregnant women and the fetus is high, but those who survive recover completely. Usually, the disorder does not recur in subsequent pregnancies.

Peripartum Cardiomyopathy: The heart's walls may be damaged late in pregnancy or after delivery, causing peripartum cardiomyopathy. The cause is unknown. Peripartum cardiomyopathy tends to occur in women who have had several pregnancies, who are older, who are carrying twins, or who have preeclampsia. In some women, heart function does not return to normal after pregnancy. They may develop peripartum cardiomyopathy in subsequent pregnancies. These women should not become pregnant again. Peripartum cardiomyopathy can result in heart failure, which is treated.

Problems With Amniotic Fluid: Too much amniotic fluid (polyhydramnios) in the membranes containing the fetus (amniotic sac) stretches the uterus and puts pressure on the diaphragm of pregnant women. This complication can lead to severe breathing problems for the women or to preterm labor.

Too much fluid tends to accumulate when pregnant women have diabetes, are carrying more than one fetus (multiple pregnancy), or produce Rh antibodies to the fetus's blood. Another cause is birth defects in the fetus, especially a blocked esophagus or defects of the brain and spinal cord (such as spina bifida). About half the time, the cause is unknown.

Too little amniotic fluid (oligohydramnios) can also cause problems. If the amount of fluid is greatly reduced, the fetus's lungs may be immature and the fetus may be compressed, resulting in deformities; this combination of conditions is called Potter's syndrome.

Too little amniotic fluid tends to develop when the fetus has birth defects in the urinary tract, has not grown as much as expected, or dies. Other causes include the use of angiotensin-converting enzyme (ACE) inhibitors, such as enalapril or captopril, in the 2nd and 3rd trimesters. These drugs are given during pregnancy only when they must be used to treat severe heart failure or high blood pressure. Taking nonsteroidal anti-inflammatory drugs (NSAIDs) late in pregnancy can also reduce the amount of amniotic fluid.

Placenta Previa: Placenta previa is implantation of the placenta over or near the cervix, in the lower rather than the upper part of the uterus. The placenta may completely or partially cover the opening of the cervix. Placenta previa occurs in 1 of 200 deliveries, usually in women who have had more than one pregnancy or who have structural abnormalities of the uterus, such as fibroids.

Placenta previa can cause painless bleeding from the vagina that suddenly begins late in pregnancy. The blood may be bright red. Bleeding may become profuse, endangering the life of the woman and the fetus.

Ultrasonography helps doctors identify placenta previa and distinguish it from a placenta that has detached prematurely (placental abruption).

When bleeding is profuse, women may be hospitalized until delivery, especially if the placenta is located over the cervix. Women who bleed profusely may need repeated blood transfusions. When bleeding is slight and delivery is not imminent, doctors typically advise bed rest in the hospital. If the bleeding stops, women are usually encouraged to walk. If bleeding does not recur, they are usually sent home, provided that they can return to the hospital easily. A cesarean section is almost always performed before labor begins. If women with placenta previa go into labor, the placenta tends to become detached very early, depriving the baby of its oxygen supply. The lack of oxygen may result in brain damage or other problems in the baby.

Placental Abruption (Abruptio Placentae): Placental abruption is the premature detachment of a normally positioned placenta from the wall of the uterus. The placenta may detach incompletely (sometimes just 10 to 20%) or completely. The cause is unknown. Detachment of the placenta occurs in 0.4 to 3.5% of all deliveries. This complication is more common among women who have high blood pressure (including preeclampsia) and among women who use cocaine.

The uterus bleeds from the site where the placenta was attached. The blood may pass through the cervix and out the vagina as an external hemorrhage, or it may be trapped behind the placenta as a concealed hemorrhage. Symptoms depend on the degree of detachment and the amount of blood lost (which may be massive). Symptoms may include sudden continuous or crampy abdominal pain, tenderness when the abdomen is pressed, and shock. Premature detachment of the placenta can lead to widespread clotting inside the blood vessels (disseminated intravascular coagulation), kidney failure, and bleeding into the walls of the uterus, especially in pregnant women who also have preeclampsia. When the placenta detaches, the supply of oxygen and nutrients to the fetus may be reduced.

Doctors suspect premature detachment of the placenta on the basis of symptoms. Ultrasonography can confirm the diagnosis.

Problems With the Placenta

Normally, the placenta is located in the upper part of the uterus, firmly attached to the uterine wall until after delivery of the baby. In placental abruption (abruptio placentae), the placenta detaches from the uterine wall prematurely, causing the uterus to bleed and reducing the fetus's supply of oxygen and nutrients. Women who have this complication are hospitalized, and the baby may be delivered early. In placenta previa, the placenta is located over or near the cervix, in the lower part of the uterus. It may cause painless bleeding that suddenly begins late in pregnancy. The bleeding may become profuse. The baby is usually delivered by cesarean section.

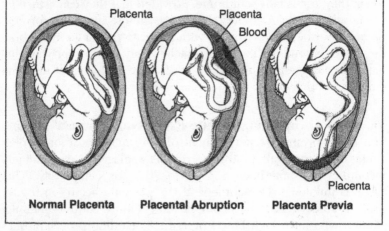

Placenta   Placenta
                          Blood

                                        Placenta

Normal Placenta   **Placental Abruption**   **Placenta Previa**

Women with premature detachment of the placenta are hospitalized. The usual treatment is bed rest. If symptoms lessen, women are encouraged to walk and may be discharged from the hospital. If bleeding continues or worsens (suggesting that the fetus is not getting enough oxygen) or if the pregnancy is near term, an early delivery is often best for the woman and the baby. If vaginal delivery is not possible, a cesarean section is performed.

Miscarriage

A miscarriage (spontaneous abortion) is the loss of a fetus due to natural causes before 24 weeks of pregnancy.

- Vaginal bleeding, a discharge, and cramping usually precede a miscarriage, although most women who have these problems have a normal pregnancy.

- Doctors examine the cervix to see if it is dilated, and ultrasonography is usually done.
- If a miscarriage seems likely and the fetus is alive, bed rest and abstinence from sexual intercourse are recommended.
- Usually after a miscarriage in which the fetus and placenta are expelled completely, no treatment is needed.

Miscarriage is a common end to a high-risk pregnancy. A miscarriage occurs in about 15% of recognized pregnancies. Many more miscarriages may be unrecognized because they occur before women know they are pregnant. About 85% of miscarriages occur during the first 12 weeks of pregnancy. Most miscarriages that occur during this time are thought to occur because something was wrong with the fetus, such as a birth defect or a genetic disorder.

The remaining 15% of miscarriages occur during weeks 13 to 24. For about one third of these miscarriages, no cause is identified. The other two thirds of them result from problems in the women. A miscarriage may occur because women have structural abnormalities of the reproductive organs, such as a double uterus or an incompetent cervix, which tends to open (dilate) as the uterus enlarges. A miscarriage can also occur if women use cocaine, are injured, or have certain disorders. These disorders include an underactive thyroid gland (hypothyroidism), diabetes, infections (such as a cytomegalovirus infection or rubella), and connective tissue disorders (such as lupus). Rh incompatibility (when a pregnant woman has Rh-negative blood and the fetus has Rh-positive blood) also increases risk. Emotional disturbances in women are not linked with miscarriages.

A miscarriage is more likely for women who have had a miscarriage or preterm labor in a previous pregnancy. For women who have had three consecutive miscarriages during the 1st trimester, the chance of having another miscarriage is about 1 in 4. Before trying to become pregnant again, women who have had repeated miscarriages may want to be checked for genetic or structural abnormalities and for other disorders that increase the risk of a miscarriage. An imaging procedure (such as hysteroscopy, hysterosalpingography, or ultrasonography) may be performed to look for structural abnormalities. If the cause of a previous miscarriage is identified, treatment may correct the problem.

Symptoms

A miscarriage is usually preceded by spotting or more obvious bleeding and a discharge from the vagina. The uterus contracts, causing cramps. About 20 to 30% of pregnant women have some bleeding or cramping at least once during the first 20 weeks of pregnancy. About half of these episodes result in a miscarriage.

Early in a pregnancy, the only sign of a miscarriage may be a small amount of vaginal bleeding. Later in a pregnancy, a miscarriage may cause profuse bleeding, and the blood may contain mucus or clots. Cramps become more severe until eventually, the uterus contracts enough to expel the fetus and placenta.

Sometimes the fetus dies but no miscarriage occurs. In such cases, the uterus does not enlarge. Rarely, the dead tissues in the uterus become infected before, during, or after a miscarriage. Such an infection may be serious, causing fever, chills, and a rapid heart rate. Affected women may become delirious, and blood pressure may fall.

DID YOU KNOW?

- Most miscarriages occur during the first 12 weeks, usually because something is wrong with the fetus.
- Emotional disturbances in women are not linked with miscarriages.
- Most women who have a miscarriage do not have problems in subsequent pregnancies.
- Repeated miscarriages may result from a structural uterine abnormality that can sometimes be corrected.

Diagnosis and Treatment

If a pregnant woman has bleeding and cramping during the first 20 weeks of pregnancy, a doctor examines her to determine whether a miscarriage is likely. The doctor examines the cervix to determine whether it is dilating. If it is not, the pregnancy may be able to continue. If it is dilating, a miscarriage is more likely.

Ultrasonography is usually also performed. It may be used to determine whether a miscarriage has already occurred or, if not, whether the fetus is still alive. If a miscarriage has occurred, ultrasonography can show whether the fetus and the placenta have been expelled.

If the fetus is alive and a miscarriage seems likely, bed rest is advised to help reduce bleeding and cramping. If possible, the woman should not work but should stay off her feet at home. Refraining from sexual intercourse is advised, although intercourse has not been definitely connected with miscarriages.

If a miscarriage has occurred and the fetus and the placenta have been expelled, no treatment is needed. If some of these tissues remain in the uterus, suction curettage (see page 44) is performed to remove them.

If the fetus dies but remains in the uterus, suction curettage is usually used to remove the fetus and the placenta. If the fetus dies

---

UNDERSTANDING THE LANGUAGE OF LOSS

Doctors may use the term *abortion* to refer to a miscarriage (spontaneous abortion) that occurs before 24 weeks of pregnancy as well as to medical termination of pregnancy (induced abortion). After 24 weeks of pregnancy, delivery of a fetus that has died is called a stillbirth. Other terms include the following:

Therapeutic (induced) abortion: An abortion that is brought about by medical means (drugs or surgery)

Threatened abortion: Bleeding or cramping during the first 24 weeks of pregnancy, indicating that the fetus may be lost

Inevitable abortion: Pain or bleeding with opening (dilation) of the cervix, indicating that the fetus will be lost

Complete abortion: Expulsion of all of the fetus and placenta in the uterus

Incomplete abortion: Expulsion of only part of the contents of the uterus

Habitual abortion: Three or more consecutive spontaneous abortions (miscarriages)

Missed abortion: Retention of a dead fetus in the uterus for 4 weeks or longer

Septic abortion: Infection of the contents of the uterus before, during, or after an abortion

late in the pregnancy, a drug that can induce labor (such as oxyto-cin) may be given intravenously instead. Oxytocin stimulates the uterus to contract and expel the fetus. Afterward, curettage may be needed to remove pieces of the placenta.

After a miscarriage, women may feel grief, sadness, anger, guilt, or anxiety about subsequent pregnancies. Grief for a loss is a natural response and should not be suppressed or denied. Talking about their feelings with another person may help women deal with their feelings and gain perspective. Women who have had a miscarriage may wish to talk with their doctor about the like-lihood of a miscarriage in subsequent pregnancies. Although having a miscarriage increases the risk of having another one, most women who have a miscarriage do not have problems in subsequent pregnancies.

CHAPTER 23

Drug Use During Pregnancy

- Women should avoid taking drugs during pregnancy if possible.
- If drugs are necessary to treat a disorder, women should talk to their doctor about the drug's benefits and risks.
- Use of tobacco or alcohol can decrease the baby's birth weight and increase the chance of birth defects and other problems.
- Smokers should stop smoking, and secondhand smoke should be avoided.
- Because experts do not know how much alcohol is safe during pregnancy, pregnant women are advised to drink none.
- Illicit drugs can cause serious problems during pregnancy and in the fetus and newborn.

More than 90% of pregnant women take prescription or non-prescription (over-the-counter) drugs or use social drugs, such as tobacco and alcohol, or illicit drugs at some time during pregnancy. In general, drugs, unless absolutely necessary, should not be used during pregnancy, because many can harm the fetus. About 2 to 3% of all birth defects result from the use of drugs.

However, drugs are sometimes essential for the health of the pregnant woman and the fetus. In such cases, a woman should talk with her doctor or other health care practitioner about the risks and benefits of taking the drugs. Before taking any drug (including nonprescription drugs) or dietary supplement (including medicinal herbs), a pregnant woman should consult her health care practitioner. A health care practitioner may recommend that a woman take certain vitamins and minerals during pregnancy.

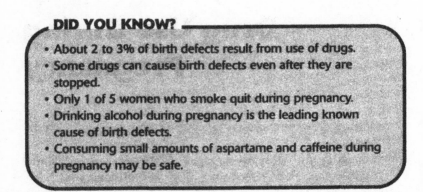

DID YOU KNOW?

- About 2 to 3% of birth defects result from use of drugs.
- Some drugs can cause birth defects even after they are stopped.
- Only 1 of 5 women who smoke quit during pregnancy.
- Drinking alcohol during pregnancy is the leading known cause of birth defects.
- Consuming small amounts of aspartame and caffeine during pregnancy may be safe.

Drugs taken by a pregnant woman reach the fetus primarily by crossing the placenta, the same route taken by oxygen and nutrients, which are needed for the fetus's growth and development. Drugs that a pregnant woman takes during pregnancy can affect the fetus in several ways:

- They can act directly on the fetus, causing damage, abnormal development (leading to birth defects), or death.
- They can alter the function of the placenta, usually by constricting blood vessels and reducing the supply of oxygen and nutrients to the fetus from the mother and thus sometimes resulting in a baby that is underweight and underdeveloped.
- They can cause the muscles of the uterus to contract forcefully, indirectly injuring the fetus by reducing its blood supply or triggering preterm labor and delivery.

How Drugs Cross the Placenta

Some of the fetus's blood vessels are contained in tiny hairlike projections (villi) of the placenta that extend into the wall of the uterus. The mother's blood passes through the space surrounding the villi (intervillous space). Only a thin membrane (placental membrane) separates the mother's blood in the intervillous space from the fetus's blood in the villi. Drugs in the mother's blood can cross this membrane into blood vessels in the villi and pass through the umbilical cord to the fetus.

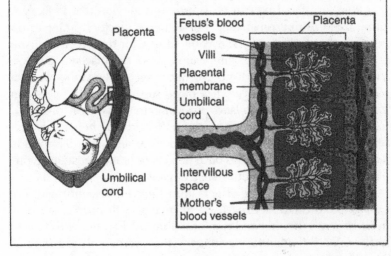

How a drug affects a fetus depends on the fetus's stage of development and the strength and dose of the drug. Certain drugs taken early in pregnancy (before the 20th day after fertilization) may act in an all-or-nothing fashion, killing the fetus or not affecting it at all. During this early stage, the fetus is highly resistant to birth defects. However, the fetus is particularly vulnerable to birth defects between the 3rd and the 8th week after fertilization, when its organs are developing. Drugs reaching the fetus during this stage may cause a miscarriage, an obvious birth defect, or a permanent but subtle defect that is noticed later in life. Drugs taken after organ development is complete are unlikely to cause obvious birth defects, but they may alter the growth and function of normally formed organs and tissues.

The Food and Drug Administration (FDA) classifies drugs according to the degree of risk they pose for the fetus if they are used during pregnancy. Some drugs are highly toxic and should never be used by pregnant women because they cause severe birth defects. One example is thalidomide. Several decades ago, this drug caused extreme underdevelopment of arms and legs and defects of the intestine, heart, and blood vessels in the babies of women who took the drug during pregnancy. Some drugs cause birth defects in animals, but the same effects have not been seen in people. One example is meclizine, frequently taken for motion sickness, nausea, and vomiting.

Often, a safer drug can be substituted for one that is likely to cause harm during pregnancy. For example, doctors prefer to use insulin rather than oral hypoglycemic drugs, for treatment of diabetes in pregnant women. Insulin cannot cross the placenta and controls diabetes better. Oral hypoglycemic drugs can cross the placenta, sometimes resulting in a very low blood sugar level in the newborn. For an overactive thyroid gland, propylthiouracil is usually preferred. For prevention of blood clots, the anticoagulant heparin is preferred. For anxiety disorders, meprobamate and chlordiazepoxide, which do not appear to cause birth defects or brain damage, are preferred. Several safe antibiotics, such as penicillin, are available.

Some drugs can cause effects after they are discontinued. For example, etretinate, a drug used to treat skin disorders, is stored in fat beneath the skin and is released slowly. Etretinate can cause birth defects 6 months or longer after women discontinue it. Therefore, women are advised to wait at least 1 year after discontinuing the drug before they become pregnant.

Unless unavoidable, vaccines made with a live virus are not given to women who are or might be pregnant. Other vaccines (such as those for cholera, hepatitis A and B, plague, rabies, tetanus, diphtheria, and typhoid) are given to pregnant women only if they are at substantial risk of developing that particular infection. However, all pregnant women should be vaccinated against the influenza virus during the influenza (flu) season.

Drugs to lower high blood pressure (antihypertensives) may be needed by pregnant women who have had high blood pressure or who develop it during pregnancy (a complication called preeclampsia—see page 318). Antihypertensives commonly used to treat preeclampsia can markedly reduce blood flow to the placenta if they lower blood pressure too rapidly in pregnant women. So pregnant women who have to take these drugs are closely monitored. Angiotensin-converting enzyme (ACE) inhibitors and thiazide diuretics are usually not given to pregnant women because these drugs can cause serious problems in the fetus.

Digoxin, used to treat heart failure and some abnormal heart rhythms, readily crosses the placenta. But it typically has little effect on the baby before or after birth.

Some Drugs That Can Cause Problems During Pregnancy[*]

TYPE	EXAMPLES	PROBLEM
Antianxiety drug	Diazepam	When the drug is taken late in pregnancy, depression, irritability, shaking, and exaggerated reflexes in the newborn
Antibiotics	Chloramphenicol	Gray baby syndrome
		In women or fetuses with glucose-6-phosphate dehydrogenase (G6PD) deficiency, the breakdown of red blood cells
	Ciprofloxacin	Possibility of joint abnormalities (seen only in animals)
	Kanamycin	Damage to the fetus's ear, resulting in deafness
	Nitrofurantoin	In women or fetuses with G6PD deficiency, the breakdown of red blood cells
	Streptomycin	Damage to the fetus's ear, resulting in deafness
	Sulfonamides	Jaundice and possibly brain damage in the newborn (much less likely with sulfasalazine)
		In women or fetuses with G6PD deficiency, the breakdown of red blood cells
	Tetracycline	Slowed bone growth, permanent yellowing of the teeth, and increased susceptibility to cavities in the baby
		Occasionally, liver failure in the pregnant woman
Anticoagulants	Heparin	When the drug is taken a long time, osteoporosis and a decrease in the number of platelets (which help blood clot) in the pregnant woman

(Continued)

Some Drugs That Can Cause Problems During Pregnancy*
(Continued)

TYPE	EXAMPLES	PROBLEM
	Warfarin	Birth defects Bleeding problems in the fetus and the pregnant woman
Anticonvulsants	Carbamazepine Phenobarbital Phenytoin	Some risk of birth defects Bleeding problems in the newborn, which can be prevented if pregnant women take vitamin K by mouth every day for a month before delivery or if the newborn is given an injection of vitamin K soon after birth Some risk of birth defects
	Trimethadione Valproate	Increased risk of miscarriage in the woman Increased risk of birth defects in the fetus, including a cleft palate and abnormalities of the heart, face, skull, hands, or abdominal organs (the risk is 70% with trimethadione and 1% with valproate)
Antihypertensives	Angiotensin-converting enzyme (ACE) inhibitors	When the drugs are taken late in pregnancy, kidney damage in the fetus, a reduction in the amount of fluid around the developing fetus (amniotic fluid), and deformities of the face, limbs, and lungs
	Thiazide diuretics	A decrease in the levels of oxygen and potassium and the number of platelets in the fetus's blood
Chemotherapy drugs	Busulfan Chlorambucil Cyclophosphamide Mercaptopurine Methotrexate	Birth defects such as less-than-expected growth before birth, underdevelopment of the lower jaw, cleft palate, abnormal development of the skull bones, spinal defects, ear defects, and clubfoot
Mood-stabilizing drug	Lithium	Birth defects (mainly of the heart), lethargy, reduced muscle tone, poor feeding, underactivity of the thyroid gland, and nephrogenic diabetes insipidus in the newborn

TYPE	EXAMPLES	PROBLEM
Nonsteroidal anti-inflammatory drugs (NSAIDs)	Aspirin Other salicylates	When the drugs are taken in large doses, a delay in the start of labor, premature closing of the connection between the aorta and artery to the lungs (ductus arteriosus), jaundice, and (occasionally) brain damage in the fetus and bleeding problems in the woman during and after delivery and in the newborn When the drugs are taken late in pregnancy, a reduction in the amount of fluid around the developing fetus
Oral hypoglycemic drugs	Chlorpropamide Tolbutamide	A very low level of sugar in the blood of the newborn Inadequate control of diabetes in the pregnant woman
Sex hormones	Danazol Synthetic progestins (but not the low doses used in oral contraceptives) Diethylstilbestrol (DES)	Masculinization of a female fetus's genitals, sometimes requiring surgery to correct Abnormalities of the uterus, menstrual problems, and an increased risk of vaginal cancer and complications during pregnancy in daughters Abnormalities of the penis in sons
Skin treatments	Etretinate Isotretinoin	Birth defects, such as heart defects, small ears, and hydrocephalus (sometimes called water on the brain)
Thyroid drugs	Methimazole Propylthiouracil Radioactive iodine	An overactive and enlarged thyroid gland in the fetus An underactive thyroid gland in the fetus
Vaccines	Live-virus vaccines such as those for measles, mumps, German measles (rubella), polio, chickenpox, and yellow fever	With rubella vaccine, potential infection of the placenta and developing fetus; with other vaccines, potential but unknown risks

*Unless absolutely necessary, drugs should not be used during pregnancy. However, drugs are sometimes essential for the health of the pregnant woman and the fetus. In such cases, a woman should talk with her health care practitioner about the risks and benefits of taking the drugs.

Most antidepressants appear to be relatively safe when used during pregnancy.

Social Drugs

Cigarette Smoking: Although cigarette smoking harms both pregnant women and the fetus, only about 20% of women who smoke quit during pregnancy. The most consistent effect of smoking on the fetus during pregnancy is a reduction in birth weight: The more a woman smokes during pregnancy, the less the baby is likely to weigh. The average birth weight of babies born to women who smoke during pregnancy is 6 ounces less than that of babies born to women who do not smoke. The reduction in birth weight seems to be greater among the babies of older smokers.

Birth defects of the heart, brain, and face are more common among babies of smokers than among those of nonsmokers. Also, the risk of sudden infant death syndrome (SIDS) may be increased. A mislocated placenta (placenta previa), premature detachment of the placenta (placental abruption), premature rupture of the membranes, preterm labor, uterine infections, miscarriages, stillbirths, and premature births are also more likely. In addition, children of women who smoke have slight but measurable deficiencies in physical growth and in intellectual and behavioral development. These effects are thought to be caused by carbon monoxide and nicotine. Carbon monoxide may reduce the oxygen supply to the body's tissues. Nicotine stimulates the release of hormones that constrict the vessels supplying blood to the uterus and placenta, so that less oxygen and fewer nutrients reach the fetus.

Pregnant women should avoid exposure to secondhand smoke because it may similarly harm the fetus.

Alcohol: Drinking alcohol during pregnancy is the leading known cause of birth defects. Because the amount of alcohol required to cause fetal alcohol syndrome is unknown, pregnant women are advised to abstain from drinking alcohol altogether. The range of effects of drinking during pregnancy is great.

The risk of miscarriage almost doubles for women who drink alcohol in any form during pregnancy, especially if they drink heavily. Often, the birth weight of babies born to women who drink during pregnancy is substantially below normal. The average birth weight is about 4 pounds for babies exposed to significant amounts of alcohol, compared with 7 pounds for all babies. Newborns of women who drank during pregnancy may not thrive and are more likely to die soon after birth.

Fetal alcohol syndrome is one of the most serious consequences of drinking during pregnancy. It occurs in about 2 of 1,000 live births. This syndrome includes inadequate growth before or after birth, facial defects, a small head (probably caused by inadequate growth of the brain), mental retardation, and abnormal behavioral development. Less commonly, the position and function of the joints are abnormal and heart defects are present.

Babies or developing children of women who drank alcohol during pregnancy may have severe behavioral problems, such as antisocial behavior and attention deficit disorder. These problems can occur even when the baby has no obvious physical birth defects.

Caffeine: Whether consuming caffeine during pregnancy harms the fetus is unclear. Evidence seems to suggest that consuming caffeine in moderation during pregnancy poses little or no risk to the fetus. Caffeine, which is contained in coffee, tea, some sodas, chocolate, and some drugs, is a stimulant that readily crosses the placenta to the fetus. Thus, it may stimulate the fetus, increasing the heart and breathing rates. Caffeine also may decrease blood flow across the placenta and decreases the absorption of iron (possibly increasing the risk of anemia—see page 316). Whether drinking more than seven or eight cups of coffee a day increases the risk of having a stillbirth, premature birth, low-birth-weight baby, or miscarriage is also unclear. Some experts recommend limiting coffee consumption to two or three cups a day and drinking decaffeinated beverages when possible.

TAKING DRUGS WHILE BREASTFEEDING

When new mothers who are breastfeeding have to take a drug, they wonder whether they should stop breastfeeding. The answer depends on how much of the drug appears in the milk, whether the drug is absorbed by the baby, how the drug affects the baby, and how much milk the baby consumes. How much milk the baby consumes depends on the baby's age and the amount of other foods and liquids in the baby's diet. Some drugs, such as epinephrine, heparin, and insulin, do not appear in breast milk and are thus safe to take. Most drugs appear in breast milk but usually in tiny amounts. However, even in tiny amounts, some drugs can harm the baby. Some drugs appear in breast milk, but the baby usually absorbs so little of them that they do not affect the baby. Examples are the antibiotics gentamicin, kanamycin, streptomycin, and tetracycline.

Drugs that are considered safe include most nonprescription (over-the-counter) drugs. Exceptions are antihistamines (commonly contained in cough and cold remedies, allergy drugs, motion sickness drugs, and sleep aids) and, if taken in large amounts for a long time, aspirin and other salicylates. Acetaminophen and ibuprofen, taken in usual doses, appear to be safe.

Drugs that are applied to the skin, eyes, or nose or that are inhaled are usually safe. Most antihypertensive drugs do not cause significant problems in breastfed babies. Warfarin is considered compatible with breastfeeding a full-term, healthy baby. Caffeine and theophylline do not harm breastfed babies but may make them irritable. Even though some drugs are reportedly safe for breastfed babies, women who are breastfeeding should consult a health care practitioner before taking any drug, even a nonprescription drug, or a medicinal herb. Drug labels should be checked because they contain warnings against use during breastfeeding, if applicable.

Some drugs require a doctor's supervision during their use. Taking them safely while breastfeeding may require adjusting the dose, limiting the length of time the drug is used, or timing when the drug is taken in relation to breastfeeding. Most antianxiety drugs, antidepressants, and antipsychotic drugs require a doctor's supervision, even though they are unlikely to cause significant problems in the baby. However, these drugs stay in the body a long time. During the first few months of life, babies may have difficulty eliminating the drugs, and the drugs may affect the baby's nervous system. For example, the antianxiety drug diazepam (a benzodiazepine) causes lethargy, drowsiness, and weight loss in breastfed babies. Babies eliminate phenobarbital (an anticonvulsant and a barbiturate) slowly, so this drug may cause excessive drowsiness. Because of these effects, doctors reduce the dose of benzodiazepines and barbiturates as well as monitor their use by women who are breastfeeding.

Some drugs should not be taken while breastfeeding. They include atropine, chemotherapy drugs (such as doxorubicin and methotrexate), chloramphenicol, ergotamine, lithium, methimazole, methysergide, radioactive drugs for diagnostic procedures, thiouracil, vaccines, and illicit drugs such as cocaine, heroin, and phencyclidine (PCP). Other drugs should not be taken because they may suppress milk production. They include bromocriptine, estrogen, oral contraceptives that contain high-dose estrogen and a progestin, and levodopa.

If women who are breastfeeding must take a drug that may harm the baby, they must stop breastfeeding. But they can resume breastfeeding after they discontinue the drug. While taking the drug, women can maintain their milk supply by pumping breast milk, which is then discarded.

Aspartame: Aspartame, an artificial sweetener, appears to be safe during pregnancy when it is consumed in small amounts, such as in amounts used in artificially sweetened foods and beverages.

Illicit Drugs

Use of illicit drugs (particularly cocaine and opioids) during pregnancy can cause complications during pregnancy and serious problems in the developing fetus and the newborn. For pregnant women, injecting illicit drugs also increases the risk of infections that can affect or be transmitted to the fetus. These infections include hepatitis and sexually transmitted diseases (including AIDS). Also, growth of the fetus is more likely to be inadequate, and premature births are more common.

Cocaine: Cocaine readily crosses the placenta and affects the fetus. It constricts blood vessels, possibly reducing blood flow (and the oxygen supply) to the fetus. The reduced blood and oxygen supply to the fetus can slow the growth of the fetus, particularly of the bones and the intestine. Babies are more likely to be small and to have a small head. Rarely, use of cocaine results in birth defects of the brain, eyes, kidneys, and genital organs.

Use of cocaine during pregnancy can also cause complications during pregnancy. Among women who use cocaine throughout pregnancy, about 31% have a preterm delivery and 15% have premature detachment of the placenta (placental abruption). The chances of a miscarriage are also increased. About 19% have a baby who did not grow as much as normally expected before birth. If women stop using cocaine after the first 3 months of pregnancy, the risks of a preterm delivery and premature detachment of the placenta are still increased, but the fetus's growth will probably be normal.

Newborns may have withdrawal symptoms. Their behavior is also affected. Newborns interact less with other people. Babies of cocaine users may be hyperactive, tremble uncontrollably, and have difficulty learning (which may continue through age 5 years or even longer).

Opioids: Opioids, such as heroin, methadone, and morphine, readily cross the placenta. Consequently, the fetus may become addicted to them and may have withdrawal symptoms 6 hours to 8 days after birth. However, use of opioids rarely results in birth defects. Use of opioids during pregnancy increases the risk of complications during pregnancy, such as miscarriage, abnormal presentation of the baby, and preterm delivery. Babies of heroin users are more likely to be small.

Amphetamines: Use of amphetamines during pregnancy may result in birth defects, especially of the heart.

Marijuana: Whether use of marijuana during pregnancy can harm the fetus is unclear. The main ingredient of marijuana, tetrahydrocannabinol, can cross the placenta and thus may affect the fetus. If marijuana is used heavily during pregnancy, newborns may have behavioral problems. Some studies have found that babies born to women who used marijuana while pregnant were smaller and, therefore, more likely to have health problems, than babies born to women who did not use marijuana.

Drugs Used During Labor and Delivery

Local anesthetics, opioids, and other analgesics usually cross the placenta and can affect the newborn. For example, they can weaken the newborn's urge to breathe. Therefore, if these drugs are needed during labor, they are given in the smallest effective doses.

CHAPTER 24

Normal Labor and Delivery

Although each labor and delivery is different, most follow a general pattern. Therefore, an expectant mother can have a general idea of what changes will occur in her body to enable her to deliver the baby and what procedures will be followed to help her. She also has several choices to make, such as whether to have the father present and where to have the baby.

DID YOU KNOW?

- Because unexpected complications can occur, experts do not recommend delivery at home.
- On average, labor lasts 15 to 16 hours in a first pregnancy and tends to be shorter, averaging 6 to 8 hours, in subsequent pregnancies.
- Such drugs should be used sparingly, particularly before contractions become effective and when delivery is imminent.
- Preparation for childbirth (for example, by attending classes) may reduce anxiety and the need for pain medicine.
- Episiotomy is not done routinely.
- Most complications in the woman and baby occur within the first 24 hours after delivery.

An expectant mother may want the baby's father to remain with her during labor. His encouragement and emotional support may help her relax, sometimes reducing her need for drugs to relieve pain. In addition, sharing the meaningful experience of childbirth has emotional and psychologic benefits, such as creating strong family bonds. Childbirth education classes prepare both father and mother for the entire process. On the other hand, an expectant mother may prefer privacy during labor, the father may not want to be present, or another partner may be more appropriate or supportive.

In the United States, almost all babies are born in hospitals, but some women want to have their babies at home. However, because unexpected complications can occur during or shortly after labor, most experts do not advise delivery at home. Women who prefer a homelike setting and fewer rules (for example, no limit on the number of visitors or on visiting hours) may choose birthing centers. Such centers provide an informal, personal experience of childbirth but are much safer than delivery at home. Birthing centers are part of a hospital or have an arrangement with a nearby hospital. Thus, birthing centers can provide a medical staff, emergency equipment, and full hospital facilities, if needed. If complications develop during labor, birthing centers immediately transfer the woman to the hospital.

Some hospitals have private rooms in which a woman stays from labor until discharge. These rooms are called LDRPs for labor, delivery, recovery, and postpartum (after delivery).

Regardless of the choices a woman makes, knowing what to expect helps prepare her for labor and delivery.

Labor

Labor is a series of rhythmic, progressive contractions of the uterus that gradually move the fetus through the lower part of the uterus (cervix) and birth canal (vagina) to the outside world.

- The main signs of labor are regular uterine contractions and back pain, sometimes with a small bloody vaginal discharge.

- A health care practitioner examines the woman to determine the position of the fetus, how dilated the cervix is, and whether the membranes around the fetus have ruptured.
- The heart rates of the woman and fetus are monitored.
- Pain relief for labor and delivery can be provided in many different ways.
- Some women choose natural childbirth and a strategy to deal with pain long before labor begins.

Stages of Labor

FIRST STAGE

   From the beginning of labor to the full opening (dilation) of the cervix—to about 4 inches (10 centimeters).

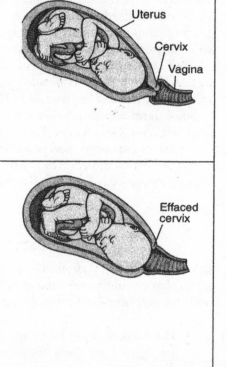

Initial (Latent) Phase

Contractions become progressively stronger and more rhythmic.

Discomfort is minimal.

The cervix thins and opens to about 1½ inches (4 centimeters).

This phase lasts an average of 12 hours in a first pregnancy and 5 hours in subsequent pregnancies.

Uterus

Cervix

Vagina

Active Phase

The cervix opens from about 1½ inches (4 centimeters) to the full 4 inches (10 centimeters).

The presenting part of the baby, usually the head, begins to descend into the woman's pelvis.

The woman begins to feel the urge to push as the baby descends.

This phase averages about 3 hours in a first pregnancy and 2 hours in subsequent pregnancies.

Effaced cervix

SECOND STAGE

From the complete opening of the cervix to delivery of the baby. This stage averages about 45 to 60 minutes in a first pregnancy and 15 to 30 minutes in subsequent pregnancies.

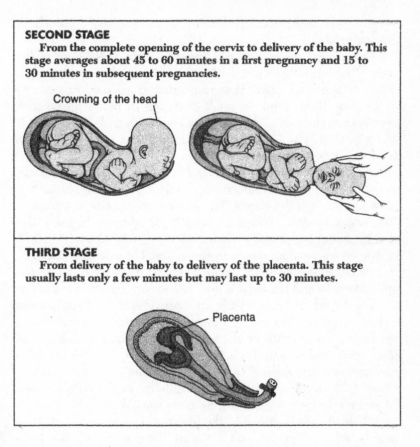

Crowning of the head

THIRD STAGE

From delivery of the baby to delivery of the placenta. This stage usually lasts only a few minutes but may last up to 30 minutes.

Placenta

Labor occurs in three main stages. The first stage (which has two phases: initial and active) is labor proper. In it, contractions cause the cervix to open gradually (dilate) and to thin and pull back (efface) until it merges with the rest of the uterus. These changes enable the fetus to pass through the vagina. The second and third stages constitute delivery of the baby and the placenta.

Labor usually starts within 2 weeks of (before or after) the estimated date of delivery. Exactly what causes labor to start is unknown. Toward the end of pregnancy (after 36 weeks), a doctor may perform a pelvic examination to try to predict when labor will start. On average, labor lasts 15 to 16 hours in a woman's first pregnancy and tends to be shorter, averaging 6 to 8 hours, in subsequent pregnancies. A woman who has had rapid deliveries in previous pregnancies should notify her doctor as soon as she thinks she is going into labor.

All pregnant women should know what the main signs of the start of labor are: contractions in the lower abdomen at regular intervals and back pain. However, other clues may precede or accompany these signs. A small discharge of blood mixed with mucus from the vagina (bloody show) is usually a clue that labor is about to start. The bloody show may appear as early as 72 hours before contractions start.

Occasionally, the fluid-filled membranes that contain the fetus (amniotic sac) rupture before labor starts, and the amniotic fluid flows out through the vagina. This event is commonly described as "the water breaks." When a woman's membranes rupture, she should contact her doctor or midwife immediately. About 80 to 90% of women whose membranes rupture before but near their due date go into labor spontaneously within 24 hours. If labor has not started after 24 hours and the baby is due, women are usually admitted to the hospital, where labor is artificially started (induced) to reduce the risk of infection. After the membranes rupture, bacteria from the vagina can enter the uterus more easily and cause an infection in the woman, the fetus, or both. Oxytocin (which causes the uterus to contract) or a similar drug, such as a prostaglandin, is used to induce labor. If the membranes rupture prematurely, doctors do not induce labor until the fetus is more mature (see page 357).

When the contractions in the lower abdomen first start, they may be weak, irregular, and far apart. They may feel like menstrual cramps. As time passes, abdominal contractions become longer, stronger, and closer together. When strong contractions occur 5 minutes apart or less and the cervix is dilated more than $1\frac{1}{2}$ inches (4 centimeters), the woman is admitted to the hospital or birthing center. The strength, duration, and frequency of contractions are noted. Her weight, blood pressure, heart and breathing rates, and temperature are measured, and samples of urine and blood are taken for analysis. Her abdomen is examined to estimate how big the fetus is, whether the fetus is facing rearward or forward (position), and whether the head, face, buttocks, or shoulder is leading the way out (presentation).

The presentation and position of the fetus affect how the fetus passes through the vagina. The most common and safest combination is facing rearward (toward the woman's back), with the face and body angled toward the right or left, and head first, with the neck bent forward, chin tucked in, and arms folded across the chest (see page 360). Head first is called a vertex or cephalic presentation. During the last week or two before delivery, most fetuses turn so that the back of the head presents first. If the presentation is buttocks first (breech) or shoulder first or the fetus is facing forward, delivery is considerably more difficult for the woman, fetus, and doctor. Cesarean delivery is recommended.

Usually, the vagina is examined to determine if the membranes have ruptured and how dilated and effaced the cervix is, but this examination may be omitted if the woman is bleeding or if the membranes have ruptured spontaneously. The color of the amniotic fluid is noted. The fluid should be clear and have no significant odor. If the membranes rupture and the amniotic fluid is green, the discoloration results from the fetus's first stool (fetal meconium).

Soon after the woman is admitted to the hospital, the doctor or another health care practitioner listens to the fetus's heartbeat directly using a fetal stethoscope (fetoscope) or uses an ultrasound device to monitor heartbeats (a procedure called electronic fetal heart monitoring).

During the first stage of labor, the heart rates of woman and fetus are monitored periodically or continuously. Monitoring the fetus's heart rate, with a fetal stethoscope or electronic fetal heart monitoring, is the easiest way to determine whether the fetus is receiving enough oxygen. An abnormal heart rate (too fast or too slow) may indicate that the fetus is in distress. During the second stage of labor, the woman's heart rate and blood pressure are monitored regularly. The fetus's heart rate is monitored after every contraction or, if electronic monitoring is used, continuously.

During labor in a hospital, an intravenous line is usually inserted into the woman's arm. This line is used to give the woman fluids to prevent dehydration and, if needed, to give drugs immediately. When fluids are given intravenously, the woman does not have to eat or drink during labor, although she may choose to drink some fluids and eat some light food early in labor. An empty stomach during delivery makes the woman less likely to vomit and to inhale vomit. Inhaling vomit, although very rare, can cause respiratory distress, a potentially life-threatening disorder in which the lungs are inflamed.

Usually, a woman is given an antacid by mouth to neutralize stomach acid when she is admitted to the hospital and every 3 hours after that. Antacids reduce the risk of damage to the lungs if vomit is inhaled.

MONITORING THE FETUS

Electronic monitoring is routinely used to monitor the fetus's heart rate and the contractions of the uterus. Certain changes in the fetus's heart rate during contractions can indicate that the fetus is not receiving enough oxygen. The fetus's heart rate can be monitored externally by attaching an ultrasound device (which transmits and receives ultrasound waves) to the woman's abdomen or internally by inserting an electrode through the woman's vagina and attaching it to the fetus's scalp. The internal approach is usually used only when problems during labor appear likely or when signals detected by the external device cannot be recorded.

In a high-risk pregnancy, electronic monitoring is sometimes used as part of a nonstress test, in which the fetus's heart rate is monitored as the fetus lies still and as it moves. If the heart rate does not increase with movement, a contraction stress test may be performed. To start uterine contractions, oxytocin (a hormone that causes the uterus to contract during labor) is usually given intravenously. The fetus's heart rate is monitored during these contractions to determine whether the fetus will be able to withstand labor.

When a problem is detected, fetal scalp blood sampling may be performed. During labor, a small amount of blood is removed from the fetus's scalp to measure the acidity (pH) of the blood. This measurement helps doctors determine whether the fetus is receiving enough oxygen.

On the basis of such tests, a doctor may allow labor to continue or may perform a cesarean section immediately.

Pain Relief: With the advice of her doctor or midwife, a woman usually plans an approach to pain relief long before labor starts. She may choose natural childbirth, which relies on relaxation and breathing techniques to deal with pain, or she may plan to use analgesics or a particular type of anesthetic (local, regional, or general) if needed. After labor starts, these plans may be modified, depending on how labor progresses, how the woman feels, and what the doctor or midwife recommends.

A woman's need for pain relief during labor varies considerably, depending to some extent on her level of anxiety. Attending childbirth preparation classes helps prepare the woman for labor and delivery. Such preparation and emotional support from the people attending the labor tend to lessen anxiety and often markedly reduce her need for drugs to relieve pain.

If a woman requests analgesics during labor, they are usually given to her. However, because some of these drugs can slow (depress) breathing and other functions of the newborn, the amount given is as small as possible. Most commonly, meperidine or morphine is given intravenously to relieve pain. These drugs can slow the initial phase of the first stage of labor, so they are usually given during the active phase of the first stage. In addition, because these drugs have the greatest effect during the first 30 minutes after they are given, the drugs are often not given when delivery is imminent. To counteract the sedating effects of these drugs on the newborn, a doctor can give the newborn the drug naloxone immediately after delivery.

Local anesthesia numbs the vagina and the tissues around its opening. Commonly, this area is numbed by injecting a local anesthetic through the wall of the vagina and around the pudendal nerve (which supplies sensation to the lower genital area). This procedure, called a pudendal block, is used only late in labor, when the baby's head is about to emerge from the vagina. Another common but less effective procedure involves injecting a local anesthetic at the opening of the vagina. With both procedures, the woman can remain awake and push, and the fetus's functions are unaffected. These procedures are useful for deliveries that have no complications.

Regional anesthesia numbs a larger area. It may be used for women who want more complete pain relief. A lumbar epidural injection is almost always used. This procedure involves injecting an anesthetic in the lower back—into the space between the spine and the outer layer of tissue covering the spinal cord (epidural space). Alternatively, a catheter is placed in the epidural space, and opioids, such as fentanyl and sufentanil, are continuously and slowly given through the catheter. Another procedure (spinal anesthesia) involves injecting an anesthetic into the space between the middle and inner layers of tissue covering the spinal cord (subarachnoid space). A spinal injection is typically used for cesarean sections when there are no complications. Neither an epidural nor a spinal

---

NATURAL CHILDBIRTH

Natural childbirth uses relaxation and breathing techniques to control pain during childbirth. Natural childbirth often helps reduce or eliminate the need for analgesics or anesthetics during labor and delivery.

To prepare for natural childbirth, a pregnant woman and her partner take childbirth classes, usually six to eight sessions over several weeks, to learn how to use the relaxation and breathing techniques. They also learn what happens in the various stages of labor and delivery.

The relaxation technique involves consciously tensing a part of the body and then relaxing it. This technique helps a woman relax the rest of her body while the uterus is contracting during labor and relax her whole body between contractions.

The breathing technique involves several types of breathing, which are used at different times during labor. During the first stage of labor, before the woman begins to push, the following types of breathing may help:

- Deep breathing to help the woman relax at the beginning and end of a contraction

- Fast, shallow breathing (panting) in the upper chest at the peak of a contraction

- A pattern of panting and blowing to help the woman refrain from pushing when she has an urge to push before the cervix is completely dilated

In the second stage of labor, the woman alternates between pushing and panting.

The woman and her partner should practice relaxation and breathing techniques regularly during pregnancy. During labor, the woman's partner can help her by reminding her of what she should be doing at a particular stage and by noticing when she is tense, in addition to providing emotional support. The partner may massage the woman to help her relax more.

The most well-known method of natural childbirth is probably the Lamaze method. Another method, the Leboyer method, includes birth in a darkened room and immersion of the baby into lukewarm water immediately after delivery.

injection prevents the woman from pushing adequately. Occasionally, use of either procedure causes a fall in blood pressure. Consequently, if one of these procedures is used, the woman's blood pressure is measured frequently.

General anesthesia makes a woman temporarily unconscious. This method is rarely necessary and infrequently used because it may slow the function of the fetus's heart, lungs, and brain. Although this effect is usually temporary, it can interfere with the newborn's adjustment to life outside the uterus. General anesthesia is typically used for emergency cesarean sections because it is the quickest way to anesthetize the woman.

Delivery

Delivery is the passage of the fetus and placenta (afterbirth) from the uterus to the outside world.

- The woman bears down and pushes with each contraction to help move the fetus's head down through her pelvis.
- A few minutes after the baby is delivered, the woman must push the placenta out.
- Unless the baby needs nursery support, the baby often stays with the woman for a few hours to allow bonding to occur.

For delivery in a hospital, a woman may be moved from a labor room to a birthing or delivery room, a room used only for deliveries. Usually, the father or other support people are encouraged to accompany her. If she is already in an LDRP (for labor, delivery, recovery, and postpartum), she remains there. The intravenous line remains in place.

When a woman is about to give birth, she may be placed in a semi-upright position, between lying down and sitting up. Her back can be supported by pillows or a backrest. The semi-upright position uses gravity: The downward pressure of the fetus helps the vagina and surrounding area stretch gradually, decreasing the risk of tearing. This position also puts less strain on the woman's back and pelvis. Some women prefer to deliver lying down. However, with this position, delivery may take longer.

As delivery progresses, the doctor or midwife examines the vagina to determine the position of the fetus's head. The woman is asked to bear down and push with each contraction to help move the fetus's head down through her pelvis and to widen the vaginal opening so that more and more of the head appears. When about 1½ to 2 inches of the head appears, the doctor or midwife places a hand over the fetus's head during a contraction to control the fetus's progress. As the head crowns (when the widest part of the head passes through the vaginal opening), the head and chin are eased out of the vaginal opening to prevent the woman's tissues from tearing.

Forceps are metal instruments, similar to tongs, with rounded edges that fit around the fetus's head (see page 366). Forceps are used when the fetus is in distress, when the woman is having difficulty pushing, or when labor is not progressing well.

An episiotomy is no longer considered a routine procedure. It is used only when necessary for immediate delivery. For this procedure, the doctor injects a local anesthetic to numb the area and makes an incision in the area between the openings of the vagina and anus. If the muscle around the opening of the anus (rectal sphincter) is damaged during an episiotomy or is torn during delivery, it usually heals well if the doctor repairs it immediately.

After the baby's head has emerged, the body is rotated sideways so that the shoulders can emerge easily, one at a time. The rest of the baby usually slips out quickly. Mucus and fluid are suctioned out of the baby's nose, mouth, and throat. The umbilical cord is clamped and cut. The baby is then wrapped in a lightweight blanket and placed on the woman's abdomen or in a warmed bassinet.

After delivery of the baby, the doctor or midwife places a hand gently on the woman's abdomen to make sure the uterus is contracting. After delivery, the placenta usually detaches from the uterus within 3 to 10 minutes, and a gush of blood soon follows. Usually, the woman can push the placenta out on her own. If she cannot and particularly if she is bleeding excessively, the doctor or midwife applies firm downward pressure on the woman's abdomen, causing the placenta to detach from the uterus and come out. If the placenta has not been delivered within 30 minutes of delivery, the doctor or midwife may insert a hand into the uterus, separating the placenta from the uterus and removing it.

After the placenta is removed, it is examined for completeness. Fragments left in the uterus prevent the uterus from contracting. Contractions are essential to prevent further bleeding from the area where the placenta was attached to the uterus. So if fragments remain, bleeding can occur after delivery and may be substantial. Infections can also occur. If the placenta is incomplete, the doctor or midwife may remove the remaining fragments by hand. Sometimes fragments have to be surgically removed.

In many hospitals, as soon as the placenta is delivered or removed, the woman is given oxytocin (intravenously or intramuscularly), and her abdomen is periodically massaged to help the uterus contract.

The doctor stitches up any tears in the cervix, vagina, or nearby muscles and, if an episiotomy was performed, the episiotomy incision. The woman is then moved to the recovery room or remains in the LDRP. Often, a baby who does not need further medical attention stays with the mother. Typically, the woman and her baby remain together in a warm, private area for 3 to 4 hours so that bonding can begin. Many women wish to begin breastfeeding soon after delivery. Later, the baby may be taken to the hospital nursery. In many hospitals, the woman may choose to have the baby remain with her—a practice called rooming-in. All hospitals with LDRPs require it. With rooming-in, the baby is usually fed on demand, and the woman is taught how to care for the baby before they leave the hospital. If a woman needs a rest, she may have the baby taken to the nursery.

Because most complications, particularly bleeding, occur within the first 24 hours after delivery, nurses and doctors carefully observe the woman and baby during this time.

CHAPTER 25

Complications of Labor and Delivery

Usually, labor and delivery occur without any problems. Serious problems are relatively rare, and most can be anticipated and treated effectively. However, problems sometimes develop suddenly and unexpectedly. Regular visits to a doctor or certified midwife during pregnancy make anticipation of problems possible and improve the chances of having a healthy baby and safe delivery.

DID YOU KNOW?

- Although most serious problems during labor or delivery can be anticipated, some occur unexpectedly in low-risk pregnancies.

Problems With the Timing of Labor

- Labor may be too early (resulting in a premature infant) or too late (resulting in a postmature infant).
- If early delivery is likely, various drugs can help the infant's organs mature more quickly.
- Medication can help with labor that's progressing too slowly.

Labor may start too early (before the 37th week of pregnancy) or may start late (after the 41st to 42nd week of pregnancy). As a result, the health or life of the fetus may be endangered. Labor may start too early or late when the woman or fetus has a medical problem or the fetus is in an abnormal position.

No more than 10% of women deliver on their specified due date (usually estimated to be about 40 weeks of pregnancy). About 50% of women deliver within 1 week (before or after), and almost 90% deliver within 2 weeks of the due date. Determining the length of pregnancy can be difficult, because the precise date of conception often cannot be determined. Early in pregnancy, an ultrasound examination, which is safe and painless, can help determine the length of pregnancy. In mid to late pregnancy, ultrasound examinations are less reliable in determining length of pregnancy.

Premature Rupture of the Membranes: In about 10% of normal pregnancies, the fluid-filled membranes containing the fetus rupture before labor begins. Contractions usually begin within 12 to 48 hours. Rupture of the membranes is commonly described as "the water breaks." The fluid within the membranes (amniotic fluid) then flows out from the vagina. The flow varies from a trickle to a gush. As soon as the membranes have ruptured, a woman should contact her doctor or midwife.

If labor does not begin within 24 to 48 hours, the risk of infection of the uterus and fetus increases. Therefore, a doctor or certified midwife usually artificially starts (induces) labor, depending on whether or not the fetus is mature enough for delivery. The doctor may analyze the amniotic fluid to determine if the fetus's lungs are mature enough. If they are, labor is induced and the baby is delivered. If they are not, the doctor usually does not induce labor.

The woman's temperature and pulse rate are usually recorded at least twice daily. An increase in temperature or pulse rate may be an early sign of infection. If an infection develops, labor is promptly induced and the baby is delivered. Very rarely, if the amniotic fluid stops leaking and contractions stop, the woman may be able to go home. In such cases, the woman should be seen by her doctor at least once a week.

Preterm Labor: Because babies born prematurely can have significant health problems, doctors try to prevent or stop labor that begins before the 34th week of pregnancy. What causes preterm labor is not well understood. However, a healthy lifestyle and regular visits to the doctor or midwife during pregnancy are helpful. Preterm labor is difficult to stop. If vaginal bleeding occurs or the membranes rupture, allowing labor to continue is often best. If vaginal bleeding does not occur and the membranes are not leaking amniotic fluid, the woman is advised to rest and to limit her activities as much as possible, preferably to sedentary ones. She is given fluids and may be given drugs that can slow labor. These measures can often delay labor for a brief time.

Drugs that can slow labor include magnesium sulfate and terbutaline. Magnesium sulfate given intravenously stops preterm labor in many women. However, if the dose is too high, it may slow the woman's heart and breathing rates. Terbutaline given by injection under the skin also can be used to stop preterm labor. However, as a side effect, it increases the heart rate in the woman, fetus, or both. Sometimes ritodrine is used instead of terbutaline.

If the cervix opens (dilates) beyond 2 inches (5 centimeters), labor usually continues until the baby is born. If doctors think that premature delivery is inevitable, a woman may be given a corticosteroid such as betamethasone. The corticosteroid helps the fetus's lungs and other organs mature more quickly and reduces the risk that after birth, the baby will have difficulty breathing (neonatal respiratory distress syndrome).

DID YOU KNOW?

- Delivery much beyond 41 to 42 weeks can be a problem because the placenta may no longer function well.

Postterm Pregnancy and Postmaturity: In most pregnancies that go a little beyond 41 to 42 weeks, no problems develop. However, problems may develop if the placenta cannot continue to maintain a healthy environment for the fetus. This condition is called postmaturity.

Typically, tests are started at 41 weeks to evaluate the fetus's movement and heart rate and the amount of amniotic fluid, which decreases markedly in postmature pregnancies. The fetus's rate of breathing and heart sounds may also be monitored. Doctors can check on the fetus's well-being with electronic fetal heart monitoring (see page 350). Typically, at 42 weeks, labor is induced, or the baby is delivered by cesarean section.

Labor That Progresses Too Slowly: If labor is progressing too slowly, the fetus may be too big to move through the birth canal (pelvis and vagina). Delivery by forceps, a vacuum extractor, or cesarean section may be necessary. If the birth canal is big enough for the fetus but labor is not progressing, the woman is given oxytocin intravenously to stimulate the uterus to contract more forcefully. If oxytocin is unsuccessful, a cesarean section is performed. If the baby is already in position to be delivered, forceps or a vacuum extractor may be used instead.

Problems Affecting the Fetus or Newborn

• Various positions and presentations of the fetus are possible; the safest is head first, facing down (toward the back).

If labor does not proceed normally, the fetus or newborn may have problems.

DID YOU KNOW?

• Many abnormal fetal heart rate patterns can be relieved by simple measures such as giving the woman oxygen, increasing the amount of fluids given intravenously to the woman, and turning the woman on her left side.
• The umbilical cord is wrapped around the baby's neck in 25% of deliveries. Normally, the baby is not harmed.

Breathing Problems: Rarely, a baby does not start to breathe at birth, even though no problems were detected before delivery.

Then the baby requires resuscitation. Personnel skilled in resuscitating babies may attend the delivery for this reason.

Abnormal Position and Presentation of the Fetus: Position refers to whether the fetus is facing rearward (toward the woman's back, or face down) or forward (face up). Presentation refers to the part of the fetus's body that leads the way out through the birth canal. The most common and safest combination is head first (called a vertex or cephalic presentation) and facing down, with the face and body angled toward the right or left and with the neck bent forward, chin tucked in, and arms folded across the chest. If the fetus is in a different position or presentation, labor may be more difficult and delivery through the vagina may not be possible.

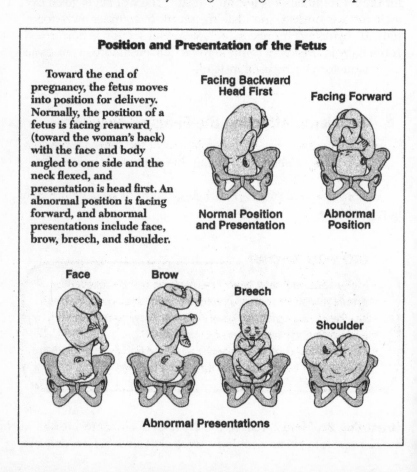

Position and Presentation of the Fetus

Toward the end of pregnancy, the fetus moves into position for delivery. Normally, the position of a fetus is facing rearward (toward the woman's back) with the face and body angled to one side and the neck flexed, and presentation is head first. An abnormal position is facing forward, and abnormal presentations include face, brow, breech, and shoulder.

Facing Backward Head First

Facing Forward

Normal Position and Presentation

Abnormal Position

Face   **Brow**   **Breech**   **Shoulder**

Abnormal Presentations

When a fetus faces up (an abnormal position), the neck is often straightened rather than bent, and the head requires more space to pass through the birth canal. Delivery by forceps, a vacuum extractor, or cesarean section may be necessary.

There are several abnormal presentations. In face presentation, the neck arches back so that the face presents first. In brow presentation, the neck is moderately arched so that the brow presents first. Usually, fetuses do not stay in these presentations; they correct themselves.

Breech presentation, in which the buttocks present first, occurs in 2 to 3% of full-term deliveries. When delivered vaginally, babies that present buttocks first are more likely to be injured than those that present head first. Such injuries may occur before, during, or after birth and include death. Complications are less likely when breech presentation is detected before labor or delivery.

Sometimes the doctor can turn the fetus to present head first by pressing on the woman's abdomen before labor begins, usually at the 37th or 38th week of pregnancy. However, if labor begins and the fetus is in breech presentation, problems may occur. The passageway made by the buttocks in the birth canal may not be large enough for the head (which is wider) to pass through. In addition, when the head follows the buttocks, it cannot be molded to fit through the birth canal, as it normally is. Thus, the baby's body may be delivered and the head may be caught inside the woman. As a result, the spinal cord or other nerves may be stretched, leading to nerve damage. When the baby's navel is first seen outside the woman, the umbilical cord is compressed between the baby's head and the birth canal, so that very little oxygen can reach the baby. Brain damage due to lack of oxygen is more common among babies presenting buttocks first than among those presenting head first. In a first delivery, these problems are worse because the woman's tissues have not been stretched by previous deliveries. Because the baby could be injured or die, delivery by cesarean section is preferred when the fetus is in breech presentation.

Occasionally, a fetus lying horizontally across the birth canal presents shoulder first. A cesarean section is performed, unless the fetus is the second in a set of twins. In such a case, the fetus may be turned to be delivered through the vagina.

Multiple Births: The number of twin, triplet, and other multiple births has been increasing during the last two decades. During pregnancy, the number of fetuses can be confirmed by ultrasonography.

Carrying more than one fetus overstretches the uterus, and an overstretched uterus tends to start contracting before the pregnancy reaches full term. As a result, the babies are usually born prematurely and are small. In some cases, the overstretched uterus does not contract well after delivery, causing bleeding in the woman after delivery. Because the fetuses can be in various positions and presentations, vaginal delivery can be complicated. Also, the contraction of the uterus after delivery of the first baby may shear away the placenta of the remaining baby or babies. As a result, the baby or babies that follow the first may have more problems during delivery and later.

For these reasons, doctors may decide in advance how to deliver twins: vaginally or by cesarean section. Occasionally, the first twin is delivered vaginally, but a cesarean section is considered safer for the second twin. For triplets and other multiple births, doctors usually perform a cesarean section.

Shoulder Dystocia: Shoulder dystocia occurs when one shoulder of the fetus lodges against the woman's pubic bone, and the baby is therefore caught in the birth canal. The head comes out, but it is pulled back tightly against the vaginal opening. The baby cannot breathe because the chest is compressed by the birth canal. As a result, oxygen levels in the baby's blood decrease. This complication is more common with large fetuses, particularly when labor has been difficult or when forceps or a vacuum extractor has been used because the fetus's head has not fully descended in the pelvis.

When this complication occurs, the doctor quickly tries various techniques to free the shoulder so that the baby can be delivered vaginally. In extreme circumstances, if the techniques are unsuccessful, the baby may be pushed back into the vagina and delivered by cesarean section.

Prolapsed Umbilical Cord: The umbilical cord precedes the baby through the vagina (prolapses) in about 1 of 1,000 deliveries. When the umbilical cord prolapses, it may constrict so that the fetus's blood supply is cut off. This complication may be obvious (overt) or not (occult).

Prolapse is overt when the membranes have ruptured and the umbilical cord protrudes into or out of the vagina before the baby emerges. Overt prolapse usually occurs when a baby emerges buttocks first (breech presentation). But it can occur when the baby emerges head first, particularly if the membranes rupture prematurely or the fetus has not descended into the woman's pelvis. If the fetus has not descended, the rush of fluid as the membranes rupture can carry the cord out ahead of the fetus. If the cord prolapses, immediate delivery, almost always by cesarean section, is necessary to prevent the blood supply to the fetus from being cut off. Until surgery begins, a nurse or doctor holds the fetus's body off the cord so that the blood supply through the prolapsed cord is not cut off.

In occult prolapse, the membranes are intact and the cord is in front of the fetus or trapped in front of the fetus's shoulder. Usually, occult prolapse can be identified by an abnormal pattern in the fetus's heart rate. Changing the woman's position or raising the fetus's head to relieve pressure on the cord usually corrects the problem. Occasionally, a cesarean section is necessary.

Nuchal Cord: The umbilical cord is wrapped around the fetus's neck in about one fourth of deliveries. Normally, the baby is not harmed. Before birth, a nuchal cord can sometimes be detected by ultrasonography, but no action is required. Doctors routinely check for it as they deliver the baby. If they feel it, they can slip the cord over the baby's head.

Problems Affecting the Woman

Preeclampsia: Preeclampsia is a complication of pregnancy. It involves high blood pressure that develops late in pregnancy or shortly after delivery. Preeclampsia may lead to premature detachment of the placenta from the uterus (placental abruption—see page 325) and problems in the newborn.

Amniotic Fluid Embolism: Very rarely, a volume of amniotic fluid—the fluid that surrounds the fetus in the uterus—enters the woman's bloodstream, usually during a particularly difficult labor.

The fluid travels to the woman's lungs and may cause the arteries in the lungs to constrict. This constriction may result in a rapid heart rate, irregular heart rhythm, collapse, shock, or even cardiac arrest and death. Widespread blood clotting (disseminated intravascular coagulation) is a common complication, requiring emergency care.

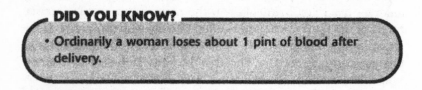

DID YOU KNOW?

- Ordinarily a woman loses about 1 pint of blood after delivery.

Uterine Bleeding: After the baby is delivered, excessive bleeding (postpartum hemorrhage) from the uterus is a major concern. Ordinarily, the woman loses about 1 pint of blood after delivery. Blood is lost because some blood vessels are opened when the placenta detaches from the uterus. The contractions of the uterus help close these vessels until the vessels can heal.

Loss of more than 1 pint of blood during or after the third stage of labor (when the placenta is delivered) is considered excessive. Severe blood loss usually occurs soon after delivery but may occur even as late as 1 month afterward.

Excessive bleeding may result when the contractions of the uterus after delivery are impaired. Then, the blood vessels that were opened when the placenta detached continue to bleed. Contractions may be impaired if the uterus has been stretched too much—for example, by too much amniotic fluid in the uterus, by several fetuses, or by a very large fetus. Contractions may also be impaired when a piece of placenta remains inside the uterus after delivery, when the labor was prolonged or abnormal, when a woman has been pregnant several times, or when a muscle-relaxing anesthetic was used during labor and delivery. Excessive bleeding can result if the vagina or cervix is torn or cut during delivery or the blood level of fibrinogen (which helps blood to clot) is low. Excessive bleeding after one delivery may increase the risk of excessive bleeding after subsequent deliveries.

Before a woman goes into labor, doctors take steps to prevent or to prepare for excessive bleeding after delivery. For example, they determine whether the woman has any conditions that increase the risk of bleeding, such as too much amniotic fluid. If the woman has an unusual blood type, doctors make sure that her type of blood is available. After delivery of the placenta, the woman is monitored for at least 1 hour to make sure that the uterus has contracted and to assess vaginal bleeding.

If severe bleeding occurs, the woman's lower abdomen is massaged to help the uterus contract, and she is given oxytocin continuously through an intravenous line to help the uterus contract. If bleeding continues, prostaglandins can be injected into the uterine muscle to help the uterus contract. The woman may need a blood transfusion.

Doctors look for the cause of excessive bleeding. The uterus may be examined for retained fragments of the placenta. Dilation and curettage may be performed to remove these fragments. In this procedure, a small, sharp instrument (curet) is passed through the cervix (which is usually still open from the delivery— see page 129). The curet is used to remove the retained fragments. This procedure requires an anesthetic. The cervix and vagina are examined for any tears.

If the uterus cannot be stimulated to contract and bleeding continues, the arteries supplying blood to the uterus may have to be closed off. The procedures used usually have no lasting ill effects, such as infertility or abnormalities in menstruation. Removal of the uterus (hysterectomy) is rarely necessary to stop the bleeding.

Inverted Uterus: Very rarely, the uterus is turned inside out, so that it protrudes through the cervix, into or through the vagina. An inverted uterus is a medical emergency that must be treated promptly. Doctors return the uterus to its normal position (reinvert it) by hand. Usually, the woman recovers fully after this procedure.

Procedures Used During Labor

Induction of labor is the artificial starting of labor. Usually, labor is induced by giving the woman oxytocin, a hormone that makes the uterus contract more frequently and more forcefully. The oxytocin given is identical to the oxytocin produced by the pituitary gland. It is given intravenously with an infusion pump, so that the amount of drug given can be controlled precisely.

Sometimes prostaglandins, which help the cervix dilate, are also given to help start labor. Throughout induction and labor, the fetus's heart rate is monitored electronically. At first, a monitor is placed on the woman's abdomen. After the membranes are ruptured, an internal monitor may be inserted through the vagina and attached to the fetus's scalp. If induction is unsuccessful, the baby is delivered by cesarean section.

Augmentation of labor is the artificial hastening of labor that is proceeding ineffectively or too slowly. Oxytocin is used to augment labor. Labor is augmented when a woman has contractions that are not effectively moving the fetus through the birth canal.

Slowing of labor is the artificial delaying of labor that is proceeding too forcefully. Very rarely, a woman has contractions that are too strong, too close together, or both. If contractions are caused by the use of oxytocin, the drug is discontinued immediately. The woman may be repositioned and given analgesics. If the contractions occur spontaneously, a drug that can slow labor (such as terbutaline or ritodrine) may be given to stop or slow the contractions.

Forceps are metal surgical instruments, similar to tongs, with rounded edges that fit around the fetus's head. Forceps are occasionally used in a normal labor to ease delivery. Forceps

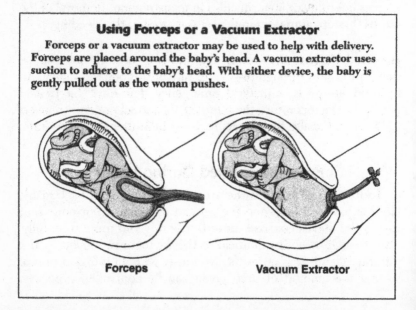

Using Forceps or a Vacuum Extractor

Forceps or a vacuum extractor may be used to help with delivery. Forceps are placed around the baby's head. A vacuum extractor uses suction to adhere to the baby's head. With either device, the baby is gently pulled out as the woman pushes.

Forceps   **Vacuum Extractor**

may be required when the fetus is in distress or abnormally positioned, when the woman is having difficulty pushing, or when labor is prolonged. (Sometimes doctors perform a cesarean section instead.) If forceps delivery is tried and is unsuccessful, a cesarean section is performed. Rarely, using forceps bruises the baby's face or tears the woman's vagina.

A **vacuum extractor** can be used instead of forceps to help with delivery. A vacuum extractor consists of a small cup made of a rubberlike material that is connected to a vacuum. It is inserted into the vagina and uses suction to attach to the fetus's head. Rarely, a vacuum extractor bruises the baby's scalp.

Cesarean section is surgical delivery of a baby by incision through a woman's abdomen and uterus. Doctors perform this procedure when they think it is safer than vaginal delivery for the woman, the baby, or both. In the United States, about one fourth of deliveries are cesarean sections. An obstetrician, an anesthesiologist, nurses, and sometimes a pediatrician are involved in this surgical procedure. Use of anesthetics, intravenous drugs, antibiotics, and blood transfusions helps make a cesarean section safe. Having the woman walk around soon after surgery reduces the risk of pulmonary embolism, in which blood clots that form in the legs or pelvis travel to the lungs and block arteries there. Compared with a vaginal delivery, delivery by cesarean section results in more overall pain afterward, a longer hospital stay, and a longer recovery time.

For a cesarean section, an incision is made in the upper or lower part of the uterus. A lower incision is more common. The lower part of the uterus has fewer blood vessels, so that less blood is usually lost. Also, the healed scar is stronger, so that it is less likely to open in subsequent deliveries. A lower incision may be horizontal or vertical. Usually, an upper incision is used when the placenta covering the cervix (a complication called placenta previa), when the fetus lies horizontally across the birth canal, or when the fetus is very premature.

The choice of having a vaginal delivery or a repeat cesarean section may be offered to women who have had a lower incision. However, a woman opting for vaginal delivery should plan to have her baby in facilities equipped to rapidly perform a cesarean section, because there is a very small chance that the incision from the previous cesarean section will open during labor.

CHAPTER 26

Postdelivery Period

The postdelivery (postpartum) period is the 6 to 8 weeks after delivery of a baby, when the mother's body returns to its prepregnancy state.

After delivery, the mother can expect to have some symptoms, but they are usually mild and temporary. Complications are rare. Nonetheless, the doctor, hospital staff members, or health care plan usually sets up a home visit or close follow-up program. The most common complications are excessive bleeding (postpartum hemorrhage—see page 364); bladder, kidney, or breast infections; problems with breastfeeding; and depression. Postpartum hemorrhage may occur soon after delivery but may occur as late as 1 month afterward.

What to Expect in the Hospital

- The new mother can resume a normal diet, sometimes shortly after delivery.
- Walking soon after delivery is encouraged.
- A new mother is encouraged to urinate regularly.

Immediately after the delivery of a baby, the mother is monitored. The hospital staff members make every effort to minimize her pain and the risk of bleeding and infection. After delivery of the placenta (afterbirth), a nurse may periodically massage the mother's abdomen to help the uterus contract. If needed, oxytocin is given to stimulate contraction of the uterus. The drug is given intravenously as a continuous infusion for 1 to 2 hours after delivery. These steps help ensure that the uterus contracts and remains contracted to prevent excessive bleeding.

When a general anesthetic (used rarely) was used during delivery, the mother is monitored for 2 to 3 hours after delivery, usually in a well-equipped recovery room with access to oxygen, blood that matches the mother's, and intravenous fluids.

Within the first 24 hours, the mother's pulse rate drops, her temperature may rise slightly, and the number of white blood cells temporarily increases. A bloody vaginal discharge occurs for 3 or 4 days. During the next 10 to 12 days, the discharge becomes pale brown, then yellowish white. The discharge may continue for up to about 6 weeks after delivery. Sanitary pads, changed frequently, may be used to absorb the discharge. Urine production often increases greatly, but temporarily, after delivery. Because bladder sensation may be decreased after delivery, a new mother should try to urinate regularly, at least every 4 hours. Doing so avoids overfilling the bladder and helps prevent bladder infections. The new mother is also encouraged to defecate before leaving the hospital. She may take laxatives, if needed, to avoid constipation, which can cause or worsen hemorrhoids. Applying warm compresses and a gel containing a local anesthetic to hemorrhoids, if present, can relieve pain.

During the early stages of milk production (lactation), the breasts become engorged with milk. Sometimes they become firm and sore. If a mother is not going to breastfeed, wearing a tight bra, applying ice packs, and taking analgesics such as aspirin or acetaminophen may help relieve the discomfort.

DID YOU KNOW?

- A low grade fever can occur during the 24 hours after delivery, even in the absence of infection.
- A woman will have a vaginal discharge for up to about 6 weeks after delivery.
- Breast engorgement affects all women who have given birth.

For mothers who are breastfeeding, feeding the baby regularly helps reduce breast engorgement. Wearing a comfortable nursing bra 24 hours a day can help relieve the discomfort. If the breasts are very swollen, the mother may have to express her milk manually just before breastfeeding to enable the baby's mouth to fit around the areola (the pigmented area of skin around the nipple). If the mother is uncomfortable between feedings, she can express milk by hand in a warm shower to relieve the pressure. However, expressing milk between feedings tends to result in continued engorgement and should be done only when necessary for relief.

After the first 24 hours, recovery is rapid. The mother can have a regular diet as soon as she wants it, sometimes shortly after delivery. She should get up and walk as soon as possible. If delivery was vaginal, a new mother can start exercises to strengthen abdominal muscles, often after 1 day. Sit-ups with bent knees, done in bed, are effective. However, most new mothers are too tired to start exercising so soon after delivery.

Before the mother leaves the hospital, she is examined. If she has never had German measles (rubella) or the German measles vaccine, she is vaccinated. If she has Rh-negative blood and the baby has Rh-positive blood, she is given $Rh_0(D)$ immune globulin within 3 days of delivery. This drug destroys any of the baby's red blood cells that may have passed to the mother and may trigger the production of antibodies by the mother. Such antibodies may endanger subsequent pregnancies (see page 322). The new mother is examined again 6 weeks later. Also before leaving the hospital, she is given information about changes to expect in her body and the type of contraception that can be used as her body recovers from having a baby.

If mother and baby are healthy, they commonly leave the hospital within 48 hours after vaginal delivery and within 96 hours after a cesarean section.

What to Expect at Home

- Contractions of the uterus after delivery help the uterus return to its normal size.
- Warm sitz baths can relieve pain resulting from an episiotomy or hemorrhoids.
- Breast milk is ideal for babies, and correctly positioning the baby to breastfeed is important.

- A woman can expect to feel very tired as she recovers from the delivery and tends to her newborn.
- Normal daily activities can be resumed as soon as the woman is ready. This includes sexual intercourse.

The uterus, still enlarged, continues to contract for some time, becoming progressively smaller during the next 2 weeks. These contractions are irregular and often painful. Contractions are intensified by breastfeeding. Breastfeeding triggers the production of the hormone oxytocin. Oxytocin stimulates the flow of milk (called the let-down reflex) and uterine contractions. Normally, after 5 to 7 days, the uterus is firm and no longer tender but is still somewhat enlarged, extending to halfway between the pubic bone and the navel. By 2 weeks after delivery, the uterus returns to its normal size. However, the new mother's abdomen does not become as flat as it was before the pregnancy for several months, even if she exercises. Stretch marks may not lighten for a year.

A new mother may take showers or baths, but she should refrain from vaginal douching for at least 2 weeks after delivery. Washing the area around the vagina with warm water 2 or 3 times a day helps reduce tenderness. Warm sitz baths can relieve pain resulting from an episiotomy or from hemorrhoids. Sitz baths are taken in a sitting position with water covering only the hips and buttocks.

DID YOU KNOW?

- Breastfeeding women need extra nutrition, especially calcium.
- Although not typical, a woman can become pregnant soon after delivering a baby; contraceptives are advised.
- A new mother who has just been vaccinated against German measles (rubella) must wait at least 1 month before becoming pregnant again to avoid endangering the fetus.

Mothers who are not breastfeeding may take drugs to help them sleep or to relieve pain. For pain, they are usually given acetaminophen or a nonsteroidal anti-inflammatory drug (NSAID). Mothers who are breastfeeding are given limited amounts of such drugs because most drugs appear in breast milk (see page 340).

Mothers who are breastfeeding need to learn how to position the baby during feeding. To begin breastfeeding, the mother settles into a comfortable, relaxed position, either seated or lying almost flat, and turns from one side to the other to offer each breast. The baby faces the mother. The mother supports her breast with her thumb and index finger on top and other fingers below and brushes her nipple against the middle of the baby's lower lip. This stimulates the baby to open his mouth—the rooting reflex—and grasp the breast. If the baby is not positioned well, the mother's nipples may become sore. Sore nipples may result from poor

Positioning a Baby to Breastfeed

The mother settles into a comfortable, relaxed position. She may sit or lie almost flat, and she may hold the baby in several different positions. A mother should find the position that works best for her and her baby. She may wish to alternate among different positions.

A common position is holding the baby on the lap so that the baby is stomach to stomach with the mother. The mother supports the baby's neck and head with her left arm when the baby is feeding on the left breast. The baby is brought to the level of the breast, not the breast to the baby. Support for the mother and the baby is important. Pillows can be placed behind the mother's back or under her arm. Placing her feet on a footstool or coffee table may help keep her from leaning over the baby. Leaning over may strain her back and result in sore nipples. A pillow or folded blanket may be placed under the baby for added support.

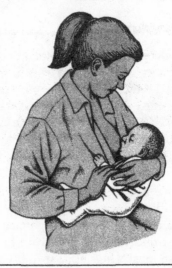

positioning and are easier to prevent than to cure. Sometimes the baby draws in its lower lip and sucks it, irritating the nipple. In such cases, the mother can ease the baby's lip out of its mouth with her thumb. After a feeding, she should let the milk dry naturally on the nipples rather than wipe or wash them. If she wishes, she can dry her nipples with a hair dryer set on low. In very dry climates, hypoallergenic lanolin or ointment can be applied to the nipples. Plastic bra liners should be avoided.

As long as a mother is breastfeeding, she needs extra nourishment, especially calcium. Dairy products are an excellent source of calcium. Nuts and green leafy vegetables may be substituted if the mother cannot tolerate dairy products. Or she may take calcium supplements. Vitamin supplements are not necessary if the mother's diet is well balanced, particularly if it includes sufficient amounts of vitamins B_6, B_{12}, and C.

A new mother may resume normal daily activities when she feels ready. She may resume sexual intercourse as soon as she desires it and it is comfortable. Use of contraceptives is recommended because pregnancy is possible as soon as the mother begins to release an egg from the ovary (ovulate) again. Mothers who are not breastfeeding usually begin to ovulate again about 4 weeks after delivery, before their first period. However, ovulation can occur earlier. Mothers who are breastfeeding tend to start ovulating and menstruating somewhat later, usually 10 to 12 weeks after delivery. The interval depends on how much food other than breast milk the baby consumes. If more than four fifths of the baby's food is breast milk, ovulation is unlikely to occur. Occasionally, a mother who is breastfeeding ovulates, menstruates, and becomes pregnant as quickly as a mother who is not breastfeeding.

Full recovery after pregnancy takes about 1 to 2 years. So doctors usually advise a new mother to wait before becoming pregnant again (although she may choose not to follow that advice). At her first doctor's appointment after delivery, a new mother can discuss contraceptive options (see page 30) with her doctor and choose one that suits her situation. A new mother who has just been vaccinated against German measles (rubella) must wait at least 1 month before becoming pregnant again to avoid endangering the fetus.

Postpartum Infections

- Postpartum infections are rare.
- A postpartum infection is usually diagnosed if more than 24 hours have passed since delivery and the woman has a fever of at least 100.4°F (38°C) on two occasions at least 6 hours apart.
- The uterus, kidneys, bladder, breasts, or lungs may be infected.

Immediately after delivery, the woman's temperature often increases. A temperature of 101°F (38.3°C) or higher during the first 12 hours after delivery could indicate an infection but usually does not. Nonetheless, in such cases, the woman should be evaluated by her doctor or midwife. A postpartum infection is usually diagnosed after 24 hours have passed since delivery and the woman has had a temperature of 100.4°F (38°C) or higher on two occasions at least 6 hours apart. Postpartum infections are rare, because doctors try to prevent or treat conditions that can lead to infections. However, infections may be serious. Thus, if a woman has a temperature of more than 100.4°F at any time during the first week after delivery, she should call the doctor.

Postpartum infections may be directly related to delivery (occurring in the uterus or the area around the uterus) or indirectly related (occurring in the kidneys, bladder, breasts, or lungs).

DID YOU KNOW?

- If a woman has a temperature of more than 100.4°F at any time during the first week after delivery, she should call the doctor.

INFECTIONS OF THE UTERUS

Postpartum infections usually begin in the uterus. If an infection of the membranes containing the fetus (amniotic sac) caused a fever during labor, an infection of the uterine lining (endometritis), uterine muscle (myometritis), or areas around the uterus (parametritis) may result.

Causes and Symptoms

Bacteria that normally live in the healthy vagina can cause an infection after delivery. Conditions that make a woman more likely to develop to infection include anemia, preeclampsia (see page 318), repeated vaginal examinations, a delay of longer than 18 hours between rupture of the membranes and delivery, prolonged labor, a cesarean section, placental fragments remaining in the uterus after delivery, and excessive bleeding after delivery (postpartum hemorrhage).

Symptoms commonly include paleness, chills, headache, a general feeling of illness or discomfort, and loss of appetite. The heart rate is rapid, and the number of white blood cells is abnormally high. The uterus is swollen, tender, and soft. Typically, there is a malodorous discharge from the vagina, which varies in amount.

When the tissues around the uterus are infected, they swell, holding the swollen, tender uterus rigidly in place. The woman has severe pain and a high fever.

The abdominal lining can become inflamed, causing peritonitis. Blood clots may form in the pelvic veins, causing pelvic thrombophlebitis. A blood clot may travel to the lung and block an artery there, causing pulmonary embolism. Some infections may cause blood pressure to fall dramatically and the heart rate to become very rapid. Severe kidney damage and even death may result.

Diagnosis and Treatment

An infection is usually diagnosed based on results of a physical examination. Samples of urine, blood, and the vaginal discharge are cultured for bacteria.

If the uterus is infected, the woman is usually given an antibiotic intravenously until she has had no fever for 48 hours. For a few days afterward, she may be given antibiotics by mouth.

BLADDER AND KIDNEY INFECTIONS

A bladder infection (cystitis) sometimes develops when a catheter is placed in the bladder to relieve a buildup of urine during and after labor. Or bacteria may be present in the bladder during pregnancy but cause no symptoms until after delivery. A kidney infection (pyelonephritis) is caused by bacteria spreading from the bladder to the kidney after delivery.

Symptoms may include a fever and painful or frequent urination. Infection that has reached the kidneys may cause pain in the lower back or side, a general feeling of illness or discomfort, and constipation.

Typically, a woman is given an antibiotic. If there is no evidence that the bladder infection has spread to the kidneys, antibiotics may be given for only a few days. If a kidney infection is suspected, antibiotics are given until the woman has had no fever for 48 hours. Urine samples are cultured to identify the bacteria. After culture results are available, the antibiotic may be changed to one that is more effective against the bacteria present. Drinking plenty of fluids helps keep the kidneys functioning well and flushes bacteria out of the urinary tract. Another urine sample is cultured 6 to 8 weeks after delivery to verify that the infection is cured.

BREAST INFECTION

A breast infection (mastitis—see page 211) can occur after delivery, usually during the first 6 weeks and almost always in women who are breastfeeding. If the skin of or around the nipples becomes cracked, bacteria from the skin can enter the milk ducts and cause an infection. An infected breast usually appears red and swollen and feels warm and tender. The woman may have a fever. A fever that develops later than 10 days after delivery is often caused by a breast infection, although it may be caused by a bladder infection.

Breast infections are treated with antibiotics. Women who have a breast infection and are breastfeeding should continue to breastfeed. Breastfeeding decreases the risk of a breast abscess (a collection of pus), which is rare. Breast abscesses are treated with antibiotics and are usually drained surgically.

Blood Clots

The risk of developing blood clots (thromboembolic disease) is increased after delivery. Typically, blood clots occur in the legs or pelvis (a disorder called thrombophlebitis). A fever that develops between 4 and 10 days after delivery may be caused by a blood clot.

Treatment consists of warm compresses (to reduce discomfort), compression bandages applied by a doctor or nurse, and bed rest with the leg elevated (by raising the foot of the bed 6 inches). Anticoagulants may be necessary.

Thyroid Disorders

In 4 to 7% of women, the thyroid gland malfunctions during the first 6 months after delivery. Thyroid hormone levels may be high or low, usually temporarily. Women who have a family history of thyroid disorders or diabetes are particularly susceptible. In women who already have a thyroid disorder, such as a goiter or Hashimoto's thyroiditis, the disorder may become worse. Treatment may be required.

Postpartum Depression

Postpartum depression is a feeling of extreme sadness and related psychologic disturbances during the first few weeks or months after delivery.

- The sudden decrease in hormone levels may contribute to postpartum depression.
- Lack of social support and marital discord increase the likelihood of postpartum depression.
- In addition to experiencing episodes of frequent crying, mood swings, and irritability, the woman may show no interest in her baby.
- Typically, a combination of counseling and antidepressants is needed.
- Postpartum psychosis (including a desire to harm the baby) may develop but is rare.

The baby blues—feeling sad or miserable within 3 days of delivery—is common after delivery. New mothers should not be overly concerned about these feelings because they usually disappear within 2 weeks. Postpartum depression is a more serious mood change. It lasts weeks or months. This form affects about 1% of women. An even more severe, very rare form, called postpartum psychosis, includes psychotic behavior.

The causes of sadness or depression after delivery are unclear. The sudden decrease in levels of hormones, particularly estrogen and progesterone, may contribute. Depression that was present before pregnancy is likely to evolve into postpartum depression. Women who have had depression before they became pregnant should tell their doctor or midwife about it during the pregnancy. The stresses of having and caring for a baby may also contribute. Such stresses include difficulties during labor and delivery, lack of sleep, and feelings of isolation and incompetence. Women who develop postpartum depression may have had depression or another psychologic disorder before pregnancy, or they may have close relatives with depression. Lack of social support and marital discord increase the likelihood of developing postpartum depression.

Symptoms may include frequent crying, mood swings, and irritability as well as feelings of sadness. Less common symptoms include extreme fatigue, difficulty concentrating, sleep problems, loss of interest in sex, anxiety, appetite changes, and feelings of inadequacy or hopelessness. These symptoms interfere with the woman's daily activities. A woman with postpartum depression may show no interest in her baby.

DID YOU KNOW?

- Many women experience a few days of the baby blues after delivery; postpartum depression is less common.

In postpartum psychosis, depression may be combined with suicidal or violent thoughts, hallucinations, or bizarre behavior. Sometimes postpartum psychosis includes a desire to harm the baby.

If the woman is sad, support from family members and friends is usually all that is needed. But if depression is diagnosed, professional help is also needed. Typically, a combination of counseling and antidepressants is recommended. A woman who has postpartum psychosis may need to be hospitalized, preferably in a unit that allows the baby to remain with her. She may need antipsychotic drugs as well as antidepressants. A woman who is breastfeeding should consult with her doctor before taking any of these drugs to determine whether she can continue to breastfeed (see page 340).

Men's Health

Part III

Men's Health

CHAPTER 27

Male Reproductive System

The external structures of the male reproductive system include the penis and scrotum. The internal structures include the vas deferens, testes (testicles), urethra, prostate gland, and seminal vesicles.

The sperm, which carries the man's genes, is made in the testes and stored in the seminal vesicles. During ejaculation, the sperm is transported along with a fluid called semen through the vas deferens and the erect penis.

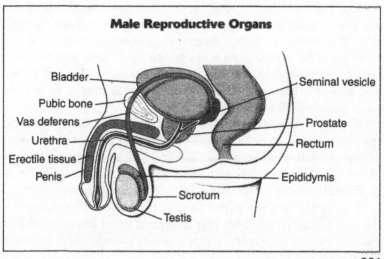

Male Reproductive Organs

Bladder

Pubic bone

Vas deferens

Urethra

Erectile tissue

Penis

Seminal vesicle

Prostate

Rectum

Epididymis

Scrotum

Testis

Structure

- The penis and the urethra are part of the urinary and reproductive systems.
- The scrotum, testes, vas deferens, and prostate gland constitute the rest of the reproductive system.

The penis consists of the root (which is attached to the abdominal wall), the body (the middle portion), and the glans penis (the cone-shaped end). The opening of the urethra (the channel that transports semen and urine) is located at the tip of the glans penis. The base of the glans penis is called the corona. In uncircumcised males, the foreskin (prepuce) extends from the corona to cover the glans penis.

The body of the penis primarily consists of three cylindrical spaces (sinuses) of erectile tissue. The two larger ones, the corpora cavernosa, occur side by side. The third sinus, the corpus spongiosum, surrounds the urethra. When these spaces fill with blood, the penis becomes large and rigid (erect).

The scrotum is the thin-skinned sac that surrounds and protects the testes. The scrotum also acts as a climate-control system for the testes, because they need to be slightly cooler than body temperature for normal sperm development. The cremaster muscles in the scrotal wall relax or contract to allow the testes to hang farther from the body to cool or to be pulled closer to the body for warmth or protection.

The testes are oval bodies the size of large olives that lie in the scrotum; usually the left testis hangs slightly lower than the right one. The testes have two functions: producing sperm and testosterone (the primary male sex hormone). The epididymis is a coiled tube almost 20 feet long. It collects sperm from the testis and provides the space and environment for sperm to mature. One epididymis lies against each testis.

The vas deferens is a firm duct that transports sperm from the epididymis. One such duct travels from each epididymis to the back of the prostate and enters the urethra. Other structures, such as blood vessels and nerves, also travel along with each vas deferens and together form an intertwined structure, the spermatic cord.

The urethra serves a dual function in males. This channel is the part of the urinary tract that transports urine from the bladder and the part of the reproductive system through which semen is ejaculated.

The prostate gland lies just under the bladder and surrounds the urethra. Walnut-sized in young men, the prostate gland enlarges with age. When the prostate enlarges too much, it can block urine flow through the urethra. The seminal vesicles, located above the prostate, join with the vas deferens to form the ejaculatory ducts. The prostate and the seminal vesicles produce fluid that nourishes the sperm. This fluid provides most of the volume of semen, the secretion in which the sperm is expelled during ejaculation. Other fluid that makes up the semen comes from the vas deferens and from mucous glands in the head of the penis.

TESTOSTERONE REPLACEMENT THERAPY

Beginning at about age 30, the production of testosterone (the main male sex hormone) in men usually decreases an average of 1 to 2% per year. This decline differs from the usually rapid and nearly universal hormonal changes of menopause in women, but the decline in testosterone is sometimes referred to as male menopause or andropause. The rate of testosterone decline also varies greatly among men; many men in their 70s have testosterone levels that match those of the average man in his 30s.

All men with low testosterone levels develop certain characteristics associated with aging, including decreased libido, decreased muscle mass, increased abdominal fat, thin bones that easily fracture, decreased energy level, slow mathematical and spatial thinking, and a low blood count. Many men are interested in taking testosterone to slow or reverse development of these characteristics, but this is only helpful for men with abnormally low levels of testosterone.

The most worrisome side effect of testosterone replacement therapy is worsening of prostate disease. Without knowing it, many men have small prostate cancers that would likely never produce symptoms. Testosterone can make prostate cancers grow, so testosterone replacement therapy could cause an unnoticed prostate cancer to produce symptoms or become lethal. Testosterone also worsens benign prostatic hyperplasia, a noncancerous enlargement of the prostate.

Testosterone replacement therapy is recommended only for men whose blood tests show low testosterone levels and who have no prostate disease. Men taking testosterone need to be checked frequently for prostate cancer. Such testing may detect cancers early, when they are more often curable.

Function

- The penis becomes erect through a complex interaction of physiologic and psychologic factors.
- Contractions during ejaculation impel semen into the urethra and out of the penis.

During sexual activity, the penis becomes erect, enabling penetration during sexual intercourse. An erection results from a complex interaction of neurologic, vascular, hormonal, and psychologic actions. Pleasurable stimuli cause the brain to send nerve signals through the spinal cord to the penis. The arteries supplying blood to the corpora cavernosa and corpus spongiosum respond by dilating. The widened arteries dramatically increase blood flow to these erectile areas, which become engorged with blood and expand. Muscles tighten around the veins that normally drain blood from the penis, slowing the outflow of blood and elevating blood pressure in the penis. This elevated blood pressure causes the penis to increase in length and diameter.

At the climax of sexual excitement (orgasm), ejaculation usually occurs, caused when friction on the glans penis and other stimuli send signals to the brain and spinal cord. Nerves stimulate muscle contractions along the seminal vesicles, prostate, and the ducts of the epididymis and vas deferens. These contractions force semen into the urethra. Contraction of the muscles around the urethra further propels the semen through and out of the penis. The neck of the bladder also constricts to keep semen from flowing backward into the bladder.

Once ejaculation takes place—or the stimulation stops—the arteries constrict and the veins relax. This reduces blood inflow and increases blood outflow, causing the penis to become limp (detumescence). After detumescence, erection cannot be obtained for a period of time (refractory period), commonly about 20 minutes in young men.

Puberty

- Puberty may begin as early as age 9 and continue until age 16.
- At puberty, the testes start to produce testosterone.

- Testosterone causes reproductive organs to mature, facial and pubic hair to appear, and the voice to deepen.

Puberty is the stage during which a person reaches full reproductive ability and develops the adult features of their gender. In boys, puberty usually occurs between the ages of 10 and 14 years.

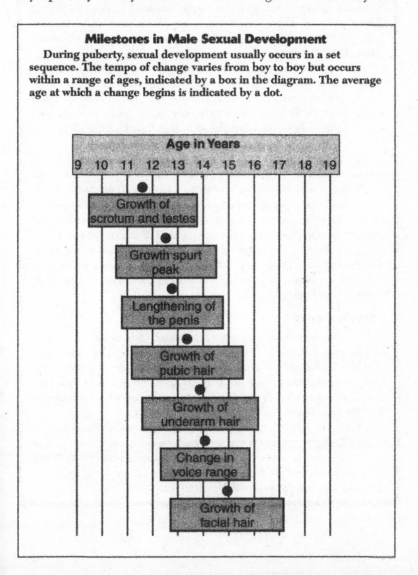

Milestones in Male Sexual Development

During puberty, sexual development usually occurs in a set sequence. The tempo of change varies from boy to boy but occurs within a range of ages, indicated by a box in the diagram. The average age at which a change begins is indicated by a dot.

Age in Years

9 10 11 12 13 14 15 16 17 18 19

Growth of scrotum and testes

Growth spurt peak

Lengthening of the penis

Growth of pubic hair

Growth of underarm hair

Change in voice range

Growth of facial hair

BREAST DISORDERS IN MEN

Breast disorders, which include breast enlargement and breast cancer, occur infrequently in men.

Breast Enlargement

Breast enlargement in males (gynecomastia) sometimes occurs during puberty. The enlargement is usually normal and transient, lasting a few months to a few years. Breast enlargement commonly takes place after age 50.

Male breast enlargement may be caused by certain diseases (particularly liver disease), certain drug therapies (including the use of female sex hormones and anabolic steroids), or heavy use of marijuana, beer, or heroin. Less commonly, male breast enlargement results from a hormonal imbalance, which can be caused by rare estrogen-producing tumors in the testes or adrenal glands.

One or both breasts may become enlarged. The enlarged breast may be tender. If tenderness is present, cancer is probably not the cause. Breast pain in men, as in women, is not usually a sign of cancer.

Generally, no specific treatment is needed. Breast enlargement often disappears on its own or after its cause is identified and treated. Surgical removal of excess breast tissue is effective but rarely necessary. Liposuction, a surgical technique that removes tissue through a suction tube inserted through a small incision, is becoming increasingly popular and sometimes is followed by additional cosmetic surgery.

Breast Cancer

Men can develop breast cancer, although 99% of all breast cancers develop in women. Because male breast cancer is uncommon, it may not be suspected as a cause of symptoms. As a result, male breast cancer often progresses to an advanced stage before it is diagnosed. The prognosis is the same as that for a woman whose cancer is at the same stage.

Treatment options are generally the same as those used for women (surgery, radiation therapy, and chemotherapy), except that breast-conserving surgery is rarely used. If an examination of tissue samples shows that sex hormones are making the cancer grow, those hormones are suppressed with the drug tamoxifen.

However, it is not unusual for puberty to begin as early as age 9 or to continue until age 16.

The pituitary gland, which is located in the brain, initiates puberty. The pituitary gland secretes luteinizing hormone and follicle-stimulating hormone, which stimulate the testes to produce testosterone. Testosterone is responsible for the development of secondary sex characteristics, such as facial hair growth and voice change.

Testosterone also produces many changes in the male reproductive organs, including elongation and thickening of the penis; enlargement of the scrotum, testes, epididymis, and prostate; darkening of the skin of the scrotum; and growth of pubic hair. Sperm usually develops by age 14. Ejaculation first occurs during late puberty.

Effects of Aging

It is not clear whether aging itself or the diseases associated with aging cause the gradual changes that occur in men's sexual functioning. The frequency, length, and rigidity of erections gradually decline throughout adulthood. Levels of the male sex hormone (testosterone) decrease also, reducing sex drive (libido). Blood flow to the penis decreases. Other changes include decreases in penile sensitivity and ejaculatory volume, reduced forewarning of ejaculation, orgasm without ejaculation, more rapid detumescence, and a longer refractory period.

CHAPTER 28

Disorders of the Penis and Testes

The penis and testes (testicles) can be affected by inflammation, scar tissue, infection (including sexually transmitted diseases), or injury. Skin cancer can also develop on the penis. Birth defects can cause difficulty in urinating and in engaging in sexual intercourse. Disorders of the penis and testes can be psychologically disturbing as well as physically damaging.

Penile Inflammation

- Inflammation can occur in several different disorders.
- Certain disorders may interfere with urination or sexual activity or increase the risk of infections or cancer.
- In certain disorders, antibacterial or anti-inflammatory creams may relieve symptoms, but in others, surgery may be needed.

Balanitis is inflammation of the glans penis (the cone-shaped end of the penis). **Posthitis** is inflammation of the foreskin. Commonly, a yeast or bacterial infection beneath the foreskin causes posthitis. Inflammation of both the glans penis and the foreskin **(balanoposthitis)** can also develop. The inflammation causes pain, itching, redness, and swelling and can ultimately lead to a narrowing (stricture) of the urethra. Men who develop balanoposthitis have an increased chance of later developing balanitis xerotica obliterans, phimosis, paraphimosis, and cancer.

In **balanitis xerotica obliterans,** chronic inflammation causes the skin near the tip of the penis to harden and turn white. The opening of the urethra is often surrounded by this hard white skin, which eventually blocks the flow of urine and semen. Antibacterial or anti-inflammatory creams may relieve the inflammation, but often the urethra must be reopened surgically.

In **phimosis,** the foreskin is tight and cannot be retracted over the glans penis. This condition is normal in a newborn or young child and usually resolves without treatment by puberty. In older men, phimosis may result from prolonged irritation or recurring balanoposthitis. The tightened foreskin can interfere with urination and sexual activity and may increase the risk of urinary tract infections. The usual treatment is circumcision.

In **paraphimosis,** the retracted foreskin cannot be pulled forward to cover the glans penis. The condition most commonly develops after a medical professional retracts the foreskin as part of a medical procedure or if someone pulls back the foreskin to clean the penis of a child and forgets to pull it back forward. The glans penis swells, increasing pressure around the trapped foreskin. The increasing pressure eventually prevents blood from reaching the penis, which could result in the destruction of penile tissue if the foreskin is not pulled back forward. Circumcision or slitting the foreskin relieves paraphimosis.

Erythroplasia of Queyrat usually occurs in uncircumcised men. It produces a discrete, reddish, velvety area on the penis, usually on or at the base of the glans penis. The cause may be long-standing irritation of the penis under the foreskin. While not cancer itself, erythroplasia of Queyrat can become cancerous if left untreated. Removal of a tissue sample for examination under a microscope (biopsy) confirms the diagnosis. Erythroplasia of Queyrat is treated with a cream containing the drug fluorouracil.

Urethral Stricture

A urethral stricture is scarring that narrows the urethra.

A urethral stricture most commonly results from previous infection or injury. A less forceful urinary stream or a double stream usually occurs with mild strictures. Severe strictures may completely block the stream of urine. The buildup of pressure behind the stricture may cause the formation of passages from the urethra into the surrounding tissues (diverticula). By decreasing the frequency or completeness of urination, strictures often lead to urinary tract infections.

A urologist diagnoses a stricture by looking directly into the urethra through a flexible viewing tube (cystoscope) after administering a lubricant containing a local anesthetic. To widen the urethra, a urologist may dilate or cut (urethrotomy) the stricture. Urethral strictures can recur and may require excision of the scar and surgical reconstruction of the urethra, sometimes with a skin graft.

Penile Growths

- Growths may be caused by sexually transmitted diseases, viral infections, or skin cancer.

Growths on the penis are sometimes caused by infections. One example is syphilis (see page 66), which may cause flat pink or gray growths (condylomata lata). Also, certain viral infections can produce one or more small, firm, raised skin growths (genital warts, or condylomata acuminata) or small, firm, dimpled growths (molluscum contagiosum).

Skin cancer can occur anywhere on the penis, most commonly at the glans penis, especially its base. Cancers affecting the skin of the penis, uncommon in the United States, are even rarer in men who have been circumcised. The cause of cancer of the penis may be long-standing irritation, usually under the foreskin. Squamous cell carcinoma occurs most commonly; less common cancers include Bowen's disease and Paget's disease. Cancer usually first appears as a painless, reddened area with sores that do not heal for weeks.

To diagnose cancer of the penis, a doctor removes a tissue sample for examination under a microscope (biopsy). To treat the cancer, a surgeon removes it and some normal surrounding tissue, sparing as much of the penis as possible. If a lot of tissue is removed, the penis can often be rebuilt surgically.

Most men with small cancers that have not spread survive for many years after treatment. Most men with cancer that has spread die within 5 years.

Priapism

Priapism is a painful, persistent erection unaccompanied by sexual desire or excitement.

- Usually, priapism is caused by taking drugs to induce erections.
- Treatment depends on the cause and may include stopping drugs that can cause erections, injecting a drug that decreases erection, draining excess blood from the penis, and surgery.

Priapism probably results from abnormalities of the blood vessels and nerves that cause blood to become trapped in the erectile tissue (corpora cavernosa) of the penis. In most cases, priapism is caused by drugs taken by mouth or injected into the penis to cause erection. Other known causes of priapism include blood clots, leukemia, sickle cell disease, a tumor in the pelvis, and an injury to the spinal cord. Sometimes, however, no cause can be found.

Several symptoms help differentiate priapism from normal erections. Priapism lasts longer, usually several hours. Sexual excitement does not accompany priapism, and the erection is painful. Also, in priapism, the glans penis may be soft.

The treatment of priapism depends on the cause. Any drug that appears to cause the priapism is discontinued immediately. Injection into the penis of a drug that decreases erection (for example, epinephrine, phenylephrine, terbutaline, or ephedrine) can relieve priapism caused by penile drug injection. Spinal anesthesia may relieve priapism caused by a spinal cord injury. If a blood clot is the probable cause, surgery to remove the clot or restore normal circulation in the penis is necessary. Usually, if other treatments are ineffective, priapism can be treated by draining excess blood from the penis with a needle and syringe and using fluid to wash out any blood clots or other blockages from the blood vessels. One or more of many possible drugs may also be used, depending on the underlying cause. Prolonged priapism usually impairs erectile function permanently.

Peyronie's Disease

Peyronie's disease is a fibrous thickening that contracts and deforms the penis, distorting the shape of an erection.

- Erections may be painful, and sexual intercourse may be impossible.

Many men have a small degree of curvature of their erect penis. Peyronie's disease produces a more severe deformity. Inflammation in the penis results in the formation of fibrous scar tissue that causes curvature in the erect penis, making penetration difficult or impossible. However, what causes the inflammation is not known.

The condition can make an erection painful. The scar tissue can extend into the erectile tissue (corpora cavernosa), preventing erection from occurring.

DID YOU KNOW?

- In many men, the penis curves slightly when it is erect.

Minor curvature or disease that does not impair sexual function does not require treatment. Peyronie's disease may resolve over several months without treatment. No treatment has proven clearly successful.

Vitamin E, which can aid wound healing and decrease scarring, may be taken by mouth. Corticosteroids or verapamil can be injected into the scar tissue to decrease inflammation and reduce scarring. Ultrasound treatments can stimulate blood flow, which may prevent further scarring. Radiation therapy may decrease pain; however, radiation often worsens tissue damage. Surgery is not recommended unless the disease has progressed and the curvature has become too severe for successful intercourse. Surgery to excise the scar may worsen the disease or result in erectile dysfunction (impotence).

Penile and Testicular Injury

- Injuries of the penis may be slight (such as scratches or irritation) or serious, sometimes requiring surgery (such as a fracture or severing).
- Injuries to the scrotum are usually caused by blunt force.

Several types of injuries can affect the penis. Catching the penis in a pants zipper is common, but the resulting cut usually heals quickly. Cuts and irritations heal quickly without treatment but may need antibiotics if they become infected. Injuries to the urethra (the opening at the end of the penis) may require other specific treatment, usually provided by a urologist (a doctor who specializes in the diagnosis and treatment of genitourinary disorders).

Fracture of the penis can occur from excessive bending of an erect penis. Pain and swelling from damage to the structures that control the erection and difficulty with intercourse or urination follow. Fractures of the penis usually occur during vigorous sexual intercourse. Emergency surgery is usually necessary to repair such a fracture to prevent abnormal curvature of the penis or permanent erectile dysfunction (impotence). The penis can also be partially or fully severed. Reattachment of a severed penis is sometimes possible, but full sensation and function are rarely recovered.

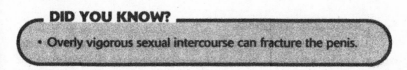

DID YOU KNOW?

- Overly vigorous sexual intercourse can fracture the penis.

The location of the scrotum makes it susceptible to injury. Blunt forces (for example, a kick or crushing blow) cause most injuries. However, occasionally gunshot or stab wounds penetrate the scrotum or testes. Rarely, the scrotum is torn off the testes. Testicular injury causes sudden, severe pain, usually with nausea and vomiting. Ultrasound may show whether the testes have ruptured. Ice packs, a jockstrap, and drugs for pain and nausea usually effectively treat internal bleeding in or around the testes. Ruptured testes require surgical repair. When the scrotum is torn off, the testes can die or lose their capacity for hormone or sperm production. Surgery to bury them under the skin of the thigh or abdomen may save the testes.

Testicular Cancer

- If the testes have not descended by age 3, the risk of cancer is increased.
- Lumps, often painless, occur in the testes or sometimes elsewhere in the scrotum.
- A physical examination, ultrasonography, and blood tests help with the diagnosis.
- Surgery to remove the affected testis and sometimes the nearby lymph nodes may be accompanied by radiation therapy or chemotherapy.

Most testicular cancers develop in men younger than age 40. Among the types of cancer that develop in the testes are seminoma, teratoma, embryonal carcinoma, and choriocarcinoma.

The cause of testicular cancer is not known, but men whose testes did not descend into the scrotum (cryptorchidism by age 3 have a greater chance of developing the disease than do men whose testes descended by that age. Cryptorchidism is best corrected surgically in childhood. Sometimes, removal of a single undescended testis in adults is recommended to reduce the risk of cancer.

Symptoms and Diagnosis

Testicular cancer may cause an enlarged testis or a lump elsewhere in the scrotum. Most lumps elsewhere in the scrotum are not caused by testicular cancer, but most lumps in the testes are. A testis normally feels like a smooth oval, with the epididymis attached behind and on top. Testicular cancer produces a firm, growing lump in or attached to the testis. With cancer, the testis loses its normal shape, becoming large, irregular, or bumpy. Although testicular cancer is often painless, the testis or lump may hurt when lightly touched and may even hurt without being touched. A firm lump on the testis requires prompt medical attention. Occasionally, blood vessels rupture within the tumor, yielding a suddenly enlarged, severely painful swelling.

Physical examination and ultrasound scanning may indicate whether a lump is part of the testis and whether it is solid (and thus more likely to be cancer) or filled with fluid (cystic). Determining the blood levels of two proteins, alpha-fetoprotein and human chorionic gonadotropin, may help in diagnosis. The levels of these proteins often increase in men with testicular cancer. If cancer is suspected, surgery to examine the testis is performed.

DID YOU KNOW?

- Because most testicular cancers develop in young men, they should examine their testes regularly.
- Loss of one testis does not impair sex drive or the ability to have children or erections.

Treatment

The initial treatment for testicular cancer is surgical removal of the entire affected testis (radical orchiectomy). The other testis is not removed, so the man retains adequate levels of male hormones and remains fertile. Infertility sometimes occurs with testicular cancer but may subside after treatment.

With certain types of cancers, lymph nodes in the abdomen are also removed (retroperitoneal lymph node dissection) because the cancer often spreads there first. Radiation therapy may also help, especially for a seminoma.

A combination of surgery and chemotherapy often cures testicular cancer that has spread. Blood levels of alpha-fetoprotein and human chorionic gonadotropin that were elevated at diagnosis decline after successful treatment. If levels rise after treatment, the cancer may have recurred. After surgery and any other necessary treatments are completed, a surgeon can replace the removed testis with an artificial one.

The prognosis for a man with testicular cancer depends on the type and extent of the cancer. Almost all men with seminomas, teratomas, or embryonal carcinomas that are not widespread survive 5 years or more. Most men with cancer that has spread survive 5 years or more. However, very few men with choriocarcinomas, which spread rapidly, survive even 5 years.

Testicular Torsion

Testicular torsion is the twisting of a testis on its spermatic cord so that the testis's blood supply is blocked.

Testicular torsion usually occurs in men between puberty and about age 25; however, it can occur at any age. Abnormal development of the spermatic cord or the membrane covering the testis makes testicular torsion possible in later life. With torsion, the testis usually dies within 6 to 12 hours after the blood supply is cut off unless it is treated.

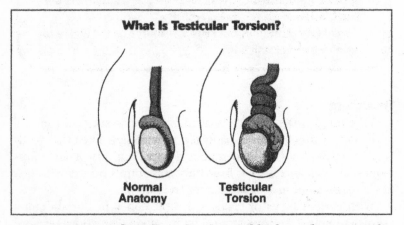

What Is Testicular Torsion?

Normal
Anatomy

Testicular
Torsion

Severe pain and swelling develop suddenly in the testis. The pain may seem to come from the abdomen, and nausea and vomiting may develop. A doctor may diagnose the condition based on the man's description of his symptoms and the physical examination findings. Alternatively, the doctor may use a scan, usually an ultrasound scan, for diagnosis. Because the testis may die rapidly, emergency surgery to untwist the spermatic cord is required. Urologists usually secure both testes during surgery to prevent future episodes of torsion.

DID YOU KNOW?

- Emergency surgery is required to prevent death of a testis that has undergone torsion.

Inguinal Hernia

An inguinal hernia is a protrusion of a piece of the intestine through an opening in the abdominal wall.

- A painless bulge may be felt in the groin or scrotum.
- If the bulge persists, part of the intestine may be trapped in the scrotum, cutting off the intestine's blood supply and requiring emergency surgery.

What Is an Inguinal Hernia?

In an inguinal hernia, a loop of intestine pushes through an opening in the abdominal wall into the inguinal canal. The inguinal canal contains the spermatic cord, which consists of the vas deferens, blood vessels, nerves, and other structures. Before birth, the testes, which are formed in the abdomen, pass through the inguinal canal as they descend into the scrotum.

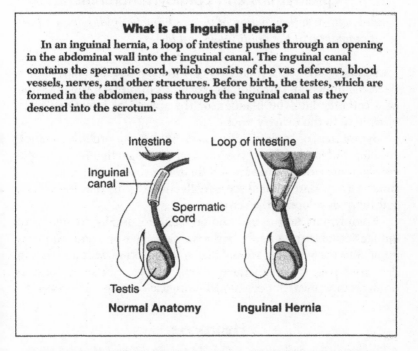

An inguinal hernia extends into the groin, and can extend into the scrotum. The opening in the abdominal wall can be present from birth or develop later in life.

Inguinal hernias usually produce a painless bulge in the groin or scrotum. The bulge may enlarge when the man stands and shrink when he lies down because the intestine slides back and forth with gravity. Sometimes a portion of the intestine is trapped in the scrotum (incarceration); this can cut off the intestine's blood supply (strangulation). Strangulated intestines may die (become gangrenous) within hours.

Surgical repair may relieve the symptoms of a hernia, depending on its size and the amount of discomfort it causes. For strangulated hernias, emergency surgery is needed to pull the intestine out of the inguinal canal and tighten the opening so the hernia cannot recur.

Epididymitis and Epididymo-orchitis

Epididymitis is inflammation of the epididymis; epididymo-orchitis is inflammation of the epididymis and testes.

Epididymitis and epididymo-orchitis are usually caused by a bacterial infection. Infection can result from surgery, the insertion of a catheter into the bladder, or the spread of infections from elsewhere in the urinary tract.

Symptoms of epididymitis and epididymo-orchitis include swelling and tenderness of the infected area, pain that may become constant and severe, fluid around the testes (hydrocele), and sometimes a fever. Rarely, an abscess (collection of pus) that feels like a soft lump develops in the scrotum.

Epididymitis and epididymo-orchitis are usually treated with antibiotics taken by mouth, bed rest, pain relievers, and ice packs applied to the scrotum. Immobilizing the scrotum with a jockstrap decreases pain from repetitive, minor bumps. Abscesses tend to drain on their own, but occasionally surgical drainage is necessary.

Hydrocele

A hydrocele is a collection of fluid in the membrane that covers the testis or testes.

A hydrocele may be present at birth or develop later in life. It is most common after age 40. Usually the cause is unknown. However, the condition occasionally results from a testicular disorder (for example, injury, epididymitis, or cancer).

Usually, a hydrocele does not cause symptoms; it is found as a painless swelling surrounding the testis. A doctor may shine a bright light on the swelling (transillumination) to confirm the diagnosis. Ultrasound examination of the testis is performed in unusual instances—for example, in a young man with no apparent cause for the hydrocele. The ultrasound may reveal an infection or tumor.

Most hydroceles need no treatment. However, surgical removal is sometimes performed for unusually large hydroceles.

Varicocele

Varicocele is a condition in which the blood supply of the testis develops varicose veins.

Veins contain valves that prevent blood from flowing backward. Faulty valves can result in a varicocele. Varicoceles usually develop on the left side of the scrotum and may produce no symptoms. Alternatively, varicoceles may cause pain and a sense of fullness that becomes bothersome. The varicocele feels like a bag of worms when the man is standing. However, the swelling usually disappears when he reclines because blood flow to the enlarged veins decreases. Rarely, a varicocele impairs fertility.

If symptoms are severe, a doctor may treat it by surgically tying off the affected veins.

Testicular Swelling

- The most common causes of testicular swelling are cancer, structural abnormalities (such as inguinal hernia, spermatocele, hydrocele, testicular torsion, varicocele, or epididymitis), cirrhosis, heart failure, and mumps.

Lymphedema causes painless swelling of the entire scrotum. Lymphedema results most often from blockage of genital blood or lymph fluid returning to the body. Cirrhosis and heart failure are common causes. Lymphedema can also result from compression of the abdominal or pelvic veins or lymph glands (for example, by a tumor). A doctor makes a diagnosis of lymphedema based on findings from a physical examination. Treating the underlying cause usually gives better results than surgery.

Mumps, a viral infection, usually affects children. If an adult contracts mumps, the testes can become painful and swollen and may sometimes shrink and stop working (atrophy). Mumps can permanently damage the ability of the testes to produce sperm but does not usually cause complete infertility unless it affects both testes.

A **spermatocele** is a collection of sperm in a sac that develops next to the epididymis. Most are painless. While most spermatoceles need no treatment, one that becomes large or bothersome can be removed surgically.

CHAPTER 29

Prostate Disorders

The prostate gland lies just under the bladder and surrounds the urethra. It produces the fluid in the semen that nourishes sperm. Walnut-sized in young men, the prostate gland enlarges with age. Three common disorders affect the prostate: benign prostatic hyperplasia, prostate cancer, and prostatitis.

Benign Prostatic Hyperplasia

Benign prostatic hyperplasia is a noncancerous (benign) enlargement of the prostate gland that can make urination difficult.

- The prostate gland enlarges as men age.
- Men may have difficulty starting urination and feel the need to urinate more often and more urgently.
- Doctors can usually diagnose the disorder during a rectal examination but may take a blood sample to help determine whether prostate enlargement is caused by prostate cancer instead.
- If treatment is needed, drugs to relax muscles of the prostate and bladder (such as terazosin, doxazosin, or tamsulosin) or to shrink the prostate (such as finasteride) are tried first, but surgery is sometimes necessary.

Benign prostatic hyperplasia (BPH) becomes increasingly common as men age, especially after age 50. The precise cause is not known but probably involves changes induced by hormones, especially testosterone.

As the prostate enlarges, it gradually compresses the urethra and blocks the flow of urine (urinary obstruction). When a man with BPH urinates, the bladder may not empty completely. Consequently, urine stagnates in the bladder, making the man susceptible to kidney stones and urinary tract infections. Prolonged obstruction can damage the kidneys.

Drugs such as over-the-counter antihistamines and nasal decongestants can increase resistance to the flow of urine or reduce the bladder's ability to contract, causing temporary urinary retention in a man with BPH.

Symptoms

BPH first causes symptoms when the enlarged prostate begins to block the flow of urine. At first, a man may have difficulty starting urination. Urination may also feel incomplete. Because the bladder does not empty completely, he has to urinate more frequently, often at night (nocturia). Also, the need to urinate becomes more urgent. The volume and force of the urinary flow may diminish noticeably, and urine may dribble at the end of urination.

Other problems can develop, but these problems affect only a small number of men with BPH. Obstruction of urine flow with urinary retention may increase the pressure in the bladder and slow the flow of urine from the kidneys, putting increased stress on the kidneys. This increased pressure may impede kidney function, although the effect is usually temporary if the obstruction is relieved early. If obstruction is prolonged, the bladder may overstretch, causing overflow incontinence. As the bladder stretches, small veins in the bladder and urethra also stretch. These veins sometimes burst when the man strains to urinate, causing blood to enter the urine. Urinary retention can develop, making urination impossible and leading to a full feeling and severe pain in the lower abdomen.

DID YOU KNOW?

- Benign prostatic hyperplasia is not treated unless symptoms or complications are bothersome.

Diagnosis

By feeling the prostate during a rectal examination, a doctor can usually determine if it is enlarged. The doctor inserts his gloved and lubricated finger into the man's rectum. The prostate can be felt just in front of the rectum. A prostate affected by BPH feels enlarged and smooth but is not painful to the touch.

A doctor may take a blood sample, which can be used to assess kidney function. A test to measure the level of prostate-specific antigen in the blood (PSA test) may also be performed in men with BPH in whom prostate cancer is suspected. A urine sample can be examined to make sure there is no infection.

Further tests are not usually needed. However, if the diagnosis is unclear or the severity of BPH is not known, other tests can be useful. An ultrasound scan can measure the size of the prostate or the amount of urine remaining in the bladder after urination. Alternatively, to check for urinary retention, a doctor can insert a catheter through the urethra after the man has tried to empty his bladder.

Treatment

Treatment is not necessary unless BPH causes especially bothersome symptoms or complications (such as urinary tract infections, impaired kidney function, blood in the urine, kidney stones, or urinary retention).

When BPH is treated, drugs are usually tried first. Alpha-adrenergic blockers (such as terazosin, doxazosin, or tamsulosin) relax certain muscles of the prostate and bladder and may ease the flow of urine. Some drugs (such as finasteride) may reverse the effects of the male hormones responsible for the prostate's growth, shrinking the prostate and helping delay the need for surgery or other treatments. However, finasteride may need to be taken for 3 months or more before symptoms are relieved. Also, many men who take finasteride never experience relief of their symptoms.

If drugs are ineffective, surgery can be performed. Surgery offers the greatest relief of symptoms but may cause complications. The most common surgical procedure is transurethral resection of the prostate (TURP), in which a doctor passes an endoscope (a flexible viewing tube) up the urethra. Attached to the endoscope is a surgical instrument that is used to remove part of the prostate. TURP is usually performed using spinal anesthesia. The procedure spares the man from a surgical incision.

TURP requires overnight hospital admission and can lead to such complications as infection and bleeding. Also, about 5% of the men who undergo the procedure have urinary incontinence afterward, which is usually temporary; permanent incontinence develops in about 1% of men. The procedure causes permanent erectile dysfunction (impotence) in about 5 to 10% of men. About 10% of men undergoing TURP need the procedure repeated within 5 years. Various alternative surgical treatments offer less symptom relief than TURP; however, the risk of complications is lower. Most of these procedures are done with instruments inserted through the urethra. These treatments destroy prostate tissue with microwave heat (transurethral thermotherapy or hyperthermia), a needle (transurethral needle ablation), ultrasound (high intensity focused ultrasound), electric vaporization (transurethral electrovaporization), or lasers (laser therapy). Inflating a balloon inserted through the urethra can also forcibly widen the prostate (transurethral balloon dilation).

Problems resulting from urine obstruction may need treatment prior to definitive treatment of BPH. Urinary retention can be treated by draining the bladder with a catheter inserted through the urethra. Infections can be treated with antibiotics.

Prostate Cancer

- The risk of prostate cancer increases as men age.
- Symptoms, such as difficulty urinating, a need to urinate frequently and urgently, and blood in the urine, usually occur only after the cancer is advanced.
- The cancer can spread, usually to the bone, kidneys, brain, or spinal cord.
- Doctors may insert a gloved, lubricated finger into the rectum and may measure prostate-specific antigen (PSA) levels in the blood to check (screen) for this cancer in men without symptoms.
- If cancer is suspected, ultrasonography and a biopsy of prostate tissue are done.

- Computer tomography or other imaging tests may be done to check for cancer spread.
- Treatment options include watchful waiting, removal of the prostate gland, radiation therapy, and hormonal drugs to slow cancer growth.

Among men in the United States, prostate cancer is the most common cancer and the second most common cause of cancer death. The chance of developing prostate cancer increases with age and is greater for African-Americans and Hispanics, men whose close relatives had the disease, and men receiving testosterone treatment. Prostate cancer usually grows very slowly and may take decades to produce symptoms. Thus, far more men have prostate cancer than die from it. Many men with prostate cancer die without ever knowing that the cancer was present.

Prostate cancer begins as a small bump in the gland. Most prostate cancers grow very slowly and never cause symptoms. Some, however, grow rapidly or spread outside the prostate. The cause of prostate cancer is not known.

Symptoms

Prostate cancer usually causes no symptoms until it reaches an advanced stage. Sometimes, symptoms similar to those of benign prostatic hyperplasia (BPH) develop, including difficulty urinating and a need to urinate frequently or urgently. However, these symptoms do not develop until after the cancer grows large enough to compress the urethra and partially block the flow of urine. Later, prostate cancer may cause bloody urine or a sudden inability to urinate.

In some men, symptoms of prostate cancer develop after it spreads (metastasizes). The areas most often affected by cancer spread are bone (typically the pelvis, ribs, or vertebrae) and the kidneys. Bone cancer tends to be painful and may weaken the bone enough for it to easily fracture. Prostate cancer can also spread to the brain, which eventually causes seizures, confusion, headaches, weakness, or other neurologic symptoms. Spread to the spinal cord, which is also common, can cause pain, numbness, weakness, or incontinence. After the cancer spreads, anemia is common.

DID YOU KNOW?

- Prostate cancer is the most common cancer among men in the United States.
- Many men with prostate cancer die without ever having known that they had the cancer.
- Whether men without symptoms should be examined and tested for prostate cancer is unclear.
- Totally eradicating prostate cancer may not be best for men whose life expectancy is short because of other reasons.
- A man's personal preferences are important in choice of treatment—for example, in exchange for peace of mind gained by eradicating a possibly nonlethal cancer, a man may have to endure certain adverse effects (such as erectile dysfunction and incontinence).

Screening

Because prostate cancer is common, many doctors check for it in men with no symptoms (screening). However, experts disagree about whether screening is helpful. In theory, screening offers the advantage of finding more prostate cancers early—when the disease is most easily cured. However, because prostate cancer grows so slowly and often never causes symptoms or death, determining the advantages of screening (and thus early treatment) is difficult. Screening may find cancers that would probably not hurt or kill a man even if they were never detected. Treating such a cancer can prove more damaging than leaving the cancer untreated. It is not clear whether the benefits of screening outweigh the harm from unnecessary treatment and testing. Additionally, screening often indicates the possibility of prostate cancer in men without the disease. When screening indicates the possibility of disease, more tests are done to find the cancer. These further tests are expensive, sometimes harmful, and often stressful.

To screen for prostate cancer, a doctor performs a blood test and a digital rectal examination. If the man has prostate cancer, a doctor sometimes feels a lump in the prostate gland. The lump is often hard. A blood test is performed to measure the level of prostate-specific antigen (PSA), a substance that is usually elevated in men with prostate cancer. PSA levels can be misleading: They can be normal when prostate cancer is present or elevated when prostate cancer is absent. PSA levels normally increase with age, but cancer increases the age-related change. Also, PSA levels can be slightly elevated in men with disorders other than prostate cancer (such as BPH or prostatitis) and in men who have undergone procedures involving the urinary tract within the previous 2 days.

Diagnosis

A doctor may suspect prostate cancer based on the man's symptoms or the results of screening tests. The first steps in diagnosing suspected cancer are digital rectal examination and measurement of PSA levels. If results of these tests suggest cancer, ultrasound scanning is usually performed. In men with prostate cancer, ultrasound scans may or may not reveal the cancer.

If the results of a digital rectal examination or PSA test suggest prostate cancer, tissue samples from the prostate are taken and analyzed (biopsy). When performing a biopsy, a doctor usually first obtains images of the prostate by inserting an ultrasound transducer, or probe, into the rectum (transrectal ultrasound). The doctor then obtains tissue samples with a needle inserted through the probe. This procedure takes only a few minutes and may be done with or without local anesthesia.

Two features help a doctor determine the likely course and the best treatment of the cancer: how distorted (malignant) the cells look under a microscope (grading) and how far the cancer has spread (staging).

Grading: Prostate cancer cells that are distorted tend to grow and spread quickly. The Gleason scoring system is the most common way to grade prostate cancer. Based on the microscopic examination and biochemical tests of tissues obtained from the biopsy, a number between 2 and 10 is assigned to the cancer. Scores between 4 and 6 are most common. The higher the number (high grade), the more likely it is that the cancer will spread. Cancers that are confined to a small area within the prostate and have

Gleason scores of 5 or lower (low grade) rarely kill a man within 15 years of diagnosis. This is true regardless of the man's age. In contrast, up to 80% of men die within 15 years if the Gleason score is higher than 7. Large, low-grade cancers are more aggressive and may require treatment.

Staging: Testing to stage the cancer often proceeds when cancer is diagnosed. However, such testing may not be necessary when the likelihood of spread beyond the prostate is extremely low.

Prostate cancers are staged according to three criteria: how far the cancer has spread within the prostate, whether the cancer has spread to lymph nodes in areas near the prostate, and whether the cancer has spread to organs far from the prostate. Results of the digital rectal examination, ultrasound scan, and biopsy reveal how far the cancer has spread within the prostate. Computed tomography (CT) or radiolabeled antibody nuclear medicine scans of the pelvis may be performed to detect spread to the lymph nodes, and bone scanning is performed to reveal spread of the cancer to bone. If spread to the brain or spinal cord is suspected, CT or magnetic resonance imaging (MRI) of those organs is performed.

Treatment

Choosing among treatment options can be complicated and often depends on the man's lifestyle preferences. For many men, doctors are uncertain about which treatments are most effective and how likely it is that a particular treatment will prolong a man's life. Some treatments can impair quality of life. For example, major surgery, radiation therapy, and hormonal therapy often cause incontinence and erectile dysfunction (impotence). When choosing among treatment options, men need to weigh the advantages and disadvantages. For these reasons, a man's preferences are a bigger consideration in choosing treatment for prostate cancer than they might be in choosing treatment for many other diseases.

Treatment for prostate cancer usually involves one of three strategies: watchful waiting, curative treatment, and palliative therapy.

Watchful waiting forgoes all treatment until symptoms develop, if they develop at all. This strategy is best for men whose cancers are unlikely to spread or cause symptoms. For example, most cancers that are confined to a small area within the prostate and have low Gleason scores grow very slowly. These cancers usually do not spread for many years. Older men are far more likely to die before such cancers kill them or cause symptoms. Watchful waiting avoids the incontinence and erectile dysfunction associated with many treatments. During watchful waiting, symptoms can be treated if necessary. Periodic testing may also be done to see if the cancer is growing rapidly or spreading. The man may later decide to pursue a cure for the cancer if testing shows growth or spread.

Curative treatment is a common strategy for men with cancers confined to the prostate that are likely to cause troublesome symptoms or death. Such cancers include any that are growing rapidly. Curative (also called definitive) therapy may also help men with small, slowly growing cancers if the man expects to otherwise live many years. Symptoms from such cancers are unlikely to develop in less than a decade and may not do so for 15 or more years. Curative therapy can also benefit men with cancers that have spread outside the prostate and thus are likely to cause symptoms in a relatively short period. However, curative therapy is likely to be successful only with cancers that are still confined to the area near the prostate. Curative therapy can prolong life and reduce or eliminate severe symptoms resulting from some cancers. However, side effects of curative therapy, most significantly permanent erectile dysfunction and incontinence, can impair quality of life.

Palliative therapy aims at treating the symptoms rather than the cancer itself. This strategy is best suited to men with widespread prostate cancer that is not curable. The growth or spread of such cancers can usually be slowed or temporarily reversed, relieving symptoms. Since these treatments cannot cure the cancer, symptoms eventually worsen. Death from the disease eventually follows.

Three forms of treatment can be used to treat prostate cancer: surgery, radiation therapy, and hormonal therapy. Chemotherapy is not usually used.

Surgery: Surgically removing the prostate (prostatectomy) is useful for cancer that is confined to the prostate. Prostatectomy is less effective in curing fast-growing cancers because they are more likely to have spread at the time of diagnosis. Prostatectomy requires general anesthesia, an overnight hospital stay, and a surgical incision, but treatment is accomplished with one procedure. Prostatectomy may lead to permanent erectile dysfunction and urinary incontinence.

There are three forms of prostatectomy: radical prostatectomy, nerve-sparing radical prostatectomy, and laparoscopic radical prostatectomy.

In radical prostatectomy, the entire prostate, the seminal vesicles, and part of the vas deferens are removed. This is the surgery most likely to cure prostate cancer. However, the procedure causes complete incontinence in about 3% of men and partial or stress incontinence in up to 20%. Temporary incontinence develops in most men and may last for several months. Incontinence is less likely in younger men. Erectile dysfunction commonly develops after radical prostatectomy. More than 90% of men with cancer confined to the prostate live at least 10 years after radical prostatectomy. Younger men who can otherwise expect to live at least 10 to 15 more years are most likely to benefit from radical prostatectomy.

Sometimes, depending on the estimated size and location of the cancer, surgery can be performed in such a way that some of the nerves needed to achieve erection are spared—this procedure is called nerve-sparing radical prostatectomy. This procedure cannot be used to treat cancer that has invaded the nerves and blood vessels of the prostate. Nerve-sparing radical prostatectomy is less likely than non-nerve-sparing radical prostatectomy to cause erectile dysfunction.

Another form of prostatectomy is laparoscopic radical prostatectomy. The advantages of this procedure are that it requires a smaller incision and produces less postoperative pain. Disadvantages include increased expense and longer operative time. Because this procedure is technically demanding, it is offered only at certain centers.

Radiation Therapy: The goal of radiation therapy is to kill the cancer and preserve healthy tissue. Radiation may cure cancers that are confined to the prostate, as well as cancers that have invaded tissues around the prostate (but not cancer that has spread to distant organs). Radiation therapy can also relieve the pain resulting from the spread of prostate cancer to bone but cannot cure the cancer itself.

For many stages of prostate cancer, 10-year survival rates with radiation therapy are nearly as high as those achieved with surgery: more than 90% of men with cancer confined to the prostate live at least 10 years after undergoing radiation therapy. Whereas surgery is accomplished in one procedure, radiation therapy usually requires many separate treatment sessions over the course of several weeks.

During traditional radiation therapy, a machine sends beams of radiation to the prostate and surrounding tissues (traditional external beam radiation). A CT scanner is used to identify the prostate and surrounding tissues that are affected by the cancer. Treatments are usually given 5 days per week for 5 to 7 weeks. Although erectile dysfunction can occur in 30% of men, it is less likely to develop after radiation therapy than after prostatectomy. Traditional external beam radiation therapy causes incontinence in fewer than 5% of men. Urethral strictures—scars that narrow the urethra and impede the flow of urine—develop in about 7% of men. Other troublesome but usually temporary side effects of traditional external radiation therapy include burning during urination, having to urinate frequently, blood in the urine, diarrhea that is sometimes bloody, irritation of the rectum and diarrhea (radiation proctitis), and sudden urges to defecate.

With recent technical advances, doctors can more precisely focus the radiation beam on the cancer (a procedure called three-dimensional conformal radiotherapy). Cure rates for traditional external beam radiation and three-dimensional conformal radiotherapy have not yet been compared. However, conformal radiotherapy causes fewer temporary side effects.

Radiation can also be delivered by inserting radioactive implants into the prostate (brachytherapy). The implants are placed using images obtained from ultrasound or CT scans. Brachytherapy offers many advantages: It can deliver high doses of radiation to the prostate while sparing healthy surrounding tissues and producing fewer side effects. Brachytherapy can be performed in a few hours, does not require repeated treatment sessions, and uses only spinal anesthesia. However, brachytherapy may cause urethral strictures in up to 20% of men. Cure rates for brachytherapy have not yet been compared to those from other treatments. Combined treatment with brachytherapy and external beam radiation is sometimes recommended.

Prostate cancer can be resistant to radiation therapy or can recur after treatment.

Hormonal Therapy: Because most prostate cancers require testosterone to grow or spread, treatments that block the effects of this hormone (hormonal therapy) can slow progression of the tumors. Hormonal therapy is commonly used to delay the spread of the cancer or to treat widespread (metastatic) prostate cancer and is sometimes combined with other treatments. Growth and spread of metastatic prostate cancer can be slowed or temporarily reversed with hormonal therapy. Hormonal therapy can prolong life as well as improve symptoms. Eventually, however, hormonal therapy becomes ineffective, and the disease progresses.

Drugs used to treat prostate cancer in the United States include leuprolide and goserelin, which prevent the pituitary gland from stimulating the testes to make testosterone. These drugs are administered by injection in a doctor's office every 1, 3, 4, or 12 months, usually for the rest of the man's life.

Drugs that block testosterone's effects (such as flutamide, bicalutamide, and nilutamide) may also be used. These drugs are taken daily by mouth. However, drugs that block testosterone produce changes associated with low testosterone levels, such as hot flashes, osteoporosis, loss of energy, reduced muscle mass, fluid weight gain, reduced libido, reduced body hair, and often erectile dysfunction and breast enlargement (gynecomastia).

The oldest form of hormonal therapy involves the removal of both testes (bilateral orchiectomy). The effects of bilateral orchiectomy on testosterone level are equivalent to those produced by leuprolide and goserelin. Bilateral orchiectomy greatly slows the growth of the prostate cancer but produces the side effects of low testosterone levels. The physical and psychologic effects of bilateral orchiectomy make the procedure difficult for some men to accept.

Hormonal therapy usually becomes ineffective within 3 to 5 years in men with widespread prostate cancer. When cancer eventually progresses despite hormonal therapy, most men die within 1 or 2 years. When hormonal therapy fails (hormone resistance), alternative hormone drugs or chemotherapy may be tried.

After all forms of treatment, PSA levels are measured at regular intervals depending on the risk for recurrence and the time from treatment completion (usually every 3 to 4 months for the first year, every 6 months for the next year, and then every year for the rest of the man's life). Increases in the PSA levels may indicate that the cancer has recurred.

Common Methods and Strategies for Treating Prostate Cancer

CHARACTERISTICS OF THE CANCER	TREATMENT STRATEGY	METHOD OF TREATMENT
Small, slow-growing cancer, confined to prostate; man expected to live many years	Definitive therapy	Surgery or radiation therapy
Small, slow-growing cancer, confined to prostate; man not expected to live many years	Watchful waiting	No treatment
Large or fast-growing cancer, confined to prostate	Definitive therapy	Surgery or radiation therapy
Cancer spread to areas around the prostate, but not to distant areas	Definitive therapy	Radiation therapy
Widespread cancer	Palliative therapy	Hormonal therapy

Prostatitis

Prostatitis is pain and swelling of the prostate gland.

- The cause is often a bacterial infection.
- Pain can occur in the area between the scrotum and anus or in the lower back, penis, or testes.
- Men feel a frequent, urgent need to urinate, and urination, erection, ejaculation, and defecation may be painful.
- Urine and sometimes fluids expressed from the prostate gland are cultured.
- Bacterial infection is treated with antibiotics.

- Symptoms of prostatitis, regardless of the cause, may be relieved with prostate massage, a warm sitz bath, relaxation techniques, and drugs.

Prostatitis usually develops for unknown reasons. Prostatitis can result from a bacterial infection that spreads to the prostate from the urinary tract or from bacteria in the bloodstream. Bacterial infections may develop slowly and tend to recur (chronic bacterial prostatitis) or develop rapidly (acute bacterial prostatitis). Rarely, fungal, viral, or protozoal infections can cause prostatitis.

Symptoms

Spasm of the muscles in the bladder and pelvis, especially in the perineum (the area between the scrotum and the anus), causes many of the symptoms of prostatitis. Prostatitis causes pain in the perineum, the lower back, and often the penis and testes. The man also may need to urinate frequently and urgently, and urinating may cause pain or burning. Pain may make obtaining an erection or ejaculating difficult or even painful. Constipation can develop, making defecation painful. Some symptoms tend to occur more often with acute bacterial prostatitis, such as fever, difficulty urinating, and blood in the urine. Bacterial prostatitis can result in a collection of pus (abscess) in the prostate or in epididymitis (inflammation of the epididymis). Chronic prostatitis can impair fertility.

Diagnosis and Treatment

The diagnosis of prostatitis is usually based on the symptoms and a physical examination. The prostate, examined through the rectum by a doctor, may be swollen and tender to the touch. Cultures are taken of urine and, sometimes, of fluids expressed from the penis after massaging the prostate during the examination. Urine cultures reveal bacterial infections located anywhere in the urinary tract. In contrast, when infection is found by culturing fluid from the prostate, the prostate is clearly the cause of the infection.

When cultures reveal no bacterial infection, prostatitis is usually difficult to cure. Most treatments for this kind of pros-

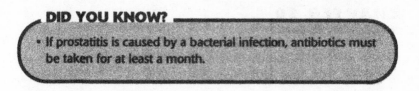

DID YOU KNOW?

- If prostatitis is caused by a bacterial infection, antibiotics must be taken for at least a month.

tatitis relieve symptoms but may not cure the prostatitis. These treatments for symptoms can also help in chronic bacterial prostatitis.

Non-drug treatments include periodic prostate massage (done by a doctor by placing a finger in the rectum), frequent ejaculation, and sitting in a warm bath. Relaxation techniques (biofeedback) may relieve spasm and pain of the pelvic muscles. Among drug therapies, stool softeners can relieve painful defecation resulting from constipation. Analgesics and anti-inflammatory drugs may relieve pain and swelling regardless of its source. Alpha-adrenergic blockers that are used to treat prostate enlargement (such as doxazosin, terazosin, and tamsulosin) may help relieve symptoms by relaxing the muscles within the prostate. For reasons that are not understood, antibiotics sometimes relieve symptoms. If symptoms are severe despite other treatments, surgery, such as partial or complete removal of the prostate, may be considered as a last resort. Destruction of the prostate by microwave or laser treatments is another alternative.

When prostatitis results from a bacterial infection, an oral antibiotic that can penetrate prostate tissue (such as ofloxacin, levofloxacin, ciprofloxacin, or trimethoprim-sulfamethoxazole) is taken for 30 to 90 days. Taking antibiotics for less time may lead to a chronic infection. Chronic bacterial prostatitis can be difficult to cure. If a prostate abscess occurs, surgical drainage is usually necessary.

CHAPTER 30

Sexual Dysfunction in Men

- Sexual dysfunction may affect the sex drive or the ability to have an erection, to ejaculate, or to have an orgasm.

In men, sexual dysfunction refers to difficulties engaging in sexual intercourse. Sexual dysfunction encompasses a variety of disorders that affect sex drive (libido), the ability to achieve or maintain an erection (erectile dysfunction, or impotence), ejaculation, and the ability to achieve orgasm.

Sexual dysfunction may result from either physical or psychologic factors; many sexual problems result from a combination of both. A physical problem may lead to psychologic problems (such as anxiety, fear, or stress), which can in turn aggravate the physical problem. Men sometimes pressure themselves or feel pressured by a partner to perform well sexually and become distressed when they cannot (performance anxiety). Performance anxiety can be troublesome and further worsen a man's ability to enjoy sexual relations.

DID YOU KNOW?

- How much of sexual dysfunction is due to physical factors and how much is due to psychologic factors can be difficult or impossible to discern.

Erectile dysfunction is the most common sexual dysfunction in men. Decreased libido also affects some men. Problems with ejaculation include uncontrolled ejaculation before or shortly after penetrating the vagina (premature ejaculation), ejaculation into the bladder (retrograde ejaculation), and blockage (obstruction) of the ejaculatory ducts.

PSYCHOLOGIC CAUSES OF SEXUAL DYSFUNCTION

- Anger toward a partner
- Anxiety
- Depression
- Discord or boredom with a partner
- Fear of pregnancy, dependence on another person, or losing control
- Feelings of detachment from sexual activities or one's partner
- Guilt
- Inhibitions or ignorance about sexual behavior
- Performance anxiety (worrying about performance during intercourse)
- Previous traumatic sexual experiences (for example, rape, incest, sexual abuse, or previous sexual dysfunction)

Normal Sexual Function

Normal sexual function is a complex interaction involving both the mind (thoughts, memories, and emotions) and the body. The nervous, circulatory, and endocrine (hormonal) systems all interact with the mind to produce a sexual response. A delicate and balanced interplay among all parts of the nervous system controls the sexual response in men.

Desire (also called sex drive or libido) is the wish to engage in sexual activity. It may be triggered by thoughts, words, sights, smell, or touch. Desire leads to the first stage of the sexual response cycle, excitement. Excitement is sexual arousal. During excitement, blood flow to the penis increases, leading to an erection. Also, muscle tension increases throughout the body. In the plateau stage, excitement and muscle tension are maintained or intensified. Orgasm is the peak or climax of sexual excitement. At orgasm, muscle tension throughout the body further increases. The man experiences contractions of the pelvic muscles followed by a release of muscle tension. Semen is usually, but not always, ejaculated from the penis. Although ejaculation and orgasm often occur nearly simultaneously, they are separate events. Ejaculation can occur without orgasm. Also, orgasm can occur in the absence of ejaculation, especially before puberty, or with the use of certain drugs (such as some antidepressants). Most men find orgasm highly pleasurable. In resolution, a man returns to an unaroused state. After orgasm, men cannot have another erection for some time (refractory period), often as short as 20 minutes or less in young men but much longer in older men. The time between erections generally increases as men age.

SEXUAL ACTIVITY AND HEART DISEASE

Sexual activity is generally less taxing than moderate to heavy physical activity and is therefore usually safe for men with heart disease. Although the risk of a heart attack is higher during sexual activity than it is during rest, the risk is still very low during sexual activity.

Still, sexually active men with diseases of the heart and cardiovascular system (which include angina, high blood pressure, heart failure, abnormal rhythms of the heart, and blockage of the aortic valve [aortic stenosis]) need to take reasonable precautions. Usually, sexual activity is safe if the disease is mild, if it causes few symptoms, and if blood pressure is normal. If the disease is moderate in severity or if the man has other conditions that make a heart attack likely, testing may be necessary to determine how safe sexual activity is. If the disease is severe or if the man has an enlarged heart that blocks the flow of blood leaving the left ventricle (obstructive cardiomyopathy), sexual activity should be deferred until after treatment reduces the severity of the symptoms. Use of sildenafil may be dangerous; men taking nitroglycerine should not use sildenafil. Sexual activity should also be deferred until at least 2 to 6 weeks after a heart attack.

Most often, testing to determine the safety of sexual activity involves monitoring the heart for signs of poor blood supply while exercising on a treadmill. If the blood supply is adequate during exercise, a heart attack during sexual activity is very unlikely.

Erectile Dysfunction

Erectile dysfunction (impotence) is the inability to achieve or maintain an erection.

- The cause may be a disorder that reduces blood flow or damages nerves to the penis, a hormonal disorder, use of certain drugs, or psychologic issues.
- In many men, sex drive also decreases.
- A physical examination (including blood pressure measurement), blood tests, and sometimes ultrasonography may detect a disorder contributing to erectile dysfunction.
- Drugs, taken by mouth or inserted or injected into the penis, may help, as may constriction and vacuum devices and psychologic therapy.

Every man is occasionally unable to achieve an erection; this is normal. Erectile dysfunction occurs when the problem is frequent or continuous.

Erectile dysfunction can range from mild to severe. A man with mild erectile dysfunction may occasionally achieve a full erection, but more often he achieves an erection that is inadequate for penetration. He may frequently be unable to achieve an erection at all. A man with severe erectile dysfunction is rarely able to achieve an erection.

Erectile dysfunction becomes more common with age but is not part of the normal aging process. About half of men 65 years of age and three fourths of men 80 years of age have erectile dysfunction.

Causes

To achieve an erection, the penis needs both an adequate inflow of blood and a slowing of blood outflow (see page 384). Disorders that narrow arteries and decrease blood inflow (such as atherosclerosis, diabetes, or a blood clot) or surgery on the blood vessels can cause erectile dysfunction. Also, abnormalities in the veins of the penis can sometimes drain blood back to the body so rapidly that erections cannot be sustained despite adequate blood inflow.

Neurologic damage is another possible cause of erectile dysfunction. Damage to the nerves leading to or from the penis produces erectile dysfunction. Such damage could result from surgery (most commonly prostate surgery), spinal disease, diabetes, multiple sclerosis, peripheral nerve disorders, stroke, alcohol, and drugs.

Occasionally, hormonal disturbances (such as abnormally low levels of testosterone) cause erectile dysfunction. Also, factors that decrease a man's energy level (such as illness, fatigue, and stress) can make erections difficult.

Many drugs can interfere with the ability to achieve an erection, especially among older men. Drugs that commonly cause erectile dysfunction include antihypertensives, antidepressants, some sedatives, cimetidine, digoxin, lithium, and antipsychotics.

Psychologic issues (such as depression, performance anxiety, guilt, fear of intimacy, and ambivalence about sexual orientation) can impair the ability to achieve erections. Psychologic causes are more common in younger men. Any new stressful situation, such as a change of sex partners or problems with relationships or at work, can also contribute.

DID YOU KNOW?

- Occasional inability to achieve an erection is normal and does not mean that a man has erectile dysfunction.
- About half of men older than 65 and one fourth of men older than 80 can still have erections.
- Low levels of testosterone tend to decrease sex drive rather than cause erectile dysfunction.
- Treatment of erectile dysfunction is often unnecessary when couples are satisfied with other forms of physical intimacy.
- Combinations of drugs injected into the penis and devices that constrict or apply suction to the penis are highly effective and lack many of the side effects of oral drugs.
- Psychologic therapies can help even when erectile dysfunction has a physical cause.

Symptoms

Sex drive (libido) often decreases in men with erectile dysfunction, although some men do maintain a normal libido. Regardless of whether libido changes, men with erectile dysfunction have difficulty engaging in intercourse either because the erect penis is not sufficiently hard, long, or elevated for penetration or because the erection cannot be sustained. Some men stop having erections during sleep or upon awakening. Others may attain strong erections sometimes but be unable to attain or maintain erections other times.

When testosterone levels are low, the result is more likely to be a drop in libido than erectile dysfunction. Low testosterone levels can cause gradual development of many symptoms, including enlargement of the breasts (gynecomastia—see page 386), raised pitch of the voice, shrinking of the testes (testicles), and loss of pubic hair. Low testosterone may also cause thinning of the bones, loss of energy, and loss of muscle mass.

Diagnosis

To diagnose erectile dysfunction, a doctor performs a general physical examination and examines the man's genitals. The doctor may also assess the function of the nerves and blood vessels that supply the genitals. Measurement of blood pressure in the legs may reveal a problem with the arteries in the pelvis and groin that supply blood to the penis. Examination of the man's rectum may reveal a problem with the nerve supply of the penis.

A blood sample is taken to measure the level of testosterone. Certain blood tests can help identify diseases that may lead to temporary or permanent erectile dysfunction. For example, blood tests can reveal evidence of diabetes (which can lead to permanent erectile dysfunction) or infection (which can lead to temporary erectile dysfunction).

If a problem with the arteries or veins is suspected, specialized tests may be performed. Ultrasound examination can reveal narrowing or blockage within the arteries of the penis.

Treatment

Some men and their partners may choose not to pursue treatment for erectile dysfunction. Physical contact without an erection may satisfy their needs for intimacy and fulfillment.

Sometimes, discontinuing use of a particular drug can improve erections.

For men who choose to pursue treatment, there are many choices.

Drug Treatment: Many drugs are used to treat erectile dysfunction. Most drugs given to treat erectile dysfunction increase blood flow to the penis. Most of these drugs are given by mouth, but some drugs can be applied locally—by injection or insertion into the penis.

Sildenafil is the drug most frequently used to treat erectile dysfunction. Sildenafil, which is taken by mouth, increases the frequency and rigidity of erections within 30 to 60 minutes; erections last about 10 to 30 minutes. The drug is effective only when the man is sexually aroused. Side effects of sildenafil include headache, flushing, runny nose, upset stomach, and vision problems. More serious side effects, including dangerously low blood pressure, can occur when sildenafil is taken with certain other drugs (such as nitroglycerin or amyl nitrite). Because of this, a man should not take sildenafil while taking drugs such as nitroglycerin. Drugs similar to sildenafil are likely to become available in the future.

Other oral drugs that have been used in the treatment of erectile dysfunction are phentolamine, yohimbine, and testosterone. Phentolamine is sometimes prescribed for erectile dysfunction but is less effective than sildenafil. Yohimbine is occasionally used to treat men whose erectile dysfunction is caused by psychologic factors, but the drug can cause side effects (including anxiety, shaking, rapid heart rate, and increased blood pressure) and is only minimally effective.

Drugs injected or inserted into the penis widen the arteries that supply blood to the penis. Men who cannot tolerate drugs taken by mouth can often be treated with these drugs.

Alprostadil, in the form of a pellet (suppository), can be inserted into the penis through the urethra. When used alone, alprostadil may result in an erection, but it is more effective when combined with another treatment, such as a binding device. Alprostadil may cause lightheadedness, a burning sensation of the penis, or, occasionally, a prolonged, painful erection (priapism— see page 391). Because these serious side effects occasionally occur, a man usually takes his first dose under observation in a doctor's office.

A man can also induce an erection by injecting drugs (such as alprostadil alone or a combination of alprostadil, papaverine, and phentolamine) into the shaft of his penis. Injection is one of the most effective ways to obtain an erection. However, many men are unwilling to inject their penis. Also, the injection can cause priapism, and repeated injections may eventually produce scar tissue.

Testosterone replacement therapy may help men whose erectile dysfunction is caused by abnormally low testosterone levels. Unlike other drugs, which work by increasing blood flow to the penis, testosterone works by correcting a hormonal deficiency. Testosterone can be taken in many forms, including pills, patches, topical creams, and injections. Side effects can include liver dysfunction, increased red blood cell counts, increased risk of stroke, and enlargement of the prostate (see page 383).

Constriction (binding) and Vacuum Devices: Most men with erectile dysfunction can achieve erections by using a constriction device with or without a vacuum device. These devices are among the least expensive treatments for erectile dysfunction, and they enable a man to avoid the side effects that can occur with drug treatment. However, the devices can cause excessive bruising in men who are taking blood-thinning (anticoagulant) drugs and in those with diseases that interfere with blood clotting. Constriction devices should not be left on for longer than 30 minutes.

Constriction devices (such as bands and rings made of metal, rubber, or leather) are placed at the base of the penis to slow the outflow of blood. These medically engineered devices can be purchased with a doctor's prescription in a pharmacy, but inexpensive versions (often called "cock rings") can be purchased in stores that sell sexual paraphernalia.

A constriction device used alone may produce an erection in a man with mild erectile dysfunction, especially when the problem is maintenance of the erection. A constriction device can also be used in combination with a vacuum device. A binding device occasionally causes pain or interferes with ejaculation.

Vacuum devices (which consist of a hollow chamber attached to a source of suction) fit over the penis, creating a seal. Suction applied to the chamber draws blood into the penis, producing an erection. Once an erection is achieved, a binding device is applied to prevent the blood from flowing out of the penis.

Surgery: When erectile dysfunction does not respond to other treatments, a device that simulates an erection (prosthesis) can be surgically implanted in the penis.

A variety of prostheses are available. One type consists of firm rods that are inserted into the penis to create a permanently hard penis. Another prosthesis is an inflatable balloon that is inserted into the penis; before having intercourse, the man inflates the balloon with a small pump (which may be part of the prosthesis). Surgical implantation of a penile prosthesis requires at least a 3-day hospitalization and a 6-week recovery before intercourse is attempted.

Psychologic Therapy: Some types of psychologic therapy (which include behavior-modification techniques, such as the sensate focus technique—see page 203) can improve the mental and emotional factors that contribute to erectile dysfunction. Psychologic therapy can even help when the erectile dysfunction has a physical cause, because psychologic factors often compound the problem.

Specific therapies are selected based on the particular psychologic cause of the man's erectile dysfunction. For example, if the man is suffering from depression, psychotherapy or antidepressants may help with erectile dysfunction. Sometimes psychotherapy can reduce anxiety about sexual performance in men with erectile dysfunction from any cause. Improvement may take a long time, and many sessions are usually required. A man, and often his partner, must be highly motivated for psychotherapy to work.

Several folk remedies for erectile dysfunction exist, but none have proven to be effective.

Decreased Libido

Decreased libido is a reduction in sex drive.

- Possible causes include psychologic factors (such as depression, anxiety, or relationship problems), drugs, and low levels of testosterone.
- Depending on the cause, doctors may suggest psychologic therapy, prescribe a different drug, or prescribe supplemental testosterone.

Sex drive (libido) varies greatly among men. Different men find different degrees of libido satisfactory. Libido may be decreased temporarily by conditions such as fatigue or anxiety. Libido also tends to gradually decrease as a man ages. Persistent low libido may cause a man and his sex partner distress.

Occasionally, libido can be low throughout a man's life. Life-long low libido can result from traumatic childhood sexual experiences or from learned suppression of sexual thoughts. Most often, however, low libido develops after years of normal sexual desire. Psychologic factors, such as depression, anxiety, and relationship problems, are often the cause. Some drugs (such as those used to treat high blood pressure, depression, or anxiety) and decreased levels of testosterone can also lower libido.

A man with decreased libido thinks less about sex. He loses interest in sexual fantasy and masturbation, and also in sexual activity. Even sexual stimulation, by sights, words, or touch, may fail to provoke interest. The man often retains the capacity for sexual function. Some men continue to engage in sexual activity to satisfy their partner.

A blood test can measure the level of testosterone in the blood. However, the diagnosis is usually based on the man's description of his symptoms.

If the cause is psychologic, various psychologic therapies—including behavioral therapies, such as the sensate focus technique (see page 203)—can help. If the testosterone level is low, testosterone can be given, usually as a patch or gel applied to the skin or as an injection. If a drug appears to be the cause, a doctor can often try treating the man with a different drug.

Premature Ejaculation

Premature ejaculation is ejaculation that occurs too early, usually before, upon, or shortly after penetration.

- The cause is most likely to be anxiety, other psychologic factors, or very sensitive penile skin.
- Behavior modification therapy, including strategies to delay ejaculation, helps most men.

Many males, especially adolescents, ejaculate sooner than they or their partners would like. Premature ejaculation is not just ejaculation that occurs before a man wants it to but rather ejaculation that occurs very soon—often within a minute or two—after penetration.

Many experts believe that premature ejaculation almost always results from anxiety or other psychologic causes. Others think that unusually sensitive penile skin may be a cause. Premature ejaculation is rarely caused by a disease, although inflammation of the prostate gland or a nervous system disorder can cause the condition.

Premature ejaculation can distress a man and his partner. If the man ejaculates too early, the partner may be left unsatisfied sexually and may become resentful.

Behavior modification therapy can help most men overcome premature ejaculation. A therapist provides reassurance, explains why premature ejaculation occurs, and teaches the man strategies for delaying ejaculation.

Other methods that can help a man delay ejaculation include drug treatment (with a selective serotonin reuptake inhibitor such as fluoxetine, paroxetine, or sertraline), application of an anesthetic to the penis, and use of condoms, which tend to decrease sensation. Sometimes a combination of drug treatment and behavioral therapy enables a man to delay ejaculation even longer than he might be able to with only one of these treatments. When premature ejaculation is caused by more serious psychologic problems, psychologic therapy may help.

THE STOP-AND-START TECHNIQUE

One technique used to treat premature ejaculation is the stop-and-start technique, which trains the man to experience high levels of excitement without ejaculating. The technique involves stimulation of the penis until the man feels that he will soon ejaculate unless the stimulation stops. He signals his partner to stop stimulation, which is resumed after 20 to 30 seconds. The partners rehearse this technique at first with hand stimulation and later during intercourse. With practice, more than 95% of the men learn to delay ejaculation for 5 to 10 minutes or even longer. The technique also helps reduce the anxiety that often aggravates the problem.

Retrograde Ejaculation

Retrograde ejaculation is a condition in which semen is ejaculated backward into the bladder rather than out through the penis.

In retrograde ejaculation, the part of the bladder that normally closes during ejaculation (the bladder neck) remains open, causing the ejaculatory fluid to travel backward into the bladder. Common causes of retrograde ejaculation include diabetes, spinal cord injuries, certain drugs, and some surgical operations (including major abdominal or pelvic surgery—one of the most common causes is transurethral resection of the prostate).

Men with retrograde ejaculation can still have orgasms. However, retrograde ejaculation decreases the amount of fluid ejaculated out of the penis; sometimes, no fluid comes out. The condition can cause infertility but is otherwise not harmful.

DID YOU KNOW?

• Insemination may be possible if infertility is caused by retrograde ejaculation.

A doctor makes the diagnosis of retrograde ejaculation by finding a large amount of sperm in a urine sample. Most men need no treatment. About one third of men with retrograde ejaculation improve after treatment with drugs that close the bladder neck (such as pseudoephedrine, phenylephrine, chlorpheniramine, brompheniramine, or imipramine). However, most of these drugs can increase heart rate and blood pressure, which can be dangerous in men with high blood pressure or heart disease.

If infertility requires treatment and drugs do not help, doctors can sometimes collect a man's sperm for insemination (see page 54).

Resources for Help and Information

AIDS
CDC National AIDS/HIV Hotline
800-342-2437
www.ashastd.org

AIDS Action
Washington, DC
202-530-8030
www.aidsaction.org

The American Foundation for AIDS Research
New York, NY
800-342-2437
212-806-1600
www.amfar.org

Gay Men's Health Crisis
New York, NY
800-243-7692
212-807-6655
212-645-7470 (TTY)
www.gmhc.org

National Association for People with AIDS
Washington, DC
202-898-0414
www.napwa.org

Project Inform
San Francisco, CA
800-822-7422
415-558-9051
415-558-8669
www.projinf.org

Universal Fellowship of Metropolitan Community Churches
AIDS Ministry
Los Angeles, CA
213-464-5100
www.thebody.com/ufmcc/ufmcc.html

Women Alive
Los Angeles, CA
800-554-4876
323-965-1564
www.women-alive.org

ALCOHOLISM
Al-Anon Family Group Headquarters
Virginia Beach, VA
888-4AL-ANON (888-425-2666)
757-563-1600
www.al-anon.org

Alcoholics Anonymous
New York, NY
212-870-3400
www.alcoholics-anonymous.org

National Clearinghouse for Alcohol & Drug Information
Rockville, MD
800-729-6686
800-487-4889 (TDD)
www.health.org

National Council on Alcoholism & Drug Dependence
New York, NY
800-622-2255
212-269-7797
www.ncadd.org

LifeRing Recovery
Oakland, CA
510-763-0779
www.lifering.org

BALDING
National Alopecia Areata Foundation
San Rafael, CA
415-472-3780
www.alopeciaareata.com

CANCER & OTHER TUMORS
American Cancer Society
Atlanta, GA
800-227-2345
404-320-3333
www.cancer.org

Cancer Care, Inc.
New York, NY
800-813-4673
212-712-8080
212-302-2400
www.cancercare.org

Livestrong
Austin, TX
866-235-7205
www.livestrong.org

National Cancer Institute
Bethesda, MD
800-422-6237
301-496-5583
www.cancer.gov

National Coalition for Cancer Survivorship
Silver Spring, MD
301-650-9127
www.canceradvocacy.org

**Patient Advocates for Advanced Cancer
Treatments, Inc.**
Grand Rapids, MI
616-453-1477
www.paactusa.org

BREAST
National Alliance of Breast Cancer Organizations
New York, NY
888-806-2226

The Susan G. Komen Breast Cancer Foundation
Dallas, TX
800-462-9273
972-855-1600
www.komen.org

Y-ME: National Breast Cancer Organization
Chicago, IL
800-221-2141
312-986-8338
www.y-me.org

PROSTATE
US-TOO International
Downers Grove, IL
800-808-7866
630-795-1002
www.ustoo.com

CARDIOVASCULAR DISORDERS

American Heart Association
Dallas, TX
800-242-8721
214-373-6300
www.americanheart.org

Heart and Stroke Foundation of Canada
Toronto, Ontario, Canada
416-489-7111
www.heartandstroke.ca

National Heart, Lung, and Blood Institute
Bethesda, MD
301-251-1222
www.nhlbi.nih.gov

National Stroke Association
Englewood, CO
800-787-6537
303-649-9299
www.stroke.org

Sister Kenny Institute
Minneapolis, MN
612-863-4457
www.sisterkennyinstitute.com

Vascular Disease Foundation
Lakewood, CO
866-723-4636 (toll free)
303-949-8337
www.vdf.org

CHILDBIRTH/PREGNANCY

America's Crisis Pregnancy Helpline
Dallas, TX
800-672-2296
www.thehelpline.org

Maternity Center Association
New York, NY
212-777-5000
www.maternitywise.org

DEATH & BEREAVEMENT

The Compassionate Friends
Oak Brook, IL
877-969-0010
630-990-0010
www.compassionatefriends.org

The Hemlock Society USA
Denver, CO
800-247-7421
www.hemlock.org

Hospice Education Institute
Machiasport, ME
800-331-1620
207-255-8800
www.hospiceworld.org

National Hospice Foundation
Alexandria, VA
703-516-4928
www.hospiceinfo.org

Partnership for Caring
Washington, DC
703-516-4928
www.partnershipforcaring.org

DEPRESSION

Depression and Related Affective Disorders Association (DRADA)
Baltimore, MD
410-955-4647
www.drada.org

National Depressive and Manic-Depressive Association
Chicago, IL
800-826-3632
312-642-0049
www.ndmda.org

Recovery, Inc.
Chicago, IL
312-337-5661
www.recovery-inc.com

DIABETES

American Diabetes Association
Alexandria, VA
800-342-2383
www.diabetes.org

DRUG ABUSE

Cocaine Anonymous World Service
Los Angeles, CA
800-347-8998
310-559-5833
www.ca.org

Hazelden
Center City, MN
800-257-7810
651-213-4000
www.hazelden.org

Narcotics Anonymous
Van Nuys, CA
818-997-3822
www.na.org

ERECTILE DYSFUNCTION (IMPOTENCE)

Impotents Anonymous
Maryville, TN
615-983-6064

FAMILY PLANNING

Planned Parenthood Federation of America
New York, NY
212-541-7800
www.plannedparenthood.org

GENERAL

American Academy of Family Physicians
Leawood, KS
www.familydoctor.org

American Medical Association
Chicago, IL
312-464-5000
www.ama-assn.org

Centers for Disease Control and Prevention
Atlanta, GA
800-311-3435
404-639-3311
www.cdc.gov

The Merck Manuals
Merck & Co, Inc.
West Point, PA
www.merckmanuals.com

National Institutes of Health
Bethesda, MD
301-496-4000
www.nih.gov

US Department of Health and Human Services
Washington, DC
877-696-6775
202-619-0257
www.os.dhhs.gov

US Food and Drug Administration
Office of Consumer Affairs Inquiry Information Line
Rockville, MD
888-463-6332
www.fda.gov

Electronic Orange Book
Approved Drug Products With Therapeutic Equivalence Evaluations
www.fda.gov/cder/ob/default.htm

GENETIC DISEASES

Alliance of Genetic Support Groups
Washington, DC
202-966-5557
www.geneticalliance.org

INCONTINENCE

National Association for Continence
Spartanburg, SC
800-252-3337
864-579-7900
www.nafc.org

The Simon Foundation for Continence
Wilmette, IL
800-237-4666

INFERTILITY

American Society for Reproductive Medicine
Birmingham, AL
202-978-5000
www.asrm.org

Ferre Institute, Inc.
Binghamton, NY
607-724-4308
www.ferre.org

Resolve: The National Infertility Association
Somerville, MA
888-623-0744
www.resolve.org

NUTRITION

American Dietetic Association
Chicago, IL
800-877-1600
312-899-0040
www.eatright.org

PROSTATE DISORDERS

The Prostatitis Foundation
Smithshire, IL
888-891-4200
www.prostatitis.org

PSYCHIATRIC DISEASE

National Alliance for the Mentally Ill
Arlington, VA
800-950-6264
703-524-7600
www.nami.org

National Institute of Mental Health
Bethesda, MD
301-443-4513
www.nimh.nih.gov

National Mental Health Association
Alexandria, VA
800-969-6642
800-443-5959 (TTY)
703-684-7722
www.nmha.org

Metanoia
800-784-2433
www.metanoia.org/suicide

Survivors of Suicide
www.thewebpager.com/sos

SEXUAL HEALTH
Answer at Rutgers University
New Brunswick, NJ
732-445-7929
www.sexetc.org

The Sexual Health Network
Shelton, CT
www.sexualhealth.com

WOMEN'S HEALTH
American College of Obstetricians and Gynecologists
Washington, DC
202-638-5577
202-863-2518
www.acog.org

National Women's Health Network
Washington, DC
202-347-1140
www.nwhn.org

Index

Note: Page numbers in *italics* refer to illustrations, sidebars, or tables.

Not sure what to read next?

Visit Pocket Books online at
www.simonsays.com

Reading suggestions for
you and your reading group
New release news
Author appearances
Online chats with your favorite writers
Special offers
Order books online
And much, much more!

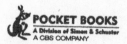

POCKET BOOKS
A Division of Simon & Schuster
A CBS COMPANY

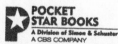

POCKET STAR BOOKS
A Division of Simon & Schuster
A CBS COMPANY

13456